T0369724

Oxford Handbook of
Epidemiology
for Clinicians

Helen Ward
Professor of Public Health
Imperial College London, UK

Mireille B. Toledano
Senior Lecturer in Epidemiology
Imperial College London, UK

Gavin Shaddick
Senior Lecturer in Statistics
University of Bath, UK

Bethan Davies
Clinical Research Fellow
Imperial College London, UK

Paul Elliott
Chair in Epidemiology and Public Health Medicine
Imperial College London, UK

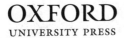

OXFORD
UNIVERSITY PRESS

Great Clarendon Street, Oxford OX2 6DP
United Kingdom

Oxford University Press is a department of the University of Oxford.
It furthers the University's objective of excellence in research, scholarship,
and education by publishing worldwide. Oxford is a registered trade mark of
Oxford University Press in the UK and in certain other countries

First edition published 2012

Impression: 4

British Library Cataloguing in Publication Data
Data available

Library of Congress Cataloging in Publication Data
Data available

ISBN 978–0–19–852988–0

Printed in China

Foreword

Now more than ever clinicians need to understand evidence. Healthcare is evolving rapidly with innovation leading to ever more effective and efficient diagnostic tools, treatments, service delivery, and preventive interventions. Being able to interpret clinical trials, meta-analyses, systematic reviews, and the results of individual investigations and apply these to the patient sitting in front of us is a greater challenge than ever given the volume of evidence being generated. Much of the evidence needed in the consulting room, as in the hospital boardroom, comes from studies of populations, and understanding these kinds of data requires good epidemiological skills and insights.

This handbook is an invaluable means for grasping the principles of epidemiology as applied to everyday clinical practice. It introduces concepts such as distribution, measurement, and risk in relation to diagnosis and management, making them very relevant for medical students and junior doctors. There is a series of helpful worked examples from diagnostics through management and discussion of prognosis which link to the later sections on study design and statistics. Doctors in training will find the very practical sections on finding and summarizing evidence through systematic review and meta-analysis, plus the step-by-step guide to clinical audit, particularly useful. The book also has a valuable reference section that medical students and others studying for professional exams will appreciate giving a structured guide to the epidemiology of some of the most common diseases.

Working with patients and communities to improve health and prevent illness is now all our business. This handbook provides an overview of the relevant evidence with reminders of how to assess risk, deliver brief interventions, and communicate risk to patients.

Many clinicians reading this book will find it opens their eyes to the widespread application of epidemiology and prevention and will embrace it in their pursuit of excellence and evidence-based practice.

Professor the Lord Darzi of Denham PC, KBE

Preface

What is a cohort study? How do I critique a scientific paper? What is the incidence of heart disease? How do I calculate relative risk? How do I plan and carry out my own study? What differentiates association from causality? These are the sorts of questions that training in epidemiology will answer but the answers may not be so readily accessible to the busy clinician or medical student. This books aims to fill that gap—to provide the basics in epidemiology for clinicians in one handy volume, following the successful Oxford Handbook format.

Unlike standard textbooks of epidemiology the focus throughout is on clinical applications of epidemiological knowledge. The book is divided into 4 sections for easy reference. In Section 1, we start by looking at how the methods used in epidemiology can be useful in the diagnostic process, clinical decision-making and the use of evidence to underpin decisions on clinical management. We also show how epidemiology can inform communication with patients about risks, and end with a practical discussion of health promotion in the clinic. In Section 2, we focus on evidence-based practice and how to obtain and summarize data, including principles of systematic review and meta-analysis. We continue with a description of preventive medicine and screening, using examples from both non-communicable and communicable disease. We complete this section with a practical guide to evaluating clinical practice and point out the similarities and differences between research and audit. In Section 3, we describe the types of study that produce epidemiological and clinical knowledge, the sources and quality of data, and how to produce, understand, and evaluate the statistics underlying research findings and their implementation into clinical practice. We conclude in Section 4 with a brief analysis of the global burden of disease and by summarizing the epidemiology of common diseases. Throughout the book we provide examples, key references, and links to other sources of information.

This book builds on our experience in the training of junior doctors and medical students to provide an understanding of key epidemiological concepts as they translate into medical practice. The application of epidemiological concepts into day-to-day practice is relevant to all clinical specialties. The book will therefore be useful to junior doctors in training and to medical students, including as they prepare for their postgraduate and undergraduate examinations.

HW
MBT
GS
BD
PE
2011

Acknowledgments

We would like to thank the many colleagues who have contributed to this book in both formal and informal ways through their advice, support, and encouragement. The book builds upon educational activities carried out at Imperial College Faculty of Medicine over many years and we are grateful to all those teachers, supervisors, trainees, and students whose work and feedback have shaped our thinking. In particular we thank Paul Aylin for contributing parts of the chapter on sources of data; and Alan Fenwick and Deirdre Hollingsworth for advice on neglected tropical disease and malaria. We would also like to acknowledge the contributions of Alex Bottle and Susan Hodgson, as well as Konrad Jamrozik, now sadly deceased, who provided valuable suggestions about the possible shape of such a book.

The editors at OUP have been both patient and supportive and we thank them for helping to bring the project to fruition, and the anonymous reviewers who commented on early drafts and provided useful feedback. Of course any remaining errors are our own. We would gratefully accept feedback from readers which we hope would benefit future editions of this Handbook.

Finally, we express our gratitude to our families, friends, and colleagues for their patience and support while we have completed the book.

HW, MBT, GS, BD, PE.

Contents

Detailed contents

Symbols and abbreviations

📖	cross reference
~	approximately
<	less than
>	greater than
ACEi	angiotensin-converting enzyme inhibitor
ACTs	artemisinin combined therapies
AIDS	acquired immune deficiency syndrome
ANOVA	analysis of variance
ARR	absolute risk reduction
ARV	anti-retroviral
BCG	Bacille Calmette-Guérin
BMI	body mass index
BP	blood pressure
CER	control event rate
CfI	Centre for Infections
CFR	case fatality rate
CHD	coronary heart disease
CI	confidence interval
CNS	central nervous system
COPD	chronic obstructive pulmonary disease
CT	computed tomography
CUSUM	cumulative sum chart
CVD	cardiovascular disease
DALY	disability-adjusted life year
DVT	deep vein thrombosis
EBH	evidence-based healthcare
EBM	evidence-based medicine
ECG	electrocardiogram
EER	experimental event rate
EID	emerging infectious disease
FAP	familial adenomatous polyposis
FOB	faecal occult blood
GBD	Global Burden of Disease (WHO)
GMC	General Medical Council (UK)
GP	general practitioner
HAART	highly active anti-retroviral therapy

HCAI	healthcare associated infection
HDL	high density lipoprotein
HES	hospital episode statistics
HIV	human immunodeficiency virus
HLA	human leukocyte antigen
HNPCC	hereditary non-polyposis colorectal cancer
HPA	Health Protection Agency
HPV	human papillomavirus
HR	hazard ratio
HRT	hormone replacement therapy
HSE	Health Survey for England
IID	infectious intestinal disease
IQR	interquartile range
ITBNs	insecticide treated bednets
ITT	intention to treat
LDL	low density lipoprotein
LR	likelihood ratio
MDA	mass drug administration
MDR	multidrug-resistant
MI	myocardial infarction
MMR	measles, mumps, rubella
MRI	magnetic resonance imaging
MSM	men who have sex with men
NCHS	National Center for Health Statistics (USA)
NHANES	National Health and Nutrition Examination Survey (USA)
NHL	non-Hodgkin lymphoma
NHS	National Health Service (UK)
NICE	National Institute for Health and Clinical Excellence (UK)
NNT	number needed to treat
NPV	negative predictive value
NRES	National Research Ethics Service (UK)
NSAID	non-steroidal anti-inflammatory drug
NTD	neglected tropical disease
OA	osteoarthritis
ONS	Office for National Statistics (UK)
OR	odds ratio
pa	per annum
PAT	Paddington Alcohol Test
PCV	packed cell volume
PDT	photodynamic therapy

PEP	postexposure prophylaxis
PPV	positive predictive value
PUD	peptic ulcer disease
RA	rheumatoid arthritis
RCT	Randomized Controlled Trial
SARS	severe acute respiratory syndrome
SBP	systolic blood pressure
SD	standard deviation
SE	standard error
SIGN	Scottish Intercollegiate Guidelines Network
SPC	statistical process control
STI	sexually transmitted infection
TB	tuberculosis
TURP	transurethral resection of prostate
UTI	urinary tract infection
UV	ultraviolet
VTE	venous thromboembolism
WHO	World Health Organization
XDR	extensively drug-resistant
YLD	years of life lost to disability

Glossary of terms

Absolute risk the probability of occurrence of a disease, death or other event over a period of time, i.e. incidence rate. (See 📖 Communicating risk, p.56.)

Absolute risk reduction the reduction in an outcome (e.g. death) comparing one group (e.g. a new drug) with a control group (placebo or standard treatment). (See 📖 How effective is the treatment, p.42 and 📖 Intervention studies and clinical trials, p.186.)

Attributable fraction the proportion of disease risk that would be prevented if the risk was changed to that of an unexposed person. (See 📖 Communicating risk, p.56.)

Attributable risk a measure of the excess risk due to the factor concerned. It is calculated by subtracting the incidence rate in the exposed from the incidence rate in the unexposed (the background risk). (See 📖 Risk factors, p.12, 📖 Communicating risk, p.56, and 📖 Cohort studies, p.178.)

Audit see 'Clinical audit'.

Basic reproductive number the number of new infections caused by one infected individual in an entirely susceptible population. (See 📖 Basic infectious disease epidemiology, p.106.)

Bias a systematic error in the design, the conduct, or the analysis (or a combination of these factors) of a study that can give rise to a false association. (See 📖 Basic concepts in epidemiological research, p.148 and 📖 Interpreting associations, p.150.)

Blinding (in a clinical trial) means that the patient does not know whether they are getting the experimental treatment or not. In a double blind trial neither the patient nor the investigator knows which treatment they are getting. (See 📖 Intervention studies and clinical trials, p.186.)

Case a person with the condition of interest either for clinical purposes or study purposes. (See 📖 Is there anything wrong? p.10, and 📖 Basic concepts in epidemiological research, p.148.)

Case–control study a design of study where people with a condition (cases) are compared with those who do not have the condition (controls) with respect to one or more exposures of interest. (See 📖 Case–control studies, p.172.)

Case fatality rate the proportion of people with a disease who die from that disease. (See 📖 Decisions, decisions … the principles of clinical management, p.28 and 📖 Prognosis: mortality, p.32.)

Chi-squared test a statistical test for comparing the proportions of outcomes in different groups.

Clinical audit a quality improvement process that seeks to improve patient care and outcomes through systematic review of care against explicit criteria and the implementation of change. (See 📖 Clinical governance and ethics, p.122 and Chapter 6.)

Clinical guidelines systematically developed statements to assist practitioner and patient decisions about appropriate health care for specific clinical circumstances. (See 📖 Clinical guidelines, p.38.)

Cohort study a study in which individuals are selected on the basis of *exposure* status and are followed over a period of time to allow the frequency of occurrence of the *outcome* of interest in the exposed and non exposed groups to be compared. (See 📖 Cohort studies, p.178.)

Confidence interval given a sample of data, the sample value e.g. mean will be the best estimate of the true population value although there will be some uncertainty associated with this. A confidence interval quantifies this uncertainty and gives a range of values in which we are confident the true population value will lie. (See 📖 Confidence intervals, p.232.)

Confounding gives rise to a false association between an exposure and disease under investigation because it distorts the observed association through a third factor known as the confounder. (See 📖 Basic concepts in epidemiological research, p.148 and 📖 Confounding, p.154.)

Confounding variable a factor that is associated with both the exposure and outcome of interest. (See 📖 Basic concepts in epidemiological research, p.148.)

Control (as opposed to a case) a person without the *outcome* under study (in a *case–control study*), or a person not receiving the intervention (in a clinical trial). (See 📖 Case–control studies, p.172 and 📖 Intervention studies and clinical trials, p.186.)

Correlation a measure of association that is used for risk factors that are continuous variables or multiple categories. A correlation coefficient (r^2) shows how much an increase in risk is explained by an increase in exposure. (See 📖 Correlation coefficients, p.262.)

Count the number of cases. The most basic measure of disease frequency. (See 📖 Measures of disease frequency, p.6.)

Critical appraisal the process of assessing the validity of research and deciding how applicable it is to the question you are seeking to answer. (See 📖 Critical appraisal, p.78.)

Critical proportion (p_c) the proportion of the population that needs to be vaccinated to control the infection, and this is dependent on the basic reproductive number R_0. (See 📖 Basic infectious disease epidemiology, p.106.)

Cross-sectional study a study that collects information on exposure and/or disease at one point in time. (See 📖 Surveys and cross-sectional studies, p.166.)

Disability-adjusted life years (DALYs) the sum of years of potential life lost due to premature mortality and the years of productive life lost due to disability. They are used in the Global Burden of Disease study. (See Chapter 11.)

Double blind see 'Blinding'.

Ecological fallacy when group level information results are inappropriately referred to individuals. (See 📖 Time trend and geographical (ecological) studies, p.162.)

Ecological study these examine the association between exposures and outcomes by using aggregate data. (See 📖 Time trend and geographical (ecological) studies, p.162.)

Endemic when there is a constant presence (or incidence) of a disease in a particular community or geographic area. (See 📖 Basic infectious disease epidemiology, p.106.)

Epidemic when the incidence of a disease rises above the expected level in a particular community or geographic area. (See 📖 Basic infectious disease epidemiology, p.106.)

Epidemiology the study of the distribution and determinants of health and illness in populations. (See 📖 Types of evidence and study designs, p.146.)

Evidence-based medicine the conscientious, explicit, and judicious use of current best evidence in making decisions about the care of individual patients. The practice of evidence-based medicine means integrating individual clinical expertise with the best available external clinical evidence from systematic research. (See 📖 Evidence-based management, p.36 and Section 2.)

Experimental event rate the incidence in the intervention arm of a study. (See 📖 Intervention studies and clinical trials, p.186.)

Exposure a factor that might affect an outcome. (See 📖 Basic concepts in epidemiological research, p.148.)

Forest plot a visual representation of the results of a meta-analysis. (See 📖 Meta-analysis, p.90.)

Frequentist statistics a method of analysis in which the data alone are used to make inferences. (See 📖 So what has my patient got? The Bayesian clinician, p.26.)

Funnel plot a visual representation to explore publication bias in a meta-analysis. Study size is plotted against the effect estimate (e.g. odds ratio). (See 📖 Meta-analysis, p.90.)

Health promotion the process of enabling people to increase control over, and to improve, their health. (See 📖 Health promotion in clinical practice, p.52.)

Herd (population) immunity the immunity of a group or population. High levels of immunity in the population protect those who are not immunized. (See 📖 Basic infectious disease epidemiology, p.106.)

Hyperendemic when there is a high constant presence (or incidence) of a disease in a particular community or geographic area. (See 📖 Basic infectious disease epidemiology, p.106.)

Hypothesis testing two alternative conclusions (hypotheses) are set up, and on the basis of the experiment one is accepted and the other rejected. This acceptance and rejection is always on the basis of some pre-specified levels of statistical confidence. (See 📖 Hypothesis tests, p.234.)

Incidence the number of new *cases* of the disease in a defined population over a defined period of time. (See 📖 Measures of disease frequency, p.6 and 📖 Cohort studies, p.178.)

Incubation period the time between initial contact with an infectious agent and the first appearance of symptoms of the disease associated with that infectious agent. (See 📖 Basic infectious disease epidemiology, p.106.)

Infant mortality rate the number of deaths of infants under age 1 per 1000 live births in a given year. (See 📖 Routine data, p.202.)

Infectious period the time during which a person is capable of transmitting the organism. (See 📖 Basic infectious disease epidemiology, p.106.)

Intention-to-treat analysis where the analysis of outcome in a clinical trial is based on the initial post-randomization treatment allocation, regardless of whether the participant ended up sticking to that protocol. (See 📖 Intervention studies and clinical trials, p.186.)

Lead time bias where survival appears to increase due to earlier detection of the disease as a result of screening. (See 📖 Evaluating screening programmes, p.116.)

Length bias occurs because cases detected through screening may be less aggressive. (See 📖 Evaluating screening programmes, p.116.)

Likelihood ratio the likelihood that a given test result would be expected in a patient with the disease compared to the likelihood that the same result would be expected in a patient without the disease. (See 📖 Likelihood ratios and post-test probabilities, p.22.)

Longitudinal study see 'Cohort study'.

Matching a method for 'controlling for' (i.e. effectively removing) the effect of *confounding* at the design stage of a *case-control study*. (See 📖 Confounding, p.154.)

Maternal mortality rate the number of maternal deaths per 100,000 births. (See 📖 Routine data, p.202.)

Measurement bias see 'Bias'.

Meta-analysis a statistical analysis of a collection of studies, often collected together through a systematic review. (See 📖 Meta-analysis, p.90.)

Morbidity the extent of disease and disability; in relation to prognosis it may include levels of disability, frequency of recurrence, etc. (See 📖 Decisions, decisions … the principles of clinical management, p.28 and Chapter 11.)

Natural history usually the course of the disease in the absence of treatment from the point of inception (or exposure to the causal agents) until recovery or death. (See 📖 Decisions, decisions … the principles of clinical management, p.28.)

Negative likelihood ratio (LR−) a measure of how much to decrease the probability of disease by if the test result is negative and is equal to 1 minus the sensitivity divided by the specificity. (See 📖 Likelihood ratios and post-test probabilities, p.22.)

Negative predictive value the probability that a person with a negative result does not have the condition. (See 📖 Validity of diagnostic tests, p.16 and 📖 Clinical uses of predictive value, p.18.)

Neonatal mortality rate the number of deaths of infants under 28 days per 1000 live births in a given year. (See 📖 Routine data, p.202.)

Normal distribution (also known as the Gaussian distribution or as a bell-shaped curve). This is the most commonly used mathematical distribution in statistics. It is defined for quantitative variables that can take any value from minus infinity to plus infinity, and is characterized by two parameters: its mean and standard deviation. (See 📖 Probability distributions, p.230.)

Null hypothesis see 'Hypothesis testing'.

Number needed to treat (NNT) a measure of how many people with an illness would need to be treated to produce one desired outcome or prevent one adverse outcome (e.g. one heart attack prevented). (See 📖 How effective is the treatment, p.42 and 📖 Interpreting reports of clinical trials, p.44.)

Observer bias see 'Bias'.

Odds another way to express probability. The mathematical relationship between odds and probability is: odds = probability / (1 − probability). (See 📖 Likelihood ratios and post-test probabilities, p.22.)

Odds ratio an estimate of relative risk obtained from case control studies where the incidence of disease is not known, but the frequency of exposure is measured in cases and controls. The *odds ratio* (of exposure) is the ratio between two odds, i.e. the *odds of exposure* in the *cases* divided by the *odds of exposure* in the *controls*. (See 📖 Risk factors, p.12, 📖 Communicating risk, p.56, and 📖 Case–control studies, p.172.)

Outbreak used interchangeably with epidemic, usually for a more localized increase in cases. (See 📖 Basic infectious disease epidemiology, p.106.)

Outcome the event or main quantity of interest in a particular study, e.g. death, contracting a disease, blood pressure. (See 📖 Basic concepts in epidemiological research, p.148.)

Pandemic when an epidemic spreads over several continents. (See 📖 Basic infectious disease epidemiology, p.106.)

Per protocol analysis see 'Intention to treat'.

Population attributable risk (also known as the population excess risk) the proportion of the disease that is due to the risk factor in the population as a whole, and thus the proportion of disease in the population that should be prevented if the risk is removed (assuming there is a causal relationship). (See 📖 Communicating risk, p.56.)

Positive likelihood ratio (LR+) a measure of how much to increase the probability of disease by if the test result is positive and is equal to the sensitivity divided by (1-specificity). (See 📖 Likelihood ratios and post-test probabilities, p.22.)

Positive predictive value the probability that a person with a positive test result has the condition. (See 📖 Validity of diagnostic tests, p.16 and 📖 Clinical uses of predictive value, p.18.)

Pre-test probability the probability of the condition disorder before a diagnostic test result is known. (See 📖 Pre-test probability, p.20 and 📖 Likelihood ratios and post-test probabilities, p.22.)

Prevalence the proportion of people with a disease at any point (point prevalence) or period (period prevalence) in time. (See 📖 Measures of disease frequency, p.6.)

Prevention paradox the fact that many people exposed to a small risk may generate more disease than the few exposed to a large risk. (See 📖 Prevention strategies, p.98.)

Primary prevention the prevention of the onset of disease. (See 📖 Levels of prevention, p.100.)

Primordial prevention the prevention of factors promoting the emergence of risk factors. (See 📖 Levels of prevention, p.100.)

Probability the chance of an event occurring, ranges from 0 (no chance) to 1 (inevitable).

Prognosis the probable course and outcome of an illness, including duration of disease, morbidity, and mortality. (See 📖 Decisions, decisions … the principles of clinical management, p.28.)

Prognostic factors variables that influence outcome, such as age, sex, disease stage. (See 📖 Decisions, decisions … the principles of clinical management, p.28.)

Protective factor something that reduces a person's chance of getting a disease. (See 📖 Risk factors, p.12.)

Publication bias the greater likelihood that research with statistically significant results will be published in the peer-reviewed literature in comparison to those with null or non-significant results. (See 📖 Analysis and interpretation of a meta-analysis, p.92.)

p-value the probability of obtaining the study result (*relative risk, odds ratio*, etc.) if the *null hypothesis* is true. The smaller the p-value, the easier it is for us to reject the *null hypothesis* and accept that the result was not just due to chance. (See Chapter 9.)

Randomization in clinical trials is done to remove bias in treatment allocation. (See 📖 Intervention studies and clinical trials, p.186.)

Recall bias see 'Bias'.

Regression a method for quantifying the relationship between a dependent variable, or response and one or more independent or explanatory variables. Often used for controlling confounding in epidemiological analysis. (See 📖 Linear regression, p.260.)

Relative risk the increase (or decrease) in probability of disease given a particular exposure or risk factor. It is estimated in cohort or follow-up studies from the incidence in the exposed (those with the risk factor) divided by the incidence in the unexposed. (See 📖 Risk factors, p.12, 📖 Communicating risk, p.56, and 📖 Cohort studies, p.178.)

Relative risk reduction the percentage reduction in an outcome (e.g. death) comparing one group with a control group. (See 📖 How effective is the treatment, p.42 and 📖 Intervention and clinical trials, p.186.)

Restriction a method for controlling the effect of *confounding* at the design stage of a study.

Risk see 'Absolute risk'.

Risk factor something that increases a person's chance of getting a disease. This definition assumes that there is a causal relationship rather than simply a statistical association. Risk factors are often described as modifiable (for example environmental exposures and behaviours) or fixed (for example genetic predisposition, age, or ethnicity). (See 📖 Risk factors, p.12.)

Risk marker a factor that is associated with an increased risk of disease but has not been shown to be causal. (See 📖 Risk factors, p.12.)

Routine health data sources of information relating to the health of the population that are collected in an ongoing way rather than for any specific research project. (See 📖 Routine data, p.202.)

Sample the subset of the population that is included in a study. (See Chapter 9 📖 Introduction, p.218.)

Screening the practice of investigating apparently healthy individuals with the object of detecting unrecognized disease or its precursors in order that measures can be taken to prevent or delay the development of disease or improve prognosis. (See 📖 Screening overview, p.112.)

Secondary prevention the halting of progression once the disease process is already established. (See 📖 Levels of prevention, p.100 and 📖 Screening overview, p.112.)

Selection bias occurs when people who participate in studies or screening programmes differ from those who do not. (See 📖 Evaluating screening programmes, p.116 and 📖 Basic concepts in epidemiological research, p.148.)

Sensitivity the ability of a diagnostic test to correctly identify people with the disease, i.e. the probability that a person with the disease will test positive. (See 📖 Validity of diagnostic tests, p.16.)

Specificity the ability of a diagnostic test to correctly identify people without the disease, i.e. the probability that a person without the disease will test negative. (See 📖 Validity of diagnostic tests, p.16.)

Standardization a method for controlling the effect of *confounding* at the analysis stage of a study. Used to produce a Standardized Mortality Ratio, a commonly used measure in epidemiology.

Stratification a method for controlling the effect of *confounding* at the analysis stage of a study. *Risks* are calculated separately for each category of *confounding variable*, e.g. each age group and each sex separately.

Survival the time from diagnosis to the outcome of interest (e.g. death). (See 📖 Decisions, decisions ... the principles of clinical management, p.28, 📖 Prognosis mortality, p.32, and 📖 Measuring survival, p.274.)

Systematic review a systematic way of drawing together and synthesizing existing evidence and producing a summary appraisal in a narrative form. (See 📖 Systematic review, p.88.)

Tertiary prevention the rehabilitation of people with established disease to minimize residual disability and complications. (See 📖 Levels of prevention, p.100.)

Under-5 mortality rate the probability that a newborn baby will die before reaching age 5, as a number per 1000 live births.

Vaccination is the introduction of a substance (vaccine) into the body in order to stimulate the production of antibodies against an infection without causing the active infection. (See 📖 Basic infectious disease epidemiology, p.106 and 📖 Vaccination, p.108.)

Validity a measure of how well a test distinguishes diseased from non-diseased individuals. The concept can be equally well applied to symptoms and signs. A completely valid test/symptom/sign will be positive for all cases and negative for all non-cases. (See 📖 Validity of diagnostic tests, p.16 and 📖 Screening overview, p.112.)

Statistical formulae

- **Sample mean and standard deviation**

Given a sample, $x_1,\ldots, x_n$, the sample mean and standard deviation (SD) are

$$\bar{x} = \frac{1}{n}\sum_{i=1}^{n} x_i \quad \text{and} \quad s = \sqrt{\frac{1}{n-1}\sum_{i=1}^{n}(x_i - \bar{x})^2}, \text{ respectively}$$

- **Pooled standard error for difference in two sample means**

If $x_{11},\ldots x_{1n_1}$ is a sample from a population with mean μ_1 and $x_{21},\ldots x_{2n_2}$ is an independent sample from a population with mean μ_2 then $(\mu_1 - \mu_2)$ can be estimated by $(\bar{x}_1 - \bar{x}_2)$, (where $\bar{x}_1$ and $\bar{x}_2$ are the means of samples 1 and 2, respectively), with standard error

$$\widehat{SE}_{\text{indep}}(\bar{x}_1 - \bar{x}_2) = \sqrt{\frac{s_1^2}{n_1} + \frac{s_2^2}{n_2}}$$

(where s_1 and s_2 are the SDs of samples 1 and 2, respectively).

An approximate 95% confidence interval for $(\bar{x}_1 - \bar{x}_2)$, when n_1 and n_2 are both large, takes the form $(\bar{x}_1 - \bar{x}_2)$, $\pm\, t_{n_1+n_2-1}\,\widehat{SE}(\bar{x}_1 - \bar{x}_2)$ where $t_{n_1+n_2-1}$ is the appropriate quantile from a t-distribution with (n_1+n_2-1) degrees of freedom (under the assumption that the variances are equal in the two groups).

- **Standard error for difference in sample means for paired sample**

If $(x_1, y_1), \ldots, (x_n, y_n)$ form a paired sample from a population whose x and y values have means μ_x and μ_y, respectively, then $(\mu_y-\mu_x)$ can be estimated by $(\bar{y}-\bar{x})$ (where $\bar{y}$ and $\bar{x}$ are the sample means of the x and y samples respectively), with standard error

$$\widehat{SE}_{\text{paired}}(\bar{y} - \bar{x}) = \frac{s_d}{\sqrt{n}}$$

(where s_d is the sample SD of the difference, $d_i = y_i - x_i$).

An approximate 95% confidence interval for $(\bar{y}-\bar{x})$ takes the form $(\bar{y}-\bar{x})\pm\, t_{n-1}\,\widehat{SE}_{\text{paired}}(\bar{y} - \bar{x})$, where t_{n-1} is the appropriate quantile from a t-distribution with $(n-1)$ degree of freedom.

- **Standard error of a proportion**

If $x_1, \ldots, x_n$ is a sample from a population which can take values in the range 0–1 then the mean, p, can be estimated by $\hat{p}=\bar{x}$, with standard error

$$\widehat{SE}(\hat{p}) = \sqrt{\frac{\hat{p}(1-\hat{p})}{n}},$$

An approximate 95% confidence interval then takes the form $\hat{p}\pm 1.96\,\widehat{SE}(\hat{p})$

- **Standard error for difference between proportions**

If $x_{11}, \ldots, x_{1n_1}$ and $x_{21}, \ldots, x_{2n_2}$ are independent sample from populations which can take values in the range 0–1 with means p_1 and p_2 respectively, then (p_1-p_2) can be estimated by $(\hat{p}_1-\hat{p}_2)$ (where $\hat{p}_1$ and $\hat{p}_2$ are the means of samples 1 and 2, respectively), with standard error

$$\widehat{SE}_{indep}(\hat{p}_1 - \hat{p}_2) = \sqrt{\frac{\hat{p}_1(1-\hat{p}_1)}{n_1} + \frac{\hat{p}_2(1-\hat{p}_2)}{n_2}}$$

An approximate 95% interval for (p_1-p_2), when n_1 and n_2 are both large takes the form, $(\hat{p}_1-\hat{p}_2) \pm 1.96\,\widehat{SE}(\hat{p}_1-\hat{p}_2)$.

Epidemiology in the clinic

Introduction

Clinical medicine involves the application of knowledge and clinical skills to a particular patient in order to make informed decisions about management. The pulling together of all the background knowledge with the specific presentation of the patient has been described as the 'art' of medicine, one that can only mature fully with experience rather than through reading books. Epidemiology is often thought of as outside of this creative process, and clinical epidemiology seen as a formulistic approach leading to automatic flowcharts rather than the interactive, skillful process that we recognize in our own clinical practice. In reality, many of the tools used in practising the 'art' of medicine are epidemiological. For example, the process of establishing a diagnosis is a series of steps that lead to an ever more specific differential diagnosis. This is essentially a risk assessment with each stage further refining the clinical options bringing you closer to the most likely diagnosis.

In this first section of the book we outline how epidemiological information, understanding, and methods can improve clinical practice in relation to setting up and refining the differential diagnosis, interpreting symptoms, signs and tests, making decisions on treatment options, and providing patients and the public with advice on prevention.

Chapter 1 starts by setting up the differential diagnosis, considering what conditions patients are likely to be presenting with based on the population they are drawn from, the clinical setting, and considers the major determinants of health that can inform your history taking. This information, based on the distribution of disease and determinants within the population, all lead to a 'pre-test probability' in relation to the patient having a specific condition. The diagnostic process then takes this one step further, narrowing the differential on the basis of reported symptoms, signs, and test results. Validity, predictive value, likelihood ratios, and post-test probabilities are explained in relation to individual patient care.

Chapter 2 considers the evidence underpinning decisions on management, including the parameters used to describe the uncertain future, i.e. the prognosis for the patient. Predictions are based on natural history studies in the population producing measures of mortality, case fatality, and morbidity. The chapter then moves onto evidence-based management, including how to find evidence, how to assess its applicability to this patient, ways of describing the pros and cons of treatment, the challenge of doing nothing, and the importance of making decisions in partnership with the patient. It includes a section on the development and use of guidelines in clinical care.

Chapter 3 concludes the section by turning towards the often overlooked part of clinical care that concerns health promotion. It starts from the patient perspective when diagnosed with a disease, the question 'Why me?' and asks whether the situation could have been avoided. Such discussions depend on epidemiological knowledge of risk factors and causal pathways, together with evidence about effectiveness of interventions. We describe how to communicate with patients about risk using terms such as relative and attributable risk appropriately, and then provide practical information on how to promote health with your patients.

The diagnostic process

Introduction: epidemiology in the clinic

Common things are common

Patients are drawn from a wider population, and through our knowledge of the distribution of disease in that population we can have an idea of the range of likely diagnoses for our patients. Before taking any history, performing an examination, or ordering investigations, you should have some background knowledge of the frequency of different conditions. This essential underpinning of clinical decision-making, rarely reflected upon, is based on epidemiology. If something is very rare, in everyday practice it will remain lower on your differential diagnosis list than if it is common. How is this distribution of disease described? How common is breast cancer, for example? There are many ways of answering this question, some being more relevant to clinical practice than others. Many people know that one in eight women will suffer from breast cancer at some point. But this does not show the probability that one of your patients has breast cancer at this time. More precise measures are needed, including prevalence and incidence, as outlined on 🕮 pp.6–8.

Index of suspicion

In addition to knowledge of disease frequency, a diagnosis is based on understanding the distribution of disease according to certain inherent criteria such as age and sex, and according to risk factors or exposures such as smoking or occupation. Again most clinicians will have an appreciation of these factors and they will adjust their differential diagnosis accordingly. Mesothelioma will be high up the differential diagnosis of a patient with pleuritic pain, cough, and weight loss who has a history of occupational exposure to asbestos, for example. Ways of quantifying the relationship of exposures to disease, as measured in epidemiological studies, are described on 🕮 pp.12–15.

Refining the diagnosis

Quantifying information on the frequency of disease in the population and the impact of different risk factors on that frequency can be used to produce a measure of the likelihood that a person will have a certain condition. This pre-test probability should be the starting point for carrying out examinations and investigations which will then aim to increase, or decrease, that probability according to their results. Each test, whether a simple examination or a complex metabolic or imaging technique, has a likelihood ratio that can be used to increase or decrease the probability of the condition according to the test result. In much clinical practice this process is carried out in a qualitative way—with a result sometimes being considered to rule in or rule out a condition, but in reality few tests carry such certainty. On 🕮 pp.22–25. we explain how to use results in a quantitative way, producing post-test probabilities of disease.

This section ends with a summary of how information can be put together to reach a diagnosis, and how to communicate this to patients ('So what have I got, doctor?'). This then forms the starting point for Chapter 2 on the management of patients.

Measures of disease frequency

In order to describe the distribution of a disease there must be an agreed definition of a case (see 📖 p.10) and this may vary according to the purpose of the measure.

Count

Definition: the number of cases:
- The most basic measure of disease frequency.
- It indicates health service needs.
- Usually not helpful in the absence of some denominator, i.e. relating it to a population of interest.
- Can be useful in monitoring disease trends in a stable population, e.g. if the condition is rare and population is stable:
  - E.g. there were 4 cases of human rabies in the UK in the 10 years from 2000–2011. Even if there has been some change in the population size, it is unnecessary to present this as incidence or a more precise rate.
- Cannot be used for comparing populations as they may differ in size.

Prevalence

See also 📖 p.167.

Definition: the proportion of people with a disease at any point (point prevalence) or period (period prevalence) in time.

$$\text{Point prevalence} = \frac{\text{Number of cases in a defined population at one point in time}}{\text{Number of persons in a defined population at the same point in time}}$$

- Measures the burden of disease in a population, and can be used to compare disease burden between populations.
- Particularly useful for chronic diseases.
- Uses are similar to count, e.g. planning healthcare resources with the additional benefit of relating these to population size.
- Can be obtained from cross-sectional studies and health service activity data (see 📖 pp.170, 206).

Incidence

See also 📖 p.179.

Definition: the number of new *cases* of the disease in a defined population over a defined period of time. *Incidence* measures events (a change from a healthy state to a diseased state).

$$\text{Incidence} = \frac{\text{Number of new cases in a defined population g over a period of time}}{\text{Number of disease-free people in a defined population g at the start of time period}}$$

- It is also referred to as *risk*, since it indicates the probability of acquisition of a disease over a period of time, or *cumulative incidence*.
- For a clinician, it can indicate the probability of diagnosing new cases for a given practice size.

- The *incidence rate* is a measure of the rate at which new cases occur, taking into account the time that each person in the population is at risk of becoming a case, and is expressed as e.g. number of new cases per person-year of follow-up. It is estimated from cohort (follow-up) studies (see ☐ p.178) or registries that include the duration of follow-up for each person.
- *How do we know?* These measures are derived from routine data of mortality, cancer registries, population surveys, or research studies. (see ☐ p.145).
- *Incidence and incidence rate* measure trends and can be used to see the impact of prevention measures or changes in risk factors.
- *Incidence* can be useful in health messages where it describes the probability, or risk, that an individual will develop the disease during a specific time period. It can be used to compare populations.

Relationship of incidence and prevalence (Table 1.1)

- Incidence measures new cases while prevalence measures all cases new and old.
- Prevalence is dependent on the incidence and the time that they remain cases (duration of disease) since people only leave the 'pool' of prevalent cases when they recover or die.
- Prevalence is the product of incidence and duration.

Table 1.1 Measures at a glance

Measure	Description	Type of measure
Count	Number of cases	Number
Prevalence	Number of cases in a population	Proportion
	Total number of people in population	
(Cumulative) incidence	New cases of disease in time period	Number per population per unit time
	Number of disease-free people in population at start of time period	
Incidence rate	Number of new cases of disease in time period	A rate
	Person-years at risk during period	

Examples (Tables 1.2 and 1.3)

Table 1.2 Relationship of incidence and prevalence in breast cancer

Measure	Breast cancer, women in UK, 2009[1]
Prevalence	550000 women are alive in UK who have had a diagnosis of breast cancer (2% of adult female population)
Incidence	47700 new cases
	124 per 100000 per year (European age-standardized incidence)
Lifetime risk	1 in 8

Table 1.3 Relationship of incidence and prevalence in genital chlamydial infection

Measure	*Chlamydia trachomatis* in 15–24-year-olds, 2009[2]
Count	482,696 cases diagnosed in sexual health clinics and community settings in the UK
Prevalence	5–7% in National Chlamydia Screening Programme, England
Incidence	2180 per 100,000 per year in England
Lifetime risk	30–50% for women by age 35 (2005 estimate)

Understanding prevalence: HIV infection

In the UK, the prevalence of HIV infection is increasing. Interpreting this finding requires an understanding of several factors:

• There has been a general increase in the numbers of people being tested for HIV leading to an increase in the proportion of people with HIV who are diagnosed. We know this from studies using anonymized testing which show that more people with HIV are aware of their status.
• There has also been an increase in the incidence of HIV in some sections of the population. This is estimated from follow-up studies of people who are repeatedly tested for HIV.
• There has been an increase in migration of people into the UK from areas of higher HIV prevalence.
• There has been a decline in mortality of people with HIV/AIDS due to the success of treatment with highly active anti-retroviral therapy (HAART). This has increased the duration of disease.
• Taken together these factors have led to a steep rise in the prevalence of HIV-positive individuals and consequently in the demand on health services (see 📖 pp.336–7).

References

1 Cancer Research UK, 2011. ॐ http://info.cancerresearchuk.org/cancerstats/types/breast
2 Health Protection Agency, 2011. ॐ http://www.chlamydiascreening.nhs.uk/ps/data/data_tables.html

Distribution of disease

Rare things can seem common

As a medical student attached to a paediatric oncology firm it seemed as if all children with a sore throat or with bleeding gums had leukaemia. Clearly the millions of children with self-limiting viral upper respiratory tract infections or gingivitis would not make it into this centre. The distribution of disease seen in clinical practice is not the same as that in the population, and therefore interpretation of signs and symptoms will depend upon where you practise.

Common things are common (but can seem rare)

Just as rare things can seem common, so some common things are rarely seen by some clinicians—the clinical iceberg. It is important to understand the background distribution of disease in the population generally, and also in the population seen in your practice (whether through referral or self-presentation).

Finding out

Finding out how common conditions are in the population is challenging. Most data are based on reported illness, which is severe, or from health-care settings which necessarily excludes all those conditions that are managed at home. Special population surveys are needed to find out the prevalence of disease, but these tend to focus on symptoms and self-report rather than confirmed diagnoses. In other words, they are measuring different things. The clinical iceberg concept indicates how little illness appears on the radar if health is measured through mortality, hospital data, or even primary care data.

Seeking advice

The 10 most common symptoms of adults seeking advice from NHS Direct in England are abdominal pain, headache, fever, chest pain, back pain, vomiting, breathing difficulties, diarrhoea, urinary symptoms, and dizziness.

Primary care consultations

The most common consultations for adults in primary care are for respiratory illness and neurological conditions.

Secondary care admissions

The most common hospital admissions in England (2009–10 data) are: cardiovascular and respiratory disease and symptoms (15%); gastrointestinal disease and symptoms (15%); and cancer (11%).

Mortality

The leading causes of death in the UK (2005 data) are circulatory disease (36%), neoplasms (27%) and respiratory disease (14%).

Is there anything wrong?

Patients are first concerned with finding out whether they have anything wrong with them, and if so, what it is, can it be cured, what the future holds, and then, often a little later, why them?

Deciding whether there is anything wrong is not always easy, since perceptions and definitions of health and disease vary. The World Health Organization (WHO) definition of health is a state of complete physical, mental, and social well-being and not merely the absence of disease or infirmity. By that definition a large proportion of people are unhealthy.

- In England, 77% of men and 74% of women consider themselves to be in good or very good health.
- 14% of men and 19% of women report acute sickness in the previous 2 weeks.

For the clinician, defining and labelling a patient with (or without) a specific disease is the key to decision-making. However, definitions are rarely clear-cut. While clinical medicine depends on distinguishing normal from diseased states, these are generally rather arbitrary distinctions since there is a range of normality and of disease which frequently overlap. In practice we are looking for a definition or cut-off which divides people into those who would benefit from treatment and those who would not, and of course such definitions may change over time.

Purpose of defining a case

The purpose of defining a case varies by setting:

- In a consultation the purpose of defining a case is to decide on management and give advice on prognosis.
- In an epidemiological study the purpose is generally to look at aetiology, and while the case definition will depend on the exact research question it is likely to be very wide to ensure all possible cases are included.
- For surveillance, case definitions must be clear and consistent to enable comparisons over time and place.
- In a clinical trial the purpose is to test a treatment and therefore the definition used should be one that can be replicated in clinical practice in order that conclusions are specific (e.g. to a certain severity of disease).
- In medico-legal situations the definition of a case may have major implications for the accused and the victim, and therefore must be precise, reproducible, and based on validated and accepted criteria.

Labels

For some conditions a diagnosis is a label with wide-ranging implications for the patient in relation to family, finances, employment, etc. Some labels carry a stigma and therefore the clinician must be particularly careful and sensitive before making the diagnosis.

Difficulties in defining a case
- Variation in normal both between and within individuals.
- Variation in the spectrum of disease, ranging from mild to severe, or continuous across the whole population (e.g. blood pressure).
- Variation in the performance of a test in both diseased and non-diseased individuals.
- Variation in the performance of a test between and within individuals.

Have I got hypertension?

Defining hypertension is important as is it relates to high levels of morbidity and mortality. But blood pressure (BP) has an essentially normal distribution in the population. At the upper end of the distribution are people with severe or 'malignant' or accelerated hypertension which is life threatening in the short term. Below this point there is no easy level at which to distinguish 'hypertensive' and 'normotensive'. In general, hypertension is defined at a level that indicates the need for treatment to reduce the risk of coronary heart disease and stroke. But the risks start to increase at a very low level, and therefore it is still somewhat arbitrary to decide that a certain amount of increased risk justifies treatment. Ideally we would define cases as those people in which intervention (e.g. antihypertensive drugs) will be more beneficial than no intervention.

Definitions of hypertension
- *Epidemiological:* studies have shown that the risk of cardiovascular disease starts to increase with a systolic BP of >115mmHg.
- *Clinical:* a persistent raised BP >140/90mmHg.[1]
- *Severe:* BP >180/110mmHg.[1]

The normal distribution
The frequency of many human characteristics in the population (height, weight, blood pressure, haemoglobin, serum albumin etc.) tends to follow a normal distribution or bell curve. For many diagnostic tests of continuously distributed variables, 'normal' is defined statistically as lying within 2 standard deviations of the mean of the distribution of variation among individuals (see 🕮 p.230). This mathematical method of defining normality is rather arbitrary and may or may not relate to disease processes.

Reference
1 National Institute for Health and Clinical Excellence. *Hypertension* (Clinical Guidelines 127). London: NICE; 2011. ℬ http://www.nice.org.uk/CG127

Risk factors

Disease is not evenly distributed across the population, and epidemiology is concerned with exploring the factors associated with that variation. Understanding the major determinants of health and disease helps clinicians in drawing up a differential diagnosis for a particular patient. For example, you are more likely to consider infective endocarditis as a diagnosis if a person presenting with fever has a prosthetic heart valve. Similarly, the possibility of bronchial carcinoma will be higher up the differential diagnosis in a smoker with haemoptysis than in a non-smoker, and Weil's disease will be more likely in a farm worker than a computer programmer if both present with headache and fever followed by jaundice. Thus understanding and quantifying risk factors can assist in the diagnostic process as well as informing preventive interventions.

Definitions

- *Risk factor*: something that increases a person's chance of getting a disease. This definition assumes that there is a causal relationship rather than simply a statistical association. Risk factors are often described as *modifiable* (e.g. environmental exposures and behaviours) or *fixed* (e.g. genetic predisposition, age, or ethnicity).
- *Risk marker*: a factor that is associated with an increased risk of disease but has not been shown to be causal.
- *Protective factor*: something that reduces a person's chance of getting a disease, e.g. high levels of high-density lipoprotein (HDL) cholesterol and high fruit and vegetable intake are protective against coronary heart disease.

Relevance to clinical practice

- Consider relevant risk factors when drawing up differential diagnosis.
- Enquire about relevant risk (or protective) factors in the history.
- Use knowledge about risk/protective factors when counselling patients about behaviours.

Quantifying risk factors

Epidemiological research is largely concerned with exploring the relationship between risk factors (exposures) and disease (outcomes). The following parameters describe the association:

- Relative risk.
- Attributable risk.
- Odds ratio.
- Correlation.

Chapter 7 includes detailed definitions and methods for measuring these parameters (see 📖 pp.145–95). In clinical practice it is useful to remember what each of them means for patients:

The relative risk (📖 pp.179–80) tells you how much more likely a disease will be in a person with a risk factor than a person without it. It is estimated in cohort or follow-up studies from the incidence in the exposed (those with the risk factor) divided by the incidence in the unexposed, i.e. I_e/I_o. Using the example in Box 1.1, a woman on hormone replacement therapy (HRT) is 2.25 times more likely to develop breast cancer than a woman who has never taken HRT.

The attributable risk (📖 pp.179–80) tells you the absolute increase in incidence of disease that is associated with the risk factor, and is also estimated from cohort studies from $I_e - I_o$. Again, the data in Box 1.1 would suggest that the woman taking HRT has an *extra risk of 2.1 cases of breast cancer per 100 women years which is equivalent to an extra 2.1% chance* of developing breast cancer each year as a result of the HRT (assuming a causal relationship).

The odds ratio (📖 pp.172–4) is an estimate of relative risk obtained from case–control studies where the incidence of disease is not known, but the frequency of exposure is measured in cases and controls. Its use with patients is the same as relative risk.

Correlation (📖 pp.162, 262) is another measure of association that is used for risk factors that are continuous variables or multiple categories. A correlation coefficient (r^2) shows how much an increase in risk is explained by an increase in exposure.

Box 1.1 Quantifying risk factors: example of breast cancer and HRT[1]

Danish women were enrolled in a cohort study, and the relationship of HRT to breast cancer incidence was explored.

The incidence of breast cancer was 1.68 per 100 women per year for those who had never used HRT, and 3.78 for those currently on HRT.

Relative risk = incidence in exposed (I_e)/incidence in unexposed (I_o)

$$= I_e/I_o$$
$$= 3.78/1.68$$
$$= 2.25$$

Attributable risk = incidence in exposed − incidence in unexposed

$$= I_e - I_o$$
$$= 3.78 - 1.68$$
$$= 2.1 \text{ per 100 women per year}$$

Reference

1 Stahlberg C et al. Breast cancer incidence, case-fatality and breast cancer mortality in Danish women using hormone replacement therapy—a prospective observational study. *Int J Epidemiol* 2005; **34**(4):931–5.

Identifying risk factors

In the consultation obtaining accurate information on relevant risk factors can help in forming a differential diagnosis. This is usually done by taking a structured history that should include demographic, occupational, social, and behavioural factors.

Taking a risk factor history

Questions must be:
- Relevant to the patient's presentation and the diagnostic process.
- Sensitive and not too intrusive.

To obtain accurate risk factor information requires skill in communication. The patient will need to understand why certain questions are being asked, and feel confident that the information is pertinent, confidential, and will not be used in any prejudicial way.

Reliable histories

Some risk factor questions are notoriously difficult to collect reliable information on. This may be due to sensitivities (see Box 1.2) or real difficulties of recall. Where possible, previous records should be consulted for exposures such as vaccinations, previous drug treatments, occupational history and possibly lifestyle (if these are routinely collected).

Box 1.2 Sensitive questions

Country of origin, nationality, ethnicity
- Rights: patients may be concerned that you may be questioning their right to healthcare rather than a risk factor.
- Racism: patients may be wary of perceived or actual discrimination on the basis of their ethnicity.

Sexual behaviour, sexuality
- Intrusion: patients may not think that their behaviour is relevant.
- Embarrassment: patients may be embarrassed disclosing multiple sex partners, particularly to a family doctor.
- Homophobia: patients may be wary of perceived or actual discrimination on the grounds of their sexual orientation.

Drug, alcohol, and tobacco use
- Law: patients reporting use of illicit drugs may fear that you will report them to the criminal justice system.
- Judgemental: patients often fear a negative response if they disclose tobacco or excessive alcohol use.

Other lifestyle factors
- Patients may be reluctant to admit to themselves or their doctor if they do not follow general advice on exercise, diet, and healthy lifestyles.

Reassurance

Improved information on sensitive issues may be obtained if:

- You explain why information is relevant to diagnosis and care.
- You explain how information will be stored and who will have access to it.
- You maintain strict patient confidentiality at all times.
- You ask in a routine and professional way, e.g. enquiring about sexual history with the same tone as questions about medical history.
- You ask yourself whether patients might feel that you are acting in a discriminatory way.
- You obtain information in an impartial way, e.g. through patient-administered questionnaire or through computer-assisted self-report.

Validity of diagnostic tests

When we order a diagnostic test, or carry out a particular examination, the intension is to make a definitive diagnosis or at least narrow the differential. Unfortunately, few if any tests are 100% correct 100% of the time.

Far from being a definitive answer, most tests require some interpretation. The key parameters for describing the validity of a test are its sensitivity and specificity. Interpreting the results of tests requires an understanding of how they perform (Tables 1.4–1.6).

Definitions
- *Validity:* a measure of how well a test distinguishes diseased from non-diseased individuals. The concept can be equally well applied to symptoms and signs. A completely valid test/symptom/sign will be positive for all cases and negative for all non-cases.
- *Gold standard:* to determine validity it is necessary to have a gold standard that distinguishes diseased from non-diseased people. The idea of a gold standard suggests a degree of certainty that is rarely found. Uncertainty exists in distinguishing diseased from normal (see 📖 Is there anything wrong?, p.10), in the interpretation of test results and the defining of cut off points. However, the concept of validity is predicated on that of a true state that can be known.

Parameters of validity
- *Sensitivity*: the ability to correctly identify people with the disease, i.e. the probability that a person with the disease will test positive.
- *Specificity*: the ability to correctly identify people without the disease, i.e. the probability that a person without the disease will test negative.
- *Positive predictive value* (PPV): the probability that a person with a positive result has the condition.
- *Negative predictive value* (NPV): the probability that a person with a negative result does not have the condition.

These parameters are also incorporated into the concept of likelihood ratios which are particularly useful in clinical practice as they can be used with pre-test probabilities in quantitative diagnostic analyses (see 📖 Likelihood ratios, p.22).

Helpful reminders
- **SpPin**: when a test has a high **Sp**ecificity a **P**ositive result tends to rule *in* the diagnosis.
- **SnNout**: when a test has a high **Sn**ositivity, a **N**egative result rules *out* the diagnosis.

Table 1.4 Calculating the parameters of a diagnostic test

Test result	Disease status[*]		
	Diseased	Non-diseased	
Positive	a	b	a+b
Negative	c	d	c+d
	a+c	b+d	N

[*]According to gold standard

- Sensitivity: a/(a+c)
- Specificity: d/(b+d)
- Positive predictive value: a/(a+b)
- Negative predictive value: d/(c+d)

Table 1.5 Alternative representation

Test result	Disease status[*]	
	Diseased	Non-diseased
Positive	True positive	False positive
Negative	False negative	True negative

[*]According to gold standard

- Sensitivity: true positive/(true positive + false negative)
- Specificity: true negative/(true negative + false positive)
- Positive predictive value: true positive/(true positive + false positive)
- Negative predictive value: true negative/(true negative + false negative)

Table 1.6 Worked example of test performance for a rapid test for genital *Chlamydia* infection

Test result	Chlamydia infection		
	Infected	Not infected	
Positive	91	14	105
Negative	18	1224	1242
	109	1238	1247

- Sensitivity: 91/109 = 83.5%
- Specificity: 1224/1238 = 98.9%
- Positive predictive value: 91/105 = 86.7%
- Negative predictive value: 1224/1242 = 98.6%

Reference

1 Mahilum-Tapay L *et al.* New point of care Chlamydia Rapid Test—bridging the gap between diagnosis and treatment: performance evaluation study. *BMJ* 2007; **335**:1190–4.

Clinical uses of predictive value

The predictive value of a symptom, sign, or test is a very useful parameter in clinical practice. It is a measure of how likely the patient is to have (or not have) a condition given that they have had a positive (or negative) result.

These values enable you to answer that common question from a patient: 'You tell me the test is positive (or negative), so have I definitely got (or not got) the disease?'

Pathognomonic?

For some conditions, a positive sign or test is said to be a definitive answer or *pathognomonic*. This can only happen when the test is completely specific, i.e. there are never any false positives, and therefore the PPV is 100%. There are probably no truly pathognomonic signs, but they were traditionally said to include rice-water stools (cholera), risus sardonicus (tetanus), Koplik's spots (measles). For a symptom, sign, or test to be fully diagnostic, then all people with the disease are positive and all those without are negative. The PPV and NPV would both be 100%, and the test would be the gold standard and a way of defining the condition. However, for the majority of conditions such simple certainty is not present, at least with preliminary tests, and we are left with interpreting differing levels of certainty.

Predictive value varies

Unlike sensitivity and specificity, predictive value is not based only on inherent test characteristics, but varies according to the prevalence of the disease in the population as well as the sensitivity and specificity of the test. This is best understood using a worked example (see Tables 1.7–1.9).

Practical use of predictive value

When a patient has had a test and the result is available, they will usually expect a definitive answer. In a number of situations you will need to discuss the uncertainty of test results in a meaningful way. Telling patients that the test has a good sensitivity or specificity is not particularly helpful as they have no way of relating that information to their own situation. Predictive value can be more useful on the proviso that it relates to a population with a similar prevalence to that of the patient in front of you.

Using the data in Tables 1.7–1.9, if you carried out a such a HIV test in a patient attending a similar primary care setting and the result was positive, you could explain to the patient that a positive test is only truly positive half of the time, and therefore they need to wait for a confirmatory test. On the other hand, if their result is negative, you could confidently say that they were free from the disease (assuming there had been sufficient time since the presumed exposure).

In the next sections (see 📖 pp.20–5) we show how knowledge about prevalence and test validity can by systematically incorporated through use of pre-test probabilities and likelihood ratios.

Predictive value varies with prevalence: worked example

Imagine that there was a new rapid test for HIV infection, and it had a sensitivity of 100% and a specificity of 99%. That means that everyone with HIV will test positive, but for every 100 people without HIV, 1 would also test positive. Tables 1.7–1.9 show the results of using the test in 3 different populations.

In these 3 different populations a test with the same sensitivity and specificity produces widely different PPV. If it were used for screening a low-prevalence population there would be a lot of false positives that would need to be subject to a confirmatory test.

Table 1.7 Test used in a sexual health clinic with a high prevalence population (prevalence = 10%)

Test result	True HIV status		
	Diseased	Non-diseased	
Positive	100	9	109
Negative	0	891	891
	100	900	1000

- Positive predictive value = 100/109 = 91.7%.

Table 1.8 Test used in a primary care setting (prevalence = 1%)

Test result	True HIV status		
	Diseased	Non-diseased	
Positive	10	10	20
Negative	0	980	980
	10	990	1000

- Positive predictive value = 10/20 = 50%.

Table 1.9 Test used in a blood donor population (prevalence = 0.1%)

Test result	True HIV status		
	Diseased	Non-diseased	
Positive	1	10	11
Negative	0	989	989
	1	999	1000

- Positive predictive value = 1/11 = 9.1%.

Pre-test probability

The process described up to now—moving towards a diagnosis based on knowledge of the distribution of disease in the population and risk factors, together with the basic history of the patient—provides a starting point for the ordering of specific investigations or tests. A test may be as simple as a physical examination or as complex as the latest imaging techniques but should be undertaken with the same purpose: to move closer to, or further from, a given diagnosis.

Definition of pre-test probability

The probability of the condition or disorder before a diagnostic test result is known.

The pre-test probability is the likelihood that the patient has the condition when you do not know the result of the test. At its broadest, this is the prevalence of the condition in the population, but in practice it should be related to the specific patient as far as possible and include the clinical setting, the age, sex, with or without known risk factors, and presenting with a particular set of symptoms or signs. In general this is unknown, and we work with a more qualitative approach based on past experience of similar patients and knowledge of risk factors, but with the growth of evidence-based clinical practice tools to quantify such information are likely to be made available.

There are a number of conditions where pre-test probabilities are well described (see Box 1.3) and these may be useful in clinical decision-making. In practice few clinicians have the time to carry out formal calculations of pre-test probabilities before deciding on investigations, but such quantitative analyses are increasingly used to inform clinical decision support tools such as algorithms and guidelines (see 📖 p.38).

Box 1.3 Pre-test probabilities

Syncope[1]

Setting: community hospitals in Italy.

Findings: of 195 patients with syncope, 35% (69) had neurovascular reflex disorders, 21% had cardiac disorders. Particular factors in the history shifted the probabilities; e.g. a lack of cardiac findings on examination and electrocardiogram (ECG) lowered the probability of cardiac disorders for this patient.

Use: such information can help in reaching diagnosis by providing a hierarchy of possibilities from the 50 or more reported causes of syncope. Investigations or, if appropriate, a trial of a treatment can then be directed to try and confirm or exclude the most likely diagnosis or diagnoses.

Chest pain[2]

A 65-year-old man comes in to see his general practitioner (GP) with chest pain

Objective of diagnostic process

Pain caused by myocardial ischaemia in impending infarction must be differentiated from non-ischaemic chest pain in order to inform management of the patient.

How do you tell if this is likely to be cardiac chest pain?

You could list all the causes of chest pain and systematically test for each one, but it is far more efficient to start by narrowing it down based on what you already know.

- You already know this is an ambulant male aged 65:
  - Male gender and increasing age are risks for coronary heart disease (CHD) so your suspicion is raised (above that of a woman, or a younger man).
- Details of the pain from the history: it has been on and off for 6 weeks, substernal, no radiation, an ache, not related to exertion or stress:
  - The pain is not characteristic of cardiac pain so CHD is less likely.
- From asking a directed history and looking at previous records you can assess some key risk factors: he has no personal history of heart disease but he has smoked 20 cigarettes a day for around 20 years:
  - The history of smoking makes it much more likely.

What do we know now?

From this information you can calculate a pre-test probability that he has CHD. This can be done qualitatively, based on 'experience' and prior knowledge, or can be done quantitatively using precise estimates based on epidemiological data. Using such a method, the authors of this example estimated a probability of 25% that this man had severe CHD (see website[2] for details and tutorial).

References

1 Ammirati F et al. Diagnosing syncope in clinical practice. *Eur Heart J* 2000; **21**:935–40.
2 National Institute of Dental and Craniofacial Research. *Symptom research: methods and opportunities.* [Interactive textbook] ♒ http://painconsortium.nih.gov/symptomresearch/index. htm. The website provides a comprehensive tutorial for use of such methods in clinical practice.

Likelihood ratios and post-test probabilities

Likelihood ratios are a useful way of quantifying results in the diagnostic process by relating the probability (p) of a result in someone with the disease to someone without it. The likelihood ratio (LR) is the likelihood that a given test result would be expected in a patient with the disease compared to the likelihood that that same result would be expected in a patient without the disease.

LR = p [test result if disease is present]/p [test result if disease is absent]

Their usefulness over and above other measures of validity is that they can be applied to a pre-test probability to produce a numeric increase or decrease in that probability given a particular test result. A LR >1 is associated with the presence of the disease, and the higher the number the stronger the association. A LR <1 is associated with the absence of the disease, with the lower the number the stronger the evidence for absence (Table 1.10).

Positive likelihood ratio (LR+) is a measure of how much to increase the probability of disease if the test result is positive:

$$LR+ = sensitivity/(1 - specificity)$$

Negative likelihood ratio (LR−) is a measure of how much to decrease the probability of disease if the test result is negative:

$$LR- = (1 - sensitivity)/specificity$$

Table 1.10 Estimated likelihood ratios for diagnosing urinary tract infection (UTI) from symptoms in previously healthy women

Symptoms	+LR	−LR
Dysuria	1.5	0.5
Frequency	1.8	0.6
Haematuria	2.0	0.9
Back pain	1.6	0.8
Vaginal discharge (absence)	3.1	0.3
Vaginal irritation (absence)	2.7	0.2
Low abdominal pain	1.1	0.9
Flank pain	1.1	0.9
Self-diagnosis	4.0	0.1
Symptom combination of +dysuria, +frequency, −discharge, −irritation	24.6	(n/a)

Estimating post-test probabilities using likelihood ratios

The calculation is done using odds rather than probabilities which can be a bit complicated and slow (see Box 1.4). In practice there are short-cuts using calculators (available online: ℘ http://www.cebm.net/index. aspx?o=1161) or a nomogram (see 📖 p.24). To do the calculations by hand you need to be able to convert probabilities (p) to odds (o) and vice versa using the following general formula:

$$o = p/(1 - p)$$
$$p = o/(1 + o)$$

Then pre-test odds are:

$$o_1 = p_1/(1 - p_1)$$

and the post-test odds, in a person with a positive test are:

$$o_2 = p_1 \times LR+$$

which can be converted back into a probability to help communicate the risk to the patient:

$$p_2 = o_2/(1 + o_2)$$

where o_1 is pre-test odds, o_2 is post-test odds, p_1 is pre-test probability and p_2 is post-test probability.

These estimates of LR are made from a systematic review of evidence applied to women presenting with possible UTI with a pre-test probability of 50%. The author concludes, 'Combinations of symptoms . . . may rule in the disease; however, no combination decreases the disease prevalence to less than 20% . . .'.[1]

Box 1.4 Example of calculating post-test probabilities

What is the role of a dipstick test in the diagnosis of UTI in symptomatic women attending GPs? The prevalence of UTI in symptomatic women (pre-test probability) was 55%, the dipstick sensitivity 90%, specificity 65%.

For a positive test:
LR+ = sensitivity/(1 − specificity) = 0.9/(1 − 0.65) = 2.57
p_1 (from prevalence) = 0.55
o_1 = 0.55/(1 − 0.55) = 1.22
o_2 = o_1 × LR+ = 1.22 × 2.57 = 3.14
p_2 = 3.14/(1 + 3.14) = 0.76

For a negative test:
LR− = (1 − sensitivity)/specificity = (1 − 0.9)/0.65 = 0.15
o_2 = o_1 × LR− = 1.22 × 0.15 = 0.18
p_2 = 0.18/(1 + 0.18) = 0.15

Conclusion
In a woman presenting in general practice with symptoms suggesting a UTI, a positive dipstick test increases the probability of a bacterial UTI from 55% to 76%, while a negative dipstick test decreases the probability to 15%.

Fagan nomogram

The Fagan nomogram allows LR to convert pre- to post-test probabilities. To use, if the pre-test probability is marked on the left axis, then a line is drawn from this point on the left side of the graph through the LR value (positive or negative) for the test. The point where the line meets the right side of the graph is the estimated post-test probability of the disease (Fig. 1.1).

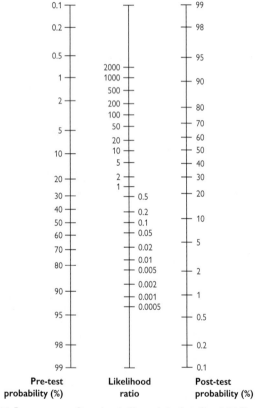

Fig. 1.1 Fagan nomogram. Reproduced with permission from Greenhalgh T. How to read a paper: Papers that report diagnostic or screening tests. *BMJ* 1997; **315**:540–3.

References

1 Aubin C. Does this woman have an acute uncomplicated urinary tract infection? *Ann Emerg Med* 2007; **49**:106–8.

Online resource

Links to a number of likelihood ratios can be found at Bandolier. ✑ http://www.medicine.ox.ac.uk/bandolier

So what has my patient got? The Bayesian clinician

The processes described in the previous sections of this chapter are all about narrowing the differential diagnosis through gathering together evidence. This is inherent in diagnostic decision-making, although we rarely think of it in these terms. The process is akin to Bayesian statistics, and if quantified through pre- and post-test probabilities and LRs it is an actual application of Bayes' theorem. Bayes' theorem states that the pre-test odds of a hypothesis being true multiplied by the weight of new evidence (LR) generates post-test odds of the hypothesis being true. Unlike 'frequentist' approaches to statistical inference, Bayesian inferences explicitly include prior knowledge, in these examples the pre-test probability. At each step in the diagnostic process you have a working idea of the probability of a diagnosis, and with the results of each question, examination and investigation you increase or decrease that probability.

In routine clinical practice this process is usually more qualitative than quantitative due to lack of relevant LR estimates, lack of time, and lack of expertise. However, quantitative estimations are important in developing clinical decision-making tools and algorithms to guide clinicians and increasingly to direct nursing and other healthcare staff in face-to-face, telephone, or online consultations. They can also be applied in clinical governance to reduce unnecessary investigations or introduce new ones.

Increasingly, new technologies are being used to improve clinical decision-making.

Clinical scoring systems

There are a large number of clinical scoring systems to assist diagnosis. Like any tool, some are better than others, and can be evaluated in terms of sensitivity and specificity.

- For example, the Alvarado scoring system for acute appendicitis uses a combination of signs and symptoms to assess the likelihood. An evaluation in children found that a score of 7 or higher had a sensitivity of 77%, and the specificity 100%.[1]
- Three different scoring systems for assessment of delirium in intensive care were compared; their sensitivities ranged from 30–83%, specificities were 91–96%.[2]
- The Manchester Self-Harm Rule had good sensitivity but poor specificity for predicting repetitions of self-harm or suicide in patients who presented to the emergency department with self-harm.[3]

References

1 McKay R, Shepherd J. The use of the clinical scoring system by Alvarado in the decision to perform computed tomography for acute appendicitis in the ED. *Am J Emerg Med* 2007; **25**:489–93.

2 Luetz A *et al.* Different assessment tools for intensive care unit delirium: which score to use? *Crit Care Med* 2010; **38**:409–18.

3 Hatcher S. The Manchester Self Harm Rule had good sensitivity but poor specificity for predicting repeat self harm or suicide. *Evid Based Med* 2007; **12**:89.

Management decisions

Decisions, decisions . . . the principles of clinical management

Once a diagnosis has been made, both doctor and patient will want to know what to do for the best to get the patient better. To recommend a course of action you need to be aware of:

- What happens in the absence of treatment (natural history and prognosis)?
- What treatments/approaches can improve the outcome?
- What is the best treatment for this patient?
- How much will this alter the natural history?
- Are there any downsides to this treatment, such as side effects?
- What treatment/course of action would the patient prefer?
- Can the patient consent to treatment?

For each of these questions it is possible to look at the evidence base from different types of study. For some conditions this may be simple, based on well-established guidelines or long-term practice. In other situations the clinician, or ideally groups of clinicians, will have to assess the evidence themselves.

For most conditions in addition to the treatment decision there are a few other considerations:

- Who should manage the treatment?
- Where should it be delivered?
- What other support will the patient need?
- Is anyone else likely to be affected?
- Does this episode present opportunities for preventing future ill health?

All of these require thought, consideration of the evidence, and discussion with the patient and possibly other people (family, carers). It is important that patients are informed and able to take part in the decisions.

What has this got to do with epidemiology?

These treatment decisions are at the heart of clinical medicine, and you may well ask what this has got to do with epidemiology. The answer is that evidence relevant to individual patients comes from looking at groups of patients with similar conditions, and therefore we need to apply the principles and methods of studying events in populations. This chapter will introduce key epidemiological measures relevant to clinical management.

Terms used in prognosis

- *Case fatality rate:* the proportion of people with a disease who die from that disease.
- *Mortality:* various measures of death, including the probability of death (within a defined time period, such as 5 years).
- *Morbidity:* the extent of disease and disability; in relation to prognosis it may include levels of disability, frequency of recurrence etc.

- *Natural history:* is usually taken to mean the course of the disease in the absence of treatment from the point of inception (or exposure to the causal agents) until recovery or death.
- *Prognosis:* is the probable course and outcome of an illness, including duration of disease, morbidity, and mortality.
- *Prognostic factors:* are variables that influence the outcome, such as age, sex, disease stage.
- *Survival:* is the opposite of mortality, and often used to describe outcomes, e.g. the 5-year survival for a particular disease means the proportion of people with this disease who are alive 5 years after diagnosis. The median survival is the length of time from diagnosis to when 50% of patients have died.

What is prognosis? Looking into the crystal ball

When a patient asks 'How long have I got, doctor?' the truthful answer is, 'I do not know as I can't see into the future'. This is not very helpful to the patient or their relatives, and would scupper the plot-line for various Hollywood films about '101 things to do in the three months before you die'. But we do provide answers, and these are based on experience of other people with similar conditions. This can be based on personal experience of similar patients, but that is not helpful if you rarely see the condition, only see a particular subset of patients with the condition (e.g. in a tertiary referral centre), if you don't routinely follow patients up (which is usually the case for specialists), or if you have a bad memory. All of these very real factors mean that estimates of prognosis based on personal clinical experience will be biased in one or more ways.

To overcome these biases and provide more accurate estimates of prognosis, studies of populations of people with the same conditions are needed.

Measures of prognosis

There is no simple measure of prognosis, since it may include the duration of the illness to recovery, progression, or death as well as the course of the illness in terms of severity. The most useful measures will depend on the type of illness (is it self-limiting, in which case an indication of duration and progress of severity may be best), the likely impact of treatment (is it 'incurable', in which case the focus will be on survival time and functional capacity), and the concerns of the patient (if they are concerned about coping with disability then they will need to know about functional capacity over the course of the disease).

Interpreting prognostic data

Since information on prognosis comes from studies of groups of people, it should be appraised using the same critical methods as for other epidemiological data with particular attention to:

- How were patients for the study selected? Were the entry criteria clearly defined with a reasonable response rate?
- Where were patients recruited? Was it a specialist centre, in which case they may have more severe or advanced disease and a worse prognosis?
- How was disease diagnosed?
- What stage were people at when they were recruited? If it varied, was this incorporated into the analysis?
- How long were patients followed for? Were they actively followed-up, or were records only kept for those who came back for treatment?
- What measures of outcome were used? Recovery, symptoms, signs, test results, standard disability/functionality measures, prescribed drugs, hospitalization, mortality?

Example of HIV—living though a changing prognosis

In the early days of the AIDS epidemic, before there was a test available for HIV, prognosis was very uncertain. The first cases of AIDS to be recognized were very ill and many died in a short space of time, so prognosis looked very poor. In the first 2 years of surveillance in the USA (to November 1984), the mortality of AIDS was 48%, based on 6993 cases. For those diagnosed for >2 years, the mortality was 73%.[1]

When HIV tests became commercially available in 1985, clinicians had to counsel patients who were HIV positive but did not have AIDS. What did the future hold for them?

• What proportion of people with HIV would get AIDS?
• What would be the average time before progressing to AIDS?

Such questions are difficult, in fact impossible, to answer accurately at the start of an epidemic. Quite simply the epidemic was too young to know what proportion of people would progress. The estimates needed to take into account that those progressing most quickly were most likely to have events (deaths or progressions) recorded. The event rate in those who progressed more slowly was still unknown.

• In 1985, it was estimated that 5–20% of people with HIV would develop AIDS within 2–5 years, and that most of these would die within 1–2 years.[2]
• In 1989, it was estimated that 45–65% of people with HIV would develop AIDS in an average (median) of 8–10 years.[3]
• In 2004, it was estimated that, in the absence of treatment, >90% of people with HIV would eventually develop AIDS over 2–20 years, and that most of these would die within 1–2 years.[4]

Once treatment became available then studies of the natural history become unethical. The information that is available on long-term outcomes in the absence of treatment is biased, coming from people who have not sought care for various reasons, or from people who do not have access to care.

References

1 Centers for Disease Control. Update: acquired immunodeficiency syndrome (AIDS) – United States. *MMWR* 1984; **33**:661–4.
2 Curran JW *et al.* The epidemiology of AIDS: current status and future prospects. *Science* 1985; **229**:1352–7.
3 Bacchetti P, Moss AR. Incubation period of AIDS in San Francisco. *Nature* 1989; 338:251.
4 Heymann DL. *Control of Communicable Diseases Manual*, 18th edn. Washington, DC: American Public Health Association; 2004.

Prognosis: mortality

Describing the mortality for patients with a disease is not as simple as it sounds. Mean survival could be used, but how would it be calculated? We could take all people diagnosed with a disease, such as breast cancer, record the time from diagnosis to death, and divide by the number of deaths. Unfortunately this would be very misleading:

- It would only include those who had died, ignoring those who had survived.
- It would depend on how long patients were followed-up.
- It depends when the clock starts, i.e. when the diagnosis is made; those who are diagnosed early through screening will automatically appear to survive longer (see 📖 p.116).

A number of measures can be used to account for these problems.

Case fatality rate (CFR)

This is not actually a rate, but is the proportion of people with a disease who die from that disease. It is useful for relatively short-term illnesses, such as acute infections, but for longer-standing conditions some kind of time period should be specified (see 📖 5-year survival, p.32). In calculating CFR it is important that the numerator is people who die from the disease in question, and that the denominator is people with the disease who die plus those who recover (or have not yet died at the end of the follow-up period). Examples:

- SARS: in the outbreak of 2003 the CFR was around 10%.
- Measles: CFR ranges from 0.02% among children in developed countries up to 20% in some poor rural areas of Africa.[1]
- Invasive breast cancer: CFR of around 30% after 11 years of follow-up.[2]

Clearly in this last example a longer period of follow-up would produce a higher CFR.

5-year survival

For most people with a potentially fatal illness the question is not so much whether they will die, but how long they will survive. For most cancers prognosis is described in terms of 5-year survival. 5-year survival can be quoted for different stages of disease, e.g. the 5-year survival rate for people with metastatic lung cancer is 2%, compared with ~50% for early disease. Other time periods may be used.

Median survival

This is the length of time by which 50% of cases have died and may be a useful way of discussing outcome with patients but, like 5-year survival rates, does not capture the variation of survival times within that summary statistic.

Survival curves

Taking survival at a single point is rather crude: a 5-year survival of 50% could occur with all the deaths in the first year and then no deaths, or there could be a steady accumulation of deaths. To provide a better picture of the pattern of mortality survival curves are used. These curves plot survival over time, usually starting with 100% at time zero and then each death is plotted as it occurs (Fig. 2.1). These are described on 📖 p.274, including methods for comparing different survival patterns. They are particularly useful in measuring the impact of treatment.

Life tables

Life tables are similar to survival curves, but take periods of time, usually a year, and calculate the proportions who survive at each point (see 📖 p.276). They can also be used to show survival at different points, for example if someone is still alive after 1 year, what is their probability of surviving the next year?

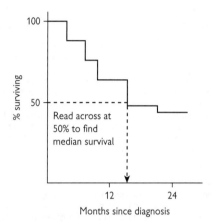

Fig. 2.1 An example of a survival curve, with median survival shown.

References

1 Dollimore N et al. Measles incidence, case fatality, and delayed mortality in children with or without vitamin A supplementation in rural Ghana. Am J Epidemiol 1997; **146**(8):646–54.
2 Starhlberg C. et al. Breast cancer incidence, case-fatality and breast cancer mortality in Danish women using hormone replacement therapy. Int J Epidemiol 2005; **34**(4):931–5.

Prognosis: morbidity

Describing morbidity shares many of the problems of mortality in terms of requiring careful attention to who is studied and time of follow-up, but with the added difficulty of defining the outcomes. Death is much easier to define than many other outcomes.

Disease course

Natural history studies provide a description of the range of patterns and outcomes following a diagnosis. They need to be treated with the same critical appraisal as any other studies (see 📖 p.78). The following factors should be considered as they could introduce bias or mean that they are not relevant to your patient:

• Was there a clearly defined sample of patients with the disease?
• Were they all at the same stage of disease—if not, was the stage included in the description of natural history?
• How long were patients followed for? Were they actively followed-up, or were records only kept for those who came back for treatment?
• What measurements were used to assess disease progression, pain, functional disability, and quality of life?

Outcome measures

Disease-free survival

This is the length of time that a person previously diagnosed with a disease remains disease free (usually after treatment). It can be measured using similar techniques as for mortality (see 📖 Prognosis: mortality, p.32) but relating to disease-free time rather than overall survival. This is used for conditions with relapse and recurrence, for assessing how well treatments work, e.g. in leukaemia or multiple sclerosis.

Progression-free survival

This is the length of time during which a patient with a disease does not progress, e.g. someone with HIV does not develop AIDS or other HIV-related disease. Progression-free survival may be used to estimate how well a new treatment works.

Non-fatal incidents

For many conditions the occurrence of non-fatal incidents may be a key outcome, e.g.:
• Non-fatal myocardial infarction.
• Hospitalization.
• Repeat surgical procedure.

Recurrent events

For intermittent conditions, e.g. migraine or epilepsy, the number of episodes over a period of time will be a useful indicator.

Symptoms

Patients with a chronic condition such as rheumatoid arthritis will want information on the likely persistence and severity of pain and stiffness. This may be expressed as days with any pain, severity of pain, analgesics required, and functional limitation. These measures may be more subjective than other outcomes but no less important. Studies of outcome need to ensure consistency of measurement using validated scales.

Disability and quality of life

There are a wide range of instruments for measuring disability ranging from simple ones used in population surveys:

- Activities of Daily Living; a series of questions such as 'How difficult is it for you to get up and down stairs or steps?' with a graded response from not difficult to impossible.
- Instrumental Activities of Daily Living: a similar set of questions but with the focus on specific functions such as 'How difficult is it for you to prepare a snack for yourself?'
- SF-36 (short form 36): this is an extensively validated instrument to measure physical, mental, and social functioning.
- EuroQol 5-dimensional Quality of Life classification of health states (EQ5D): this simple and validated questionnaire categorizes people in 5 domains: mobility, self-care, usual activities, pain, anxiety/depression.

Communicating prognosis to patients

The different measures outlined so far can be useful in comparing disease course and outcome in trials, but may not always be the most useful in counselling patients about the likely future. Usually some kind of aggregate picture is required, and this may come through contact with other people with the same condition. This may occur through:

- Patient groups.
- Online chatrooms.
- Repositories for patient narratives, e.g. ✍ http://www.healthtalkonline.com.

Communicating prognosis to patients with a life-threatening illness is very challenging. One review makes recommendations with an acronym:

- **P**repare for the discussion.
- **R**elate to the person with rapport, empathy, care and compassion.
- **E**licit patient and caregiver preferences for information.
- **P**rovide information tailored to individual needs.
- **A**void being too exact with timeframes unless in the last few days.
- (Foster) **R**ealistic hope.
- **E**xplore and facilitate realistic goals and wishes and ways of coping.
- **D**ocument the discussion and communicate with other professionals.

Further reading

Clayton JM et al. Clinical practice guidelines for communicating prognosis and end-of-life issues with adults in the advanced stages of a life-limiting illness, and their caregivers. *MJA* 2007; **186**(12 Suppl):S77–S108.

Parker S et al. *Communication of prognosis and issues surrounding end-of-life (EOL) in adults in the advanced stages of a life-limiting illness: a systematic review.* University of Sydney: NHMRC Clinical Trials Centre, 2006.

Evidence-based management

Where can you find out what is the best management for this patient?
You can base your decisions on:
- Your own experience.
- Asking colleagues.
- Referring to local or national guidelines.
- Carrying out your own structured literature search (in the absence of guidelines or to supplement guidelines relevant to your own particular patient).

This is how we do it here

Basing decisions on your own experience or that of colleagues is the traditional way of practising medicine, but has not always resulted in the best outcomes for the patient. You and your colleagues will find it very hard to keep up with all the evidence from other centres and trials, and may be unduly influenced by your own experience or the convincing data of the latest drug rep.

Guidelines

Provided they are evidence-based, guidelines from professional organizations can be helpful. But they may not relate to your particular patient with a specific problem. In this situation you may need to answer questions that are not covered in the guidelines, or you may be part of a team developing new guidelines (see 📖 p.38).

Evidence-based medicine

Evidence-based medicine (EBM), or the slightly broader evidence-based healthcare (EBH) is important for all clinical decisions, but is particularly relevant to decisions on the management of patients.

Definition of EBM

'Evidence-based medicine is the conscientious, explicit and judicious use of current best evidence in making decisions about the care of individual patients. The practice of evidence-based medicine means integrating individual clinical expertise with the best available external clinical evidence from systematic research.' (Sackett et al. 1996)[1]

The 5 steps

- Question: translate clinical uncertainty into an answerable question.
- Search: systematically retrieve the best evidence.
- Appraise: critically appraise evidence for validity, clinical relevance, and applicability.
- Apply: apply the results to your practice.
- Evaluate: evaluate the process and assess its impact.

Define the question
Many questions will arise in the course of your clinical practice. The key thing is to turn general uncertainty—What should I do for this patient?— into a precise question. The question should cover who the patients are, what you want to do to them, and what you are trying to achieve. This will then help you to find the relevant evidence. To help specify the question try using another acronym, PICO:
● **P**opulation—which patients are you interested in?
● **I**ntervention—what treatment do you want to explore?
● **C**ontrol or comparison—what do you want to compare it to?
● **O**utcome—what outcome are you interested in?

Search for the evidence
Once you have a precise question it will help define your search terms. For more information on searching the literature see 🕮 p.74. If possible, find a reputable organization that has done the work for you in the form of guidelines (from a professional organization, for example) or systematic reviews. But you should still apply your critical faculties.

Appraise the evidence
As with other parts of life, don't believe everything you read in the (scientific) papers! You need to look closely at the aims, methods, and results to see that they are valid and appropriate for your particular enquiry. Sift papers for relevance and validity. Check for author conflicts that may affect the way the data are reported (see Chapter 4).

Apply the results
EBM is not intended to be an academic exercise but to improve practice, so once you have gathered and appraised the evidence you should make a decision about changing practice. This may be for an individual patient, or a policy change that will require discussion with colleagues and perhaps patient groups.

Evaluate
Once implemented, the impact of the change should be evaluated. This may be in terms of reviewing the progress of a patient, or auditing the impact of a policy change (see Chapter 6).

Reference
1 Sackett *et al.* Evidence based medicine: what it is and what it isn't. *BMJ* 1996; **312**:71–2.

Further reading
Dawes M *et al.* Sicily statement on evidence-based practice. *BMC Med Educ* 2005, **5**:1.
Henghan C, Badenoch D. *Evidence-Based Medicine Toolkit*, 2nd edn. Oxford: Blackwell 2006.

Clinical guidelines

Clinical guidelines are regularly produced by local, national and international bodies to try and help practitioners apply the evidence contained within the large and growing medical literature.

Definition

'Clinical guidelines are systematically developed statements to assist practitioner and patient decisions about appropriate health care for specific clinical circumstances.' (Scottish Intercollegiate Guidelines Network, SIGN)[1]

Purpose

Guidelines are not merely a synthesis of evidence but they are also supposed to produce practical recommendations for particular situations.

Development

Guidelines need to be based on reviews of evidence, carried out in a systematic and open way. To be practical the evidence must be considered by clinicians who can assess the practical implications.

Evidence-base

Guidelines should always include a guide to the level of evidence for each statement made (Fig. 2.2). There are several methods for grading evidence statements. They need to reflect

- The quality of the evidence, with well conducted randomized controlled trials as the highest, observational studies lower.
- The magnitude and clinical importance of the effect.
- The consistency of findings.
- The likelihood of significant bias in the studies or their reporting.

Many organizations have now adopted the GRADE system for rating quality of evidence and strength of recommendations (see Box 2.1).

Stakeholders

There should be widespread buy-in to the guidelines, and the development and review team needs to include representation from appropriate professional bodies, healthcare organizations, and patients.

Implementation

There is little point in developing guidelines if they remain hidden and un-used. They should be widely available, publicized, and implemented.

Review

All guidelines need regular and planned review that includes detailed evaluation of their uptake and impact. A method for assessing guidelines themselves is shown in Box 2.2.

Box 2.1 Quality of evidence definitions for use in guidelines, GRADE* 2008[2]

High quality—further research is very unlikely to change our confidence in the estimate of effect.

Moderate quality—further research is likely to have an important impact on our confidence in the estimate of effect and may change the estimate.

Low quality—further research is very likely to have an important impact on our confidence in the estimate of effect and is likely to change the estimate.

Very low quality—any estimate of effect is very uncertain.

*GRADE is Grading of Recommendations Assessment, Development and Evaluation.

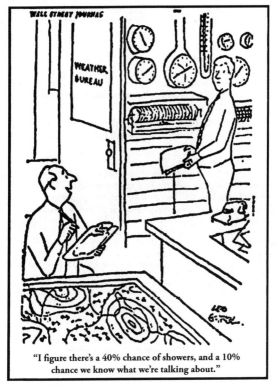

"I figure there's a 40% chance of showers, and a 10% chance we know what we're talking about."

Fig. 2.2 Reproduced with permission from BMJ Publishing Group Ltd. Guyatt, G. H. *et al.* GRADE: an emerging consensus on rating quality of evidence and strength of recommendations. *BMJ* 2008; **336**:924–6.

Box 2.2 Criteria of high quality clinical practice guidelines: the AGREE criteria[3]

1. Scope and purpose
Contains a specific statement about the overall objective(s), clinical questions, and describes the target population.

2. Stakeholder involvement
Provide information about the composition, discipline, and relevant expertise of the guideline development group and involve patients in their development. Also clearly define the target users and ensure guidelines have been piloted prior to publication.

3. Rigour of development
Provide detailed information on the search strategy, the inclusion and exclusion criteria for selecting the evidence, and the methods used to formulate the recommendations. The recommendations are explicitly linked to the supporting evidence and there is a discussion of the health benefits, side effects, and risks. They have been externally reviewed before publication and provide detailed information about the procedure for updating the guideline.

4. Clarity and presentation
Contain specific recommendations on appropriate patient care and consider different possible options. The key recommendations are easily found. A summary document and patients' leaflets are provided.

5. Applicability
Discuss the organizational changes and cost implications of applying the recommendations and present review criteria for monitoring the use of the guidelines.

6. Editorial independence
Include an explicit statement that the views or interests of the funding bodies have not influenced the final recommendations. Members of the guideline group have declared possible conflicts of interest.

Reproduced from Quality & Safety in Health Care, **12**:18–23, 2003, with permission from BMJ Publishing Group Ltd.

References

1 SIGN: ℔ http://www.sign.ac.uk/about/introduction.htm
2 Guyatt, G. H. *et al.* GRADE: an emerging consensus on rating quality of evidence and strength of recommendations. *BMJ* 2008; **336**:924–6.
3 The AGREE Collaboration. Development and validation of an international appraisal instrument for assessing the quality of clinical practice guidelines: the AGREE project. *Qual Saf Health Care* 2003; **12**:18–23.

Online resources

National Guideline Clearinghouse (USA): ℔ http://www.guideline.gov
National Institute for Health and Clinical Excellence: ℔ http://www.nice.org.uk
National Library for Health: ℔ http://www.library.nhs.uk/guidelinesfinder
Scottish Intercollegiate Guidelines Network: ℔ http://www.sign.ac.uk

How effective is the treatment?

Patients will want to know how much difference a treatment will make to their prognosis—any treatment compared with none, one treatment compared with another. To answer these questions you need to know about the natural history of the condition (see 📖 p.30) and have ways of describing the difference introduced by treatment.

The impact of treatment is measured in clinical trials (see 📖 pp.186–93 for details on trials and their methods), but the skill is in translating their results into meaningful information for patients.

Measures of treatment effect (see 📖 p.188)

The outcome of these trials is expressed as
• Relative risk reduction (or hazard ratio, odds ratio).
• Absolute risk reduction.
• Number needed to treat.

Relative risk reduction is the percentage reduction in an outcome (e.g. death) comparing one group (e.g. a new drug) with a control group (placebo or standard treatment). If there are variable times in follow-up (rather than a single measurement time) then this is properly estimated as a hazard ratio, or an odds ratio if estimated through a case–control design.

Absolute risk reduction (ARR) is the reduction in an outcome (e.g. death) comparing one group (e.g. a new drug) with a control group (placebo or standard treatment).

Number needed to treat (NNT) is a measure of how many people with an illness would need to be treated to produce *one desired outcome or prevent one adverse outcome (e.g. one heart attack prevented)*. This is a simple way of describing the effectiveness of a treatment or intervention. It is the inverse of the absolute risk reduction. The 'number needed to harm' is the same measure used to describe adverse outcomes such as side effects.

Communicating results with a patient

For a drug that improves outcome, the relative risk reduction may sound more impressive than the absolute risk reduction or NNT, for the simple reason that the denominator is not everyone taking the drug but is restricted to those who have the adverse outcome.

A hypothetical example

There is a new pill that is said to be better for athlete's foot. It is given to 100 people with the condition, while 100 controls with the same condition are given an old treatment. The numbers cured at 1 month are 10 in the intervention and 5 in the control group.

The relative risk reduction $(10 - 5)/10 = 50\%$; i.e. 50% fewer people were cured in the control than the intervention group, or put another way, you were twice as likely to be cured if you took the new pill. That sounds very impressive.

But the absolute risk reduction is $10\% - 5\% = 5\%$; a mere 5% fewer people had athlete's foot at follow-up compared with the old treatment.

The number needed to treat $(1/ARR = 1/5\%) = 20$. That means you need to treat 20 people with the new pill to cure one more person than with the old treatment.

NNT can be a useful way of describing outcomes for patients. See ✎ http://www.nntonline.net for more on this, including visual charts.

Which outcomes?
It is essential to consider what outcome you are interested in achieving, and to discuss this with the patient. Is it longer life, less time off work, better pain control, less disturbed sleep? Trials tend to look at the big clinical end-points such as death or significant event (see examples in 📖 Interpreting reports of clinical trials, p.44), but patients may have different short-term goals, including the avoidance of side effects.

Outcomes to consider include:
- Disease-specific mortality.
- All-cause mortality.
- Survival.
- Aggregate end-point (e.g. any vascular event or death).
- Hospital admissions.
- Symptomatic relief (e.g. measured by need for analgesia).

Adverse events
It is essential to look at all outcomes, including negative ones, and be able to discuss these with the patient.

Examples of NNTs*

Study	Outcome	NNT
Statins for primary prevention	Death (MI)	931 (78) for 5yrs
Statins for secondary prevention (4S)	Death (MI)	30 (15) for 5.4yrs
Mild hypertension (MRC trial)	Stroke	850 for 1yr
Systolic hypertension in elderly (SHEP)	Stroke	43 for 4.5yrs
Aspirin in acute MI (ISIS-1)	Death	40
Streptokinase in acute MI (ISIS2)	Death	40
ACEi for CCF (NYHA class IV)	Death	6 for 1yr

Keep your eye on the question NNTs can vary markedly if the question is slightly rephrased—e.g. from being about primary prevention to being about secondary prevention (as in the statin example in this box).

NNT confidence intervals Get these by taking reciprocals of the values defining the confidence interval for the ARR. If ARR ~10% with a 95% confidence interval of 5–15%, NNT ~10 (i.e. 100/10) and the 95% NNT-confidence interval ~6.7–20 (i.e. 100/15 to 100/5). Non-significant treatment effects are problematic as NNTs can only be positive; here, give NNT without confidence intervals (Altman's rule).

*Reproduced from Longmore M *et al*. *Oxford Handbook of Clinical Medicine*, 7th edn. Oxford: Oxford University Press; 2007, p.651.

Interpreting reports of clinical trials

Example 1: the JUPITER trial[1]

This trial compared treatment with the statin rosuvastatin with placebo in 18000 people with high C-reactive protein (2.0mg per litre or higher) and low density lipoprotein (LDL) levels <3.4mmol per litre (130mg per decilitre). It was stopped after a median of 2 years' follow-up when it showed a highly significant improvement in the primary end-point with rosuvastatin (hazard ratio 0.56; 95% confidence interval 0.46–0.69; P <0.00001). The primary end-point they were looking at was any vascular event (myocardial infarction, stroke, arterial revascularization, hospital admission for unstable angina, or death from cardiovascular causes).

What do these figures mean?

The hazard ratio (HR) is equivalent to the relative risk where events occur over time. So the HR of 0.56 means there was a 44% reduction in risk in those taking rosuvastatin compared with placebo.

There were 8901 people in each arm.

Control (placebo) event rate (CER) (251 events) = 1.36 per 100 person yrs.

Experimental (rosuvastatin) event rate (EER) (142) = 0.77 per 100 person yrs.

$$\text{Relative risk reduction} = \frac{\text{CER} - \text{EER}}{\text{CER}} = \frac{1.36 - 0.77}{1.36} = 44\%$$

Absolute risk reduction (ARR) = 1.36 − 0.77 = 0.59 per 100 person years.

NNT* = 1/ARR = 1/0.59 = 1.69 per 100 person years = 169 person years to prevent 1 vascular event.

*The paper quotes an NNT of 95 people treated for 2 years (based on survival analysis).[1]

These different ways of presenting the data can be confusing, and certainly controversial. As a potential patient, or prescribing GP, a drug that promises a 44% reduction in vascular events after 2 years sounds very attractive. But put in absolute terms, it means that for 100 people taking it for 1 year, there would be <1 (0.6) fewer vascular events. And 170 people would have to take the drug, including any side effects, for 1 year to prevent 1 event.

Example 2: ACCOMPLISH hypertension treatment trial[2]

The ACCOMPLISH (Avoiding Cardiovascular Events through Combination Therapy in Patients Living with Systolic Hypertension) trial compared the use of an angiotensin-converting–enzyme inhibitor (ACEi) with a dihydropyridine calcium-channel blocker (benazepril plus amlodipine, the intervention) to an ACEi plus a thiazide diuretic (benazepril plus hydrochlorothiazide, the control) in the treatment of hypertension in 11,000 patients. The primary end-point was any of the following vascular events: death from cardiovascular causes, nonfatal myocardial infarction, nonfatal stroke, hospitalization for angina, resuscitation after sudden cardiac arrest, and coronary revascularization.

Results

There were 5744 people in the intervention and 5762 in the control arm, followed for a mean of 36 months.

EER (552 events) = 9.6%

CER (679) = 11.8%

$$\text{Relative risk reduction} = \frac{\text{CER} - \text{EER}}{\text{CER}} = \frac{11.8 - 9.6}{11.8} = 19.6\%$$

ARR = CER − EER = 2.2%

NNT^* = 1/ARR = 45 people (meaning 45 people would need to take the new combination for an average of 3 years to avoid 1 vascular event).

Fig. 2.3 gives a visual presentation of how outcome diverged in the 2 groups.

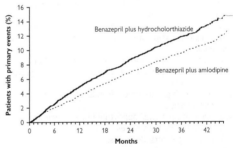

No. at Risk							
Benazepril plus amlodipine	5512	5317	5141	4959	4739	2826	1447
Benazepril plus hydrochlorothiazide	5483	5274	5082	4892	4655	2749	1390

Fig. 2.3 Kaplan–Meier curves for time to first primary end-point. Reproduced with permission from Jamerson K. et al. Benazepril plus amlodipine or hydrochlorothiazide for hypertension in high-risk patients. *N Engl J Med* 2008; **359**:2417–28.

References

1 Ridker PM *et al.* Rosuvastatin to prevent vascular events in men and women with elevated C-reactive protein. *N Engl J Med* 2008; **359**:2195–207.
2 Jamerson K *et al.* Benazepril plus amlodipine or hydrochlorothiazide for hypertension in high-risk patients. *N Engl J Med* 2008; **359**:2417–28.

How appropriate is the treatment?

Clinical trials are the mainstay of evidence-based medicine, providing data on efficacy. *Efficacy* is the impact of treatment in the controlled conditions of a trial. *Effectiveness* is a measure of the impact in 'real life', and takes into account implementation and adherence to treatment. It is important to recognize that quantitative studies are not the only form of evidence that should inform decision-making. Patient experience is generally not well captured in clinical trials and the collection of biological outcomes needs to be complemented/understood through qualitative methods. Patient narratives are an underused form of evidence.

Do no harm

In discussing treatment options with a patient it is important to consider the potential harms as well as benefits. Will this individual patient benefit more than they will suffer from this treatment?

GMC guidance[1]

'All healthcare involves decisions made by patients and those providing their care. This guidance sets out principles for good practice in making decisions. The principles apply to all decisions about care: from the treatment of minor and self-limiting conditions, to major interventions with significant risks or side effects. The principles also apply to decisions about screening.

Whatever the context in which medical decisions are made, you must work in partnership with your patients to ensure good care. In so doing, you must:

(a) listen to patients and respect their views about their health
(b) discuss with patients what their diagnosis, prognosis, treatment and care involve
(c) share with patients the information they want or need in order to make decisions
(d) maximize patients' opportunities, and their ability, to make decisions for themselves
(e) respect patients' decisions.'

(General Medical Council 2008)[1]

Reference

1 General Medical Council. *Consent: patients and doctors making decisions together.* London: GMC; 2008.

Patient-centred decision-making

Decisions about management are made by patients, since they are able to agree to or refuse a recommendation, and even if they agree may not adhere, particularly if they are unconvinced. Therefore decisions should be made in a collaborative way that provides maximum autonomy to the patient and respects their rights as an individual.

- Discuss patients' needs and preferences.
- Outline options with the best available evidence in a way that the patient can understand.
- Evidence-based information should be available in accessible formats suited to people with different abilities.
- Involve families and carers if the patient agrees.
- Comply with regulations/legislation in relation to children and people who do not have the capacity to make decisions/consent.

Not prescribing

Doctors find it very hard not to provide some intervention when someone presents with a problem, and patients may find it even harder. However, many conditions are self-limiting and can be managed with reassurance and support for symptomatic relief but this is not the same as doing nothing. Indeed, as the NICE guidance on respiratory tract infections shows, not prescribing involves quite a lot (Box 2.3)!

Box 2.3 NICE guidance on respiratory tract infections

The 2008 NICE guideline on the prescribing of antibiotics for respiratory tract infections in primary care recommends 3 strategies depending on presentation:
- No antibiotics.
- Deferred antibiotics.
- Immediate antibiotics.

For *all* antibiotic prescribing strategies, patients should be given:
- Advice about the usual natural history of the illness, including the average total length of the illness.
- Advice about managing symptoms (analgesics and antipyretics).

When the *no antibiotic prescribing strategy* is adopted, patients should be offered:
- Reassurance that antibiotics are not needed immediately because they are likely to make little difference to symptoms and may have side effects, for example, diarrhoea, vomiting and rash.
- A clinical review if the condition worsens or becomes prolonged.

When the *deferred antibiotic prescribing strategy* is adopted, patients should be offered:
- Reassurance (as for no antibiotic prescribing strategy).
- Advice about using the deferred prescription.
- Advice about re-consulting if there is a significant worsening of symptoms despite using the deferred prescription.

A deferred prescription with instructions can either be given to the patient or left at an agreed location to be collected at a later date.

More than pills

Patient management is about more than prescribing pills or surgery. You also need to consider:

- Social situation.
- Work.
- Psychological impact.
- Practical issues.
- Impact on other people.
- Follow-up.

Consent

In English law, consent is required for any intervention or treatment, including examination, phlebotomy, physiotherapy, drug treatment and surgery. In practice this is often implied from the context, such as attending for a blood test, but in all situations the patient should be informed and have the ability to decline. Written consent is advised for surgical procedures; always consider making a record of consent to other interventions/treatments by writing in the notes or through obtaining written consent. 'You must work in partnership with your patients. You should discuss with them their condition and treatment options in a way they can understand, and respect their right to make decisions about their care. You should see getting their consent as an important part of the process of discussion and decision-making, rather than as something that happens in isolation.' You must follow the GMC guidance in *Consent: patients and doctors making decisions together*.[1]

Impact on others

Patients may also want to know about the impact on other people, including family. This depends on the condition, e.g.:

Communicable disease

- Transmissibility.
- Contagiousness.
- Secondary attack rate.

Non-communicable disease

- Genetic transmission.
- Shared exposures/risks (e.g. clusters of cancers).

'There are facts from history: the desire to treat on the one hand; and the desire to be treated on the other'*

Archie Cochrane, the pioneer of evidence-based medicine, argued that there was far too little evidence that treatments being used were effective. His ideas were clearly influenced by his own experience.

During the Second World War he was in a prisoner of war (POW) camp. As the only doctor there he was the chief medical officer responsible for 20,000 POWs. They lived on very limited food rations, had widespread diarrhoea, and 'severe epidemics of typhoid, diphtheria, infections, jaundice and sand-fly fever'. His resources were a 'ramshackle hospital', aspirin, antacids, antiseptics, and some caring orderlies. He expected many deaths due to the lack of specific therapies. Yet over the course of 6 months only 4 people died—and 3 of them were from German-inflicted gun shots.

Cochrane uses this example to suggest that most illness is self-limiting, and goes on to look at evidence of harm, either direct from medical interventions, or indirect from the waste of resources in treating self-limiting conditions.

(*Cochrane 1999)[3]

References

1 General Medical Council. *Consent: patients and doctors making decisions together.* London: GMC; 2008. ᔎ http://www.gmc-uk.org/guidance/ethical_guidance/consent_guidance_contents.asp
2 NICE *Respiratory tract infections* (Clinical Guideline 69). London: NICE. ᔎ http://www.nice.org.uk/CG069
3 Cochrane AL. *Effectiveness and Efficiency: Random Reflections on Health Services,* London: RSM Press; 1999 (first published 1972).

Risk communication and promoting health

Health promotion in clinical practice

'It is better to be healthy than ill or dead', wrote Geoffrey Rose in *Rose's Strategy of Preventive Medicine*.[1] Few people would disagree, including most patients diagnosed with a new illness. Promotion of good health is a major focus of public health and epidemiological practice, but is also increasingly central to the practice of clinical medicine. Primary care practitioners are expected to contribute to the health of their patients, to reduce their risks of disease, as well as identifying and treating abnormalities at an early stage to improve outcome. All of these are part of the broad picture of prevention (see 📖 p.54). In secondary and tertiary care we are also expected to identify and tackle risks that will worsen outcomes for patients with existing disease, e.g. to advocate and support smoking cessation in people with cardiovascular disease.

In this chapter we describe the elements of promoting good health that are most relevant to clinical practice. These need to be informed by broad principles and information about prevention, so we include sections on how to discuss these issues with patients and the key activities of clinicians in this area. Later chapters in Section 2 (see 📖 pp.97–118) cover screening and preventive medicine at the population level including detailed discussion on the prevention and control of communicable and non-communicable disease.

Why me?

People who have been diagnosed with a disease will want to know 'Why me?'. They will ask whether or not it could have been averted by either a change in their own behaviour, a change in some external factor, or by a change in your activity as a doctor. In some cases it may be clear:

- A woman has a broken leg after being knocked off her bike by a speeding motorist. The cause of her injury is relatively clear: the immediate (or proximate) cause is reckless driving by the driver of the car. Of course there are many other steps along the causal pathway including her decision to cycle along that route on that day (intermediate cause), and the lack of safe cycle tracks or effective speed restrictions (distal causes).
- A man is diagnosed with lung cancer after smoking for 30 years. The proximate cause is likely to be the smoking; more distal causes include social pressures to smoke, tobacco advertising, and social determinants of smoking such as social class. Inadequate smoking cessation services locally may have played a role, and perhaps there were some missed opportunities for intervention at earlier consultations with his GP.

Generally causation is complex with a web of determinants that are:
- Social
- Genetic
- Behavioural
- Environmental.

Preventive interventions can be directed towards all levels, many of which can involve clinicians.

The role of the clinician in prevention

- Helping patients avoid future problems through providing general advice about a healthy lifestyle (see Box 3.1).
- Identifying specific risk behaviours and advising/supporting patients to reduce or avoid them.
- Ensuring specific preventive interventions are made available to patients, e.g. vaccination.
- Identifying early disease or its precursors and offering early treatment or risk reduction, e.g. monitoring and treating hypertension.
- Counselling patients with a condition about possible causes and explanations as to why them, and why now, e.g. explaining that diabetes may relate to obesity.
- Advising patients with a condition about how to reduce poor outcomes, e.g. by weight loss, exercise, diet, and smoking cessation after a myocardial infarction.
- Exploring whether anyone else is at risk through common environmental, genetic, or infectious exposures, e.g. identifying which contacts need following-up in tuberculosis (TB), or whether future children of a woman with breast cancer are at risk of inheriting *BRCA2*.
- Lobbying for policies that promote and improve health.

Box 3.1 Sensible guidelines for patients (and yourself!)

There is a mountain of material and advice available to professionals and the public on what constitutes a healthy lifestyle. A number of evidence-based guidelines have been produced, but the following are widely agreed:

- Don't smoke.
- Eat a healthy diet:
  - Eat more fruit, vegetables, and fibre.
  - Cut down on saturated fat, red meat, salt, and sugar.
- Not too much alcohol, but 1 or 2 units a day may be beneficial.
- Exercise regularly—recommendations change but all agree that any is better than none, and generally the more and more intense the better.
- Avoid being overweight or obese.
- Avoid sunburn.
- Use condoms and effective contraception to reduce the risk of unwanted pregnancy and sexually transmitted infections (STIs).
- Keep up to date with vaccinations.
- Attend for screening when invited.

Reference

1 Rose G. *Rose's Strategy of Preventive Medicine*. Oxford: Oxford University Press; 2008, p.38.

Could it have been prevented?

Once diagnosed, patients will ask whether anything else could have been done to prevent them having succumbed to this disease. Identifying specific risk factors may help to answer this question, and this requires reference to the epidemiological literature on causation. We outline research methods appropriate to the study of aetiology of disease elsewhere in the book (see 📖 p.197), and show that even at the population level, causation requires the demonstration of a complex set of criteria (see 📖 pp.156–61). At this point the focus is on the individual, and while often it is impossible to identify causation, there are examples where it is both possible and useful.

Why me and why now?

If a woman presents with an unplanned pregnancy and requests a termination, it would be useful to discuss why she became pregnant and how she can avoid this in future. This appears rather obvious, but is inconsistently done by clinicians, leading to repeat presentations and terminations in some women.

The causation may be complex and relate to:
• Lack of knowledge (e.g. of contraception, sexual health services).
• Incorrect knowledge (e.g. about ways of avoiding pregnancy).
• Inadequate provision of services (e.g. inaccessible, unacceptable).
• Contraceptive failure.

Considering which of these may have been contributory and which can be addressed may help prevent future episodes.

Extent of preventable illness

There are many other preventable diseases, with varying degrees of intervention available to the individual clinician, but consideration of determinants should be a routine part of any consultation with a view to informing future preventive interventions. Box 3.2 shows how 4 determinants—smoking, alcohol, diet, and exercise—are estimated to be responsible for 29.5% of morbidity in Europe[1].

Box 3.2 Morbidity from selected causes, DALYs* Europe (high income countries)

• Smoking: 11.2%
• Alcohol consumption: 6.4%
• Diet (overweight, obesity, low fruit/vegetables): 7.5%
• Physical inactivity: 4.4%

*Disability-adjusted life years, see 📖 p.286.

Routinely identifying these and other risk factors—such as hypertension, raised serum cholesterol—can be used to focus consultations on preventive behaviours in the future. This should include a focus on the underlying behavioural/lifestyle 'causes of the causes' of disease–e.g. high salt intake, an important cause of raised BP.

The evidence base for prevention

Preventive messages should be based on:
- Evidence of the causes of a disease.
- Evidence of the efficacy of an intervention to reduce disease by addressing that cause.

Inferring causation is arguably the most complex part of epidemiology which requires a rigorous scientific interpretation of the evidence from different modalities (including observational and animal evidence as well as clinical trials) and a sound theoretical framework for that interpretation. A detailed discussion of this is beyond the scope of this book (see 📖 Further reading, p.55) but in clinical practice it is useful to understand some of the criteria used to assess causation and these are outlined in Chapter 7 (see 📖 p.156).

Evidence of effective interventions

Providing evidence of efficacy of preventive interventions can be equally challenging.
- Randomized controlled trials (see 📖 p.186) of preventive interventions are the gold standard, and can be used to show the effectiveness of a range of different interventions from vaccinations, to dietary interventions, to smoking cessation support.
- Community randomized trials: these can be used to test more complex interventions, particularly those that address community- or population-level determinants. The unit of randomization and intervention is the community rather than the individual. These are more difficult to carry out and to interpret than individual-level trials but nonetheless can give valuable information to guide policy. For example, the Portuguese salt prevention trial[2] compared the effects on community blood pressure levels of dietary intervention to lower salt intakes in one village compared to another village (control) without the intervention.

Reference

1 WHO 2009. Global health risks: mortality and burden of disease attributable to selected major risks.
2 Forte JG et al. Salt and blood pressure: a community trial. *J Hum Hypertens* 1989; **3**:179–84.

Further reading

Bhopal R. *Concepts of Epidemiology: Integrating the ideas, theories, principles and methods of epidemiology.* Oxford: Oxford University Press; 2008.
Bibbins-Domingo et al. Projected effect of dietary salt reductions on future cardiovascular disease. *NEJM* 2010; **362**:590–9.
Bradford Hill A. The environment and disease: association or causation? *Proc Royal Soc Med* 1965; **58**:295–300. ℘ http://www.edwardtufte.com/tufte/hill

Communicating risk

Individual patients diagnosed with a disease, and those who seek to avoid disease, may want you to quantify different risk factors for them. The different measures of risk each have different uses in epidemiology and in communication. Common measures that are used are defined here with a focus on how they might be used in communication between clinicians and patients. Methods for measuring and analysing them are covered in Chapter 7 (see 📖 p.145).

Probability

This is the chance of an event occurring, and ranges from 0 (no chance) to 1 (inevitable).

Absolute risk (incidence rate)

- The probability of occurrence of a disease, death, or other event over a period of time, i.e. Incidence rate.
- For a patient, absolute risk tells them the probability that they will develop a disease in the future.
- Since the outcome can rarely be known with certainty for an individual, the best indicator is the incidence rate in similar people.
- Absolute risk estimates are now used extensively for cardiovascular disease in order to indicate appropriate risk reduction interventions.

Relative risk

- The increase (or decrease) in probability of disease given a particular exposure or risk factor.
- Calculated by dividing the incidence rate in the exposed (I_e) by the incidence rate in the unexposed (I_o) (see 📖 p.179) RR = I_e/ I_o.
- Odds ratio is an estimate of relative risk and can be used in the same way (unless the incidence of the disease is >10%).
- Relative risk can be easily translated into health messages: 'If you smoke you are 20 times more likely to die from lung cancer than if you do not'.
- It can be unhelpful if the background risk is very low.

Attributable risk

- A measure of the excess risk due to the factor concerned.
- Calculated by subtracting the incidence rate in the unexposed (the background risk) from the incidence rate in the exposed, i.e. $I_e - I_o$ (see 📖 p.179).
- It can be useful in counselling individual patients about why they have become ill, or how they can reduce future risks.

Attributable fraction

- Attributable fraction = attributable risk ÷ incidence rate in exposed, i.e. $(I_e - I_o)$/ I_e = (RR − 1)/RR (by dividing top and bottom by I_o).
- Assuming the factor is causal, then the attributable risk fraction is the proportion of disease risk that would be prevented/avoided if the risk was changed to that of an unexposed person.

Population attributable risk (PAR)

PAR = attributable risk × prevalence of risk factor in population
This is the proportion of the disease that is due to the risk factor in the population as a whole, and thus the proportion of disease in the population that should be prevented if the risk factor is removed.

Example 1: the Pill 'doubles risk of clots'

In 1995 the UK Committee on the Safety of Medicines issued an urgent letter advising doctors of an increased risk of venous thromboembolism (VTE) for 3rd- compared with 2nd-generation oral contraceptive pills (OCP). The letter reported a relative risk of 2, i.e. a doubling in the risk of VTE for women on 3rd-generation compared with 2nd-generation pills. This was widely reported in the press, and thousands of women stopped taking their pills. There was an increase in unplanned pregnancies and subsequent termination referrals. Many women were frightened by the idea of a doubling in risk. Was there a better way of communicating the findings? Look at the data:

The absolute risk of VTE in women on 3rd-generation OCP (incidence rate in exposed, I_e) was 3 per 10,000 person-years while the absolute risk in women taking the 2nd-generation OCP (incidence rate in unexposed, I_o) was 1.5 per 10,000 person-years.

$$\text{Relative risk} = I_e \div I_o = 3 \div 1.5 = 2$$

It may have been better to explain the attributable risk: there is a small risk of VTE for women on the 2nd-generation pill: if 10,000 women took them for a year, between 1 and 2 would have a VTE. If instead they take a 3rd-generation pill, this increases to 3 women, i.e. the increased risk attributable to the 3rd-generation pill is 1.5 per 10,000 woman years.

Example 2: use of attributable risk in explaining causation (data in this example are for illustration only)

A woman aged 34 presents with a deep vein thrombosis (DVT). She has been taking the 3rd-generation oral contraceptive pill and asks whether that was to blame. Let's assume that the background incidence rate of DVT in people under the age of 40 is around 1 per 10,000 per year, and that women taking the combined pill for oral contraception have an incidence rate of DVT of approximately 3 per 10,000 per year.

$$\text{Relative risk} = I_e \div I_o = (3/10,000) \div (1/10,000) = 3$$

This means that for women taking the OCP, there is a 3-fold increase in the risk of DVT.

$$\text{Attributable risk} = I_e - I_o = (3/10,000) - (1/10,000) = 2/10,000$$

This means that the increased probability of a DVT increases by 2 per 10,000 per year to an absolute risk of 3 per 10,000 women per year. This can then be used to calculate the likelihood that the OCP contributed to the DVT in this woman:

$$\text{Attributable fraction} = (I_e - I_o) \div I_e = 2/3 = 0.67$$

Therefore in women like this (under 40 who have a DVT and are on this OCP), two-thirds of DVT cases would be attributable to the OCP.

Health promotion in the clinic

Definition
Health promotion is the process of enabling people to increase control over, and to improve, their health (see Box 3.3[1]).

What does health promotion involve?
- Public policy.
- Supportive environments.
- Community action.
- Personal skills.
- Health services.

Why clinicians?
Specific responsibility
- Clinicians have a specific responsibility for promoting and protecting health for their own patients.
- In the UK the GMC's list of duties of a doctor includes the statement that you must 'protect and promote the health of patients and the public'.

Unique position to promote health
- Access to people: the majority of people will consult their GP at least once a year, >90% over a 5-year period. Other people will be in contact with clinicians in community clinics, hospitals, accident and emergency departments, and sexual health clinics.
- Receptive audience: with almost all of these clinician–patient contacts there is an opportunity for health promotion, and people are often receptive in these situations.
- Effective interventions: many clinicians are sceptical, but the evidence shows that clinician interventions can be effective (see 📖 p.60).

How to do it (see 📖 pp.60–7)
- Advocate (and offer if appropriate) vaccination and screening.
- Ask about/identify risks (e.g. obesity, problem alcohol or drug use, smoking).
- Advise on reducing these risks.
- Assist people to reduce risks (through referral, prescription, etc.).
- Arrange follow-up.
- Don't assume someone else will do it!

Reference
1 WHO. Ottawa Charter for Health Promotion. Geneva: WHO; 1986. 🔗 http://www.euro.who. int/__data/assets/pdf_file/0004/129532/Ottawa_Charter.pdf

Box 3.3 Ottawa Charter for Health Promotion (WHO 1986)[1]

Health promotion

Health promotion is the process of enabling people to increase control over, and to improve, their health. To reach a state of complete physical mental and social wellbeing, an individual or group must be able to identify and to realize aspirations, to satisfy needs, and to change or cope with the environment. Health is, therefore, seen as a resource for everyday life, not the objective of living. Health is a positive concept emphasizing social and personal resources, as well as physical capacities. Therefore, health promotion is not just the responsibility of the health sector, but goes beyond healthy lifestyles to wellbeing.

Prerequisites for health

The fundamental conditions and resources for health are peace, shelter, education, food, income, a stable ecosystem, sustainable resources, social justice and equity. Improvement in health requires a secure foundation in these basic prerequisites.

Advocate

Good health is a major resource for social, economic and personal development and an important dimension of quality of life. Political, economic, social, cultural, environmental, behavioural and biological factors can all favour health or be harmful to it. Health promotion action aims at making these conditions favourable through advocacy for health.

Enable

Health promotion focuses on achieving equity in health. Health promotion action aims at reducing differences in current health status and ensuring equal opportunities and resources to enable all people to achieve their fullest health potential. This includes a secure foundation in a supportive environment, access to information, life skills and opportunities for making healthy choices. People cannot achieve their fullest health potential unless they are able to take control of those things which determine their health. This must apply equally to women and men.

Mediate

The prerequisites and prospects for health cannot be ensured by the health sector alone. More importantly, health promotion demands coordinated action by all concerned: by governments, by health and other social and economic sectors, by non-governmental and voluntary organizations, by local authorities, by industry and by the media. People in all walks of life are involved as individuals, families and communities. Professional and social groups and health personnel have a major responsibility to mediate between differing interests in society for the pursuit of health.

Health promotion strategies and programmes should be adapted to the local needs and possibilities of individual countries and regions to take into account differing social, cultural and economic systems.

Reproduced from The Ottawa Charter for Health Promotion, First International Conference on Health Promotion, Ottawa, 21 November 1986, http://www.who.int/healthpromotion/conferences/previous/ottawa/en/, with kind permission from WHO.

Smoking and alcohol advice

Generic advice on the advantages of adopting a healthy lifestyle are mainly considered relevant to primary care and community health services, but there is evidence that patients are also receptive when they are in contact with secondary care. Indeed, patients may think it odd if they do not receive advice on remaining healthy when they are discharged after an acute episode.

Smoking

The evidence base for clinician interventions for smoking is strong. In a general setting, brief advice can motivate people to try and stop. It is important to assess their willingness to try and quit, and if they are interested then they should be provided with appropriate support, including nicotine-replacement therapy (NRT) and, if required, referral to smoking cessation services.

The evidence-based guidance on smoking cessation includes 4 essential

'On its own, brief advice from a doctor increases the chance of a person quitting (odds ratio 1.69, 95% confidence interval 1.45 to 1.98) compared with no advice' (Lancaster et al. 2000).[1]

features (the 4 As):
- **A**sk (about smoking at every opportunity).
- **A**dvise (all smokers to stop).
- **A**ssist (the smoker to stop, depending on their readiness to change).
- **A**rrange (follow-up).

Pharmacological interventions are a key and effective part of smoking cessation strategies; clinicians should offer NRT, varenicline, or bupropion, to people who are planning to stop smoking.

For full guidance refer to NICE.[2,3]

Alcohol

Screening for potentially harmful or hazardous alcohol use should also be carried out in primary care and in an opportunistic way in other clinical settings, particularly where the episode may be alcohol-related.

In the UK, NICE has developed guidance[4] that includes screening of new patients registering in primary care, undergoing reviews or health checks, presenting with sexual health concerns, for antenatal care and with minor injuries. A simple screening tool such as AUDIT (Alcohol Use Disorders Identification Test) can be used.[4]

Where problems are identified the clinician should carry out a brief intervention—immediately if possible or through a referral. The exception to this is if a person is dependent on alcohol in which case they should be referred for specialist treatment. NICE recommend that the brief intervention should last 5–15min and cover:
- Potential harm from their current level of drinking.
- The potential benefits to health and well-being of reducing alcohol intake.
- Discuss barriers to change and develop practical strategies to reduce consumption.
- Produce a set of goals and arrange for these to be reviewed.

These, followed by an appropriate brief intervention have been found to be effective in reducing alcohol intake in some settings.[5]

Alcohol risk assessment tools
- Paddington Alcohol Test (for use in emergency departments, see Box 3.4).
- Alcohol Use Disorders Identification Test (AUDIT).

Box 3.4 The Paddington alcohol test[6]

Anyone attending with 1 or more of a list of 'trigger conditions' (such as a fall, collapse, head injury, assault, etc.) or people with obvious intoxication are given the screening test in which the patient is asked:
- Do you drink alcohol?
- What is the most you will drink in any 1 day?
- How often do you drink this much?
- Do you feel your attendance at A&E is related to alcohol?

Patients are considered 'PAT +ve' based on the amount they drink in a day (8 or more units in men and 6 or more in women); if they drink this level every day they are considered a dependent drinker, less than that a hazardous drinker, and potentially PAT +ve. PAT +ve patients are offered the following verbal advice:

'We advise you that this drinking is harming your health. The recommended daily limits are 4 for men, 3 for women with two drink free days per week'.

They are then offered a referral to the alcohol nurse specialist.

References

1 Lancaster T *et al.* Effectiveness of interventions to help people stop smoking: findings from the Cochrane Library. *BMJ* 2000; **321**:355–8.
2 NICE. *Brief interventions and referral for smoking cessation.* London: NICE; 2006. ℘ http://www.nice.org.uk/guidance/PH01
3 NICE. *Smoking cessation services.* London: NICE; 2008. ℘ http://www.nice.org.uk/guidance/PH10
4 NICE. *Alcohol-use disorders: preventing the development of hazardous and harmful drinking.* London: NICE; 2010. ℘ http://www.nice.org.uk/guidance/PH24
5 Crawford MJ *et al.* Screening and referral for brief intervention of alcohol misusing patients in an emergency department: a pragmatic randomised controlled trial. *Lancet* 2004; **364**:1334–9.
6 Alcohol Learning Centre. ℘ http://www.alcohollearningcentre.org.uk

Exercise, weight, and dietary advice

Exercise

Patients should also be assessed for their level of physical activity with the aim of identifying people who could benefit from advice and support. The General Practice Physical Activity Questionnaire (GPPAQ) is one way of quickly screening people and is available online.

The standard advice is for people to do at least 30min exercise on 5 or more days each week. If they need to lose weight then a longer duration of exercise may be advised. Where possible, exercise should be integrated into regular daily activities such as cycling or walking to work. Recommended methods for increasing physical activity include brief interventions in primary care (advice and discussion), exercise referral schemes, the use of pedometers, and community schemes to promote walking and cycling.[1]

Weight and diet

There are wide-ranging health benefits from maintaining a healthy weight and good diet. Screening for overweight and obesity should be carried out sensitively based on clinical judgement.

The basic indicator of whether intervention is required is body mass index (BMI), the weight (in kg) divided by height (in m) squared. Classification by BMI (Table 3.1).

Decisions about whether to offer brief advice, refer for weight loss support, use drugs, or refer for surgery should be based on a broader risk assessment that includes comorbidities such as diabetes, waist circumference, and motivation for change.

Interventions to reduce weight and maintain weight loss are complex; referral to specialist counsellors or weight loss organizations can help.

The basic intervention should include a discussion of the health risks of overweight and obesity, discussion of targets (aim for maximum of 0.5–1kg weight loss per week), the importance of weight loss and maintenance of that loss, and the importance of using exercise and diet.

It is important to consider the wider social setting and encourage partners and other family members to be involved.

In people who struggle to lose weight and who continue to be at risk of adverse health outcomes drug treatment (with orlistat) or bariatric surgery should be considered. Dietary advice is appropriate for everyone, whether or not they are overweight or obese. There are many resources available to help people maintain a healthy diet. The general recommendations are shown in Table 3.2.[2]

Table 3.1 Classification BMI (kg/m^2)

Underweight	less than 18.5
Healthy weight	18.5–24.9
Overweight	25–29.9
Obesity I	30–34.9
Obesity II	35–39.9
Obesity III	40 or more

Table 3.2 General dietary advice: recommendations[2]

Nutrient/food	Recommendation
Total fat	Reduce to no more than 35% food energy
Saturated fat	Reduce to no more than 11% food energy
Total carbohydrate	Increase to more than 50% food energy
Sugars (added)	Reduce to no more than 11% food energy
Dietary fibre	Increase non-starch polysaccharides to 18 g per day
Salt	Reduce to no more than 6 g salt per day[*]
Fruit and vegetables	Increase to at least 5 portions of a variety of fruit and vegetables per day

[*]The maximum amount of salt recommended for children is less than that for adults—see
🖱 http://www.salt.gov.uk

References

1 NICE. *Four commonly used methods to increase physical activity.* London: NICE; 2006. 🖱 http://www.
nice.org.uk/guidance/PH02
2 NICE. *Obesity: recommendations for the NHS.* London: NICE; 2006. 🖱 http://www.nice.org.uk/
guidance/CG43

Sexual health

Interventions to prevent unplanned pregnancy and STIs are highly effective and should be delivered in a range of clinical settings.

As with other interventions to promote health, the first step is a risk assessment, in this case a good sexual history. This will establish whether someone is sexually active and who with, identify recent partner change, numbers of partners, whether sex is unprotected or not. It should also include contraceptive and reproductive history.

In the clinic setting, promotion of good sexual health should include the following:
- Advice on safer sex, recommendation of condom use for protection against STI and pregnancy.
- Advice and provision of contraception from a range of options.
- People at increased risk (those with multiple partners, who have recently had a STI, etc.) should be offered one-to-one counselling to reduce risk (NICE guidelines).[1]
- Tailored advice for the individual, e.g. men who have sex with men, sex workers and their clients.

In addition the following needs to be undertaken for specific groups:
- Screening for STIs: sexually active people <25 years should be offered *Chlamydia* screening in accordance with local guidelines.
- Testing for HIV in line with national guidelines (for UK in 2008—see 📖 UK National Guidelines on HIV testing, p.64).
- Partner notification for people with a diagnosed STI including HIV.

UK National Guidelines on HIV testing[2]

Universal HIV testing is recommended for all patients in:
- Sexual health clinics.
- Antenatal services.
- Termination of pregnancy services.
- Drug dependency programmes.
- Healthcare services for those diagnosed with TB, hepatitis B, hepatitis C, and lymphoma.

In areas with a local prevalence of 2 in 1000 or higher, an HIV test should be offered to all new patients registering with a GP, and all general medical admissions.

HIV testing should also be routinely offered and recommended to:
- Patients where HIV enters the differential diagnosis (see table of indicator diseases in guidelines[2]).
- Patients diagnosed with a STI.
- Sexual partners of men and women known to be HIV positive.
- People reporting specific risk factors—men who have sexual contact with other men, people with a history of injecting drug use, people from a country of high HIV prevalence (>1%) and their sexual partners.

References

1 NICE. *Prevention of sexually transmitted infections and under 18 conceptions.* London: NICE; 2007. 🔗 http://www.nice.org.uk/guidance/PH3
2 UK National Guidelines for HIV Testing 2008. 🔗 http://www.bhiva.org/HIVTesting2008

Outbreak investigation

An outbreak is the same as an epidemic, i.e. an increase in the number of cases above the expected level in a particular community or geographic area, but is usually applied to a localized increase. Outbreaks can be either infectious or non-infectious (environmental) in origin, but usually they are due to infectious disease. At the outset of an investigation of an outbreak both possibilities need to be borne in mind.

Types of outbreak

Common source
- Exposure to common factor.
- Can be over a prolonged time.

Point source
- Exposure to common factor.
- All exposed at same time, e.g. wedding reception meal.

Propagated
Where there is transmission from person to person.

Why investigate outbreaks?
- To stop the outbreak.
- To understand what happened and why.
- To prevent future outbreaks.
- To improve our knowledge.
- To improve surveillance and outbreak detection.
- For training.

Steps in an outbreak investigation
- Preliminary assessment:
  - Is it an outbreak?
  - Are these cases of the same condition?
  - Are there any immediate control measures required?
- Set up investigation:
  - Define cases.
  - Establish case finding methods.
  - Diagnostic processes.
  - Data collection procedures.
- Descriptive epidemiology in order to generate hypotheses:
  - Time: draw an epidemic curve.
  - Person: include relevant history of exposure.
  - Place: draw a map of the cases.
- Analytic epidemiology to test hypotheses:
  - Cohort study: identify subset of population (cohort) exposed to factor and compare incidence in them compared with those not exposed to calculate a relative risk.
  - Case–control study: identify cases and enquire about exposure; identify controls and enquire about exposure; calculate odds ratio (as an estimate of relative risk).

- Introduce control measures:
  - Remove source.
  - Isolate/treat case.
  - Destroy/treat food or other source.
  - Protect persons at risk.
  - Hygiene/prophylaxis.
  - Prevent recurrence.
  - Make recommendations.
  - Produce guidelines/change law.

Breaking the chain of infection

With any case of an infectious disease it is important to try and identify the likely source and any possible chains for onward transmission in order to try and prevent other cases. In clinical practice it is easy to forget this aspect of 'protecting and promoting the health of patients and the public', or to assume that someone else will do it. Don't.

Identifying the source (this often helps with diagnosis as well)

Ask appropriate questions (dependent on condition), e.g.
- Food.
- Travel.
- Contacts with similar symptoms.
- Sexual contacts.

If the source is likely to be in the community and putting others at risk (i.e. not within the household) you need to inform the local public health department to arrange for investigation.

Contact tracing

Who is involved?
Ask the patient about other people who may be 'involved', e.g.
- The source (in person–to–person spread).
- Subsequent contacts.
- Others exposed to the same source (e.g. same food).

How will they be told?
Establish a method for informing and managing contacts, e.g.:
- Patient referral: a person with a STI informs their contacts and suggests that they attend for screening and treatment.
- Provider referral: the clinician (or other member of the team) obtains contact details from the patient and notifies the contacts directly. Care must be taken to protect the confidentiality of the index patient.
- Outbreak investigation: where multiple people may have been exposed, it is appropriate to ask the local public health authorities to investigate and take responsibility to informing people (see 🕮 p.66).

How will they be managed?
This depends on the infection. They may be offered screening, presumptive treatment, vaccination (if available), or simply provided with information on how to recognize symptoms and what to do if they develop.

Preventing further transmission

Patients may provide an ongoing risk of infection to others depending on the specific infection. Think about who may be at risk and how that can be reduced/eliminated. For example:
- *Quarantine*: in the case of some infections this may be effective. This was key to limiting the transmission of SARS (severe acute respiratory syndrome) in 2003. For many infectious diseases it is ineffective since the maximum period of infectiousness is prior to the onset of symptoms.
- *Advice* to the patient (e.g. avoid sexual contact, no food handling).
- *Specific precautions* depending upon infection.

Appropriate precautions

It is crucial to reduce the risk of onward transmission in hospital and in the community. Universal precautions aim to reduce transmission of all agents, while specific precautions relate to the mode of transmission.
- Respiratory precautions.
- Enteric precautions (see Box 3.5 and 📖 Further reading, p.70).

Box 3.5 Enteric infections

Enteric precautions include:
- Handwashing.
- Safe disposal of excretions and soiled materials.
- Disinfection of toilet seats, flush handles, wash-hand basin taps, and toilet door handles.
- Education on personal hygiene.
- Hygienic preparation and serving of food.

Identify upstream and downstream contacts
- Identify others who may be involved as a source of infection, linked to common exposure, or who could have been infected by the patient.
- For food poisoning history to include travel, eating in different places and events, contact with anyone who was ill, food preparation for others.

Specific groups
Some people may pose a particular risk to others, and if they have an enteric infection with diarrhoea they should be prevented from resuming activity until 48 hours after their first normal stool:
- Food handlers.
- Staff of healthcare facilities who have direct contact, or contact through serving food, with susceptible patients.
- Children <5 years who attend nurseries or other groups.
- Older children and adults where hygiene is difficult (includes people with learning disabilities or special needs, residents in hostels or temporary camps, etc.).

Respiratory precautions (e.g. TB)

If a patient with smear positive respiratory TB is admitted to hospital then they should be kept with respiratory precautions:
- Single room, negative pressure where possible.
- Use of a fine mask.

Additional precautions for patients with multidrug-resistant TB (MDRTB) or extensively drug-resistant (XDRTB)
- Staff and visitors should wear dust/mist masks during patient contact while the patient is considered infectious.
- The patient should remain in isolation in a negative pressure room until assessed to be non-infectious.
- Before a discharge from hospital is made, secure arrangements for the supervision and administration of all therapy should have been made and agreed with the patient and carers.

Management of contacts
- Identify potentially exposed contacts.
- Close contacts of someone with pulmonary TB should be identified and asked about previous BCG.
- Close contacts in household are people who share a kitchen.
- Other people with symptoms.
- Others in the household.
- Close work colleagues.

Notification
- All forms of TB are compulsorily notifiable.
- The doctor making or suspecting the diagnosis is legally responsible for notification.

Further reading

Health Protection Agency. *Health Protection Report: Enteric.* ℘ http://www.hpa.org.uk/cdr/pages/enteric.htm

Evidence-based practice

Introduction

Section 1 focused on how epidemiological methods and knowledge are used in the clinic with individual patients. This section addresses how evidence is used to inform practice more generally.

Chapter 4 details how to find, assess, and summarize existing evidence. The amount of information available to clinicians and to patients continues to grow rapidly and we all need methods to sift and synthesize it. This chapter starts with a very practical introduction to searching the medical literature, using different resources such as online databases and bibliographic software, then introduces the essential elements of critical appraisal and how to assess the quality of papers, finishing with a description of how to conduct a systematic review and meta-analysis.

Chapter 5 turns to the kind of evidence underpinning preventive medicine. In Section 1 we looked at how risk can be communicated and health promotion supported in the clinic, but these are only part of wider approaches to the control of disease in the population. It is often intuitive to target interventions towards those at highest risk, but we also make the case for addressing risk factors across the whole population. Often these 'high-risk' and 'population' approaches should be undertaken hand in hand. We review the different levels of prevention—primary, secondary, and tertiary—and then provide more detail on preventing non-communicable disease, using the example of cardiovascular disease, followed by prevention of infectious disease, including vaccination. We complete this chapter with an overview of prevention through screening.

Chapter 6 concludes this section with a very practical guide to evaluating clinical practice. Ensuring that practice is carried out effectively is now part of all our roles. Research is essential to informing the evidence base, but most clinicians will be more actively involved in audit. This chapter describes the similarities and differences between research and audit, briefly explains clinical governance and ethics, and then provides a step-by-step guide to audit practice including choice of question and standards, how to choose an appropriate sample, data collection, storage, analysis, and dissemination.

Finding and summarizing evidence

Finding and evaluating existing evidence

There is an enormous amount of information available to clinicians and patients. Finding, sifting, and turning it into evidence is a major challenge.

In this chapter we introduce the skills that are needed to find existing evidence, read papers, assess the quality of the literature, and then summarize it in a systematic review and meta-analysis.

Finding evidence: overview

Evidence can be found in a wide range of sources. PubMed, a leading portal for databases like Medline, includes >20 million citations to journal articles and books. Unless you use a systematic method to find your evidence, you will waste a lot of time, and potentially miss a great deal of important work.

Defining the question

You must begin with a clearly defined clinical or research question and some idea of which information source you will use to search for evidence. Even if you define your research question thoroughly, you may have to modify your search strategy after your initial review.

Searching

- Use a bibliographic database such as PubMed and enter your search terms.
- Use specific search terms such as MeSH (Medical Subject Headings, a catalogue of terms managed by the National Library of Medicine).
- Combine terms with Boolean operators 'AND', 'OR', and 'NOT'.
- Limit your search (by year of publication, language, only those that are full text, review articles, etc.).

If you are not familiar with how to do this then make use of the online tutorials (PubMed), or contact your local librarian.

Refining the search

If your search produces 2000 articles, you may need to refine it to make the results more manageable or focused; while if only 5 articles are found, you may want to consider broadening the search terms you used. It is always essential to go back to your defined research question and use the details in the question you are attempting to answer to guide your search strategy and its criteria.

Keeping records

This is perhaps the most important adjunct to your literature review. Accurate bibliographic details, search histories, critique details, key information from papers, etc. will help you find things again quickly. Reference Manager, Endnote and Mendeley are useful electronic systems.

Finding and evaluating evidence: worked example

A 76-year-old man has been diagnosed with inoperable intra-hepatic cholangiocarcinoma and has been advised that his prognosis is poor, 6 months at best. He asks you (his GP) whether he should have photodynamic therapy (PDT) which he has heard may prolong his survival. How do you find out whether it would be appropriate for him?

Define the question (see 📖 p.74)
'In a 76-year-old man who has been diagnosed with inoperable intra-hepatic cholangiocarcinoma, will PDT increase his survival compared with palliative care alone?'

Search

In a search engine such as PubMed, type your keywords, e.g.:
• Cholangiocarcinoma AND Photodynamic.

The search engine will then translate these:
• ('cholangiocarcinoma' [MeSH Terms] OR 'cholangiocarcinoma' [All Fields] AND 'photodynamic' [All Fields].)

This produces 109 results (search performed March 2011). If you are looking for a quick answer you are likely to want a review article. You can limit your results to review, or you can add systematic review into the search, producing 9 articles.

Select

If you are doing a more thorough search (e.g. if you are doing a research project, or preparing a journal club) you should look at all 109 of these titles and abstracts to select those that are relevant. In a formal systematic review (see 📖 p.88) you would define inclusion and exclusion criteria for the papers.

Appraise

You then read the selected papers in detail to see if they are:
• Relevant (to your question).
• Valid (methodologically sound, well analysed).
• Applicable (to your patient).

Methods for assessing these are covered in detail in this chapter. In this case, a brief search identifies a recent, high-quality systematic review that concludes there is some limited evidence that PDT may improve survival,[1] but this is based on 2 small randomized controlled trials (RCTs) and some observational studies of varied quality. A firm conclusion was not possible.

Apply

If you find appropriate evidence then you should apply it. In this case, current evidence is not sufficient to make a strong recommendation. However, you would discuss this with your patient, and contact the oncologist to see if there might be ongoing trials that he could enter.

Review

As a GP you are unlikely to have another patient with this condition in the future, but you may still be interested and return to the literature in a couple of years to see if the evidence has changed.

Reference

1 Fayter D et al. A systematic review of photodynamic therapy in the treatment of pre-cancerous skin conditions, Barrett's oesophagus and cancers of the biliary tract, brain, head and neck, lung, oesophagus and skin. Health Technol Assess 2010; **14**(37):1–129.

Electronic resources

There are numerous e-resources available to help you identify information and search for up-to-date medical evidence. Any library will be able to provide a list of the key resources that you can use, including details of which ones they have free access to.

Reference databases

Some databases are simply a way of organizing information on all relevant publications in the field. Medline, Embase, and PsychInfo include articles from biomedical journals and some books and other publications. Where they cover the same broad topic, e.g. Medline and Embase, the majority of their content will overlap, but with some key areas of difference. It is always advisable to search at least 2 databases to ensure that you are not missing articles.

Some databases help to do this for you. For example, PubMed is a way of accessing several databases, and it also provides links to the publishers and to full-text articles where these are available.

Citation data

A citation is a reference to another article or source of information. Information about citations can be useful in looking for the most influential articles which are generally cited many times. There are many ways of accessing citation data now, but the most comprehensive is the Citation Indices published by the ISI Web of Science. Citation information is also provided through Google Scholar.

Conference abstracts

Information is sometimes published first at conferences where it may appear in official conference proceedings. These can be accessed through another index, the Conference Proceedings Citation Index, available through the Web of Knowledge.

Open access resources

Publicly funded research is increasingly published in open-access journals to ensure that everyone benefits from the findings. For example *UK PubMed Central (UKPMC)* provides free access to peer-reviewed research papers in the medical and life sciences. It includes over 2 million full-text journal articles, access to 24 million abstracts, and clinical guidelines (from NHS).

Evidence-based medicine resources

If you are looking for answers to a specific medical query it is best to see if the literature has already been reviewed by a reputable group. Evidence-based reviews can be found in a number of places including:

- *The Cochrane Library*: a collection of databases with results of systematic reviews, clinical trials, health technology assessments, economic evaluations, etc.
- *BMJ Clinical Evidence*: this is a journal publishing systematic reviews, but links to various resources designed to help clinicians in their evidence-based practice.
- *TRIP Database:* another database of EBM resources available on the Internet.

Bibliographic software

When you search for articles it is essential to keep good records and be able to manage the data. Bibliographic software packages allow you to manage all the referenced evidence you find by enabling you to store it in your own personal database or library. In general, these packages are designed to assist in the following tasks:

- Manual cataloguing of bibliographic references relating to particular research areas/topics.
- Automated collection and organization of references from bibliographic databases, library catalogues, etc.
- Quick searches for a particular reference.
- Search and retrieval of bibliographic subsets.
- Print or save a list of references.
- Integration with word-processing software to automatically insert and format citations and bibliographies.
- Formatting of references according to particular bibliographic styles (e.g. Chicago, Harvard, individual journals' styles) and also formats for exporting to other packages and for data-sharing.
- Find, import, and save full-text articles and access them from anywhere online.

There are many packages, including:

- Endnote: http://www.endnote.com
- Mendeley: http://www.mendeley.org
- Reference Manager: http://www.refman.com
- RefWorks: http://www.refworks.com
- Zotero: http://www.zotero.org

Critical appraisal

Critical appraisal is the process of assessing the validity of research and deciding how applicable it is to the question you are seeking to answer. This section will cover how to read a paper with these aims in mind.

- *Validity*: are the results of the study valid? Are the conclusions justified by the description of the methodology and the findings? Is the methodology sound, have the authors made reasonable assumptions, are there confounding factors they have failed to consider? If they are using a sample, has it been selected in a way that avoids bias?
- *Applicability*: will the results help locally? Are the problems I deal with sufficiently like those in the study to extrapolate the findings? Can I generalize from this study to my clinical practice?

In subsequent sections we describe tools available to support appraisal of papers reporting different types of study.

Appraising a paper: summary checklist

- Summarize the evidence you have read:
  - Why did they do it?
  - What did they do?
  - What did they find?
  - What did they conclude?
- Consider the following:
  - Question.
  - Design.
  - Population.
  - Methods.
  - Data management.
  - Analysis.
  - Confounders.
  - Bias.
  - Ethics.
  - Patient engagement.
  - Interpretation.
  - Applicability.

Question

- What is the question the researchers are trying to answer?
- How does the question relate to evidence from earlier studies? Is it original or a 'me too' study (asking a question that has been asked and answered before in other populations perhaps)?
- Is there a hypothesis and is it clearly stated?
- Is the question relevant, focused and carefully formulated?

Design

- What type of study design was used? Is it a case report/case series, ecological, time trend, cross-sectional, case–control, cohort, RCT, or is it a systematic review or meta-analysis?
- Is that study design appropriate to the question? (See 📖 p.194.)
- Where does the study design fit in the hierarchy of evidence? (See 📖 p.147.)

Population

- Which population was used? Is it relevant to my question? Are results generalizable to other populations? E.g. findings from a clinical trial conducted only in men, or adults, or people with a particular stage of disease may not be generalizable to women, children, or people with different disease stages.
- Sample size: how many people were included? Has a power calculation been conducted (see 📖 p.240) and did the researchers reach the numbers required? If not, then the study may not have sufficient power to detect differences even when they exist (see 📖 p.240).
- How were the participants recruited?
  - Were all people in the target population invited to participate or a random sample of these?
  - What was the response rate? What evidence has been provided to show how responders differed from non-responders? Could this non-response have introduced bias?
  - Participation of volunteers without reference to a target population may introduce bias, as only people with a particular interest in the research question may be motivated to respond.
  - Inclusion criteria: these will define the population to which results can be extrapolated.
  - Exclusion criteria: these refine the target population and remove avoidable sources of bias e.g. excluding patients with a coexisting illness that may make results difficult to interpret.
  - Cases: how were cases defined and where were they recruited?
  - Controls: how were they defined and where were they recruited? Are they representative of people without the disease?
  - Setting: were the subjects studied in 'real life' circumstances such as a clinical setting, or at home? These factors will affect whether results can be replicated in other settings.

Methods

- What specific intervention was being considered and what was it being compared with? Which exposure/risk factor was being studied in association with which outcome?
- What exposures and confounders were measured and how? Were they measured in the same way in all groups? Is there any potential for bias?
- What outcome was measured and how?
  - Was the outcome obtained by an objective measure, e.g. biochemical tests, or a more subjective method, e.g. symptoms, pain, psychological measures through a questionnaire?
  - Was measurement the same in all groups? Were the researchers blinded to the exposure/ treatment allocation?
- Follow-up:
  - Has the study continued for long enough to detect the effect of the intervention or followed the cohort for long enough for cases of disease to accrue? Has there been loss to follow up which may bias the results?

Data management
- Were data managed appropriately?
- Was data entry checked (e.g. by double entry) and cleaned prior to analysis (see 📖 p.220)?
- How were data stored? Was this secure and confidential?
- Who had access to the data?
- Is there any possibility that personal information could be disclosed?
- Is any data linkage described and was it likely to miss links?

Analysis
- Were primary and secondary end-points described in advance?
- Was there an explicit framework for the analysis—based on hypothesis testing, and were subgroup analyses planned, or were the data 'mined' for any associations?
- Were appropriate statistical tests carried out to evaluate probabilities of a chance finding and to adjust for confounding?
- Were statistical methods adequately described? If multivariate analysis was carried out were the steps clearly defined (e.g. how regression models were constructed and how decisions were made about which variables to include or exclude)?

Confounders
Were potential confounders (see 📖 p.148) measured and adjusted for?

Bias
- Is there a systematic error in the study design, data collection/ measurement procedures, analyses, reporting, or a combination of these factors that has led to conclusions that are systematically different from the truth?
  - e.g. measurement bias could be introduced if a thermometer was incorrectly calibrated 3° lower than the actual temperature.
  - e.g. in a RCT, if participants with more severe disease were allocated non-randomly to treatment vs placebo groups.
  - e.g. selection bias could occur if there was high participation by health-conscious people in voluntary cancer screening, or if there was low participation by heavy smokers in studies investigating the association between smoking and cancer.
- Completeness of follow-up:
  - Has any assessment been made of those who dropped out of the study? If, for example, drop-out rates were related to treatment e.g. due to adverse side effects associated with the treatment, this might bias the results.
- Was assessment blinded?
  - In interventional studies (RCTs) it is preferable that both the participants and the researchers are unaware of whether or not the participant has received the trial drug or placebo. If, for example, patients were applying cream to a wound and nurses were measuring their improvement, knowledge of who got cream with active ingredients could potentially bias the recorded results.

Ethics

- Has the study been reviewed and approved by an independent Ethics Committee or Institutional Review Board (IRB)?
- Has appropriate consent been obtained from participants?
- Are there any obvious ethical challenges, e.g. if people were tested (screened) for a condition were they provided with counselling, results, and appropriate management?

Patient engagement

Were any patients consulted or involved in any way in the design, management, analysis, or interpretation of the study?

Interpretation

- Do the authors interpret their findings appropriately?
- Are there other possible interpretations?
- Do the authors situate their results appropriately alongside other research findings?
- Do they make a causal inference? Think over the Bradford-Hill criteria (see 📖 p.156)

Applicability

Applicability is, in some ways, the hardest to judge in a rigidly scientific manner and decisions in this area may still be an art.

Ask yourself: are the problems I deal with sufficiently like those in the study to extrapolate the findings? Can I generalize from this study to my own practice?

Examples to consider:

If a doctor were to locate a paper that is scientifically faultless, he may be left pondering questions like, if the selection criteria only included 'patients between 70 and 80 years old' can I use the conclusions for patients in the 65 to 70 age group, and what about the relatively fit and 'biologically young' 81-year-olds?

Can studies on urban Americans be extrapolated from, say, Birmingham, Alabama, to Birmingham, West Midlands, and are rural practices in Norway different to those in Wales?

Similarly a teacher might ask 'Are teaching practices that have been shown to be effective in 5- to 8-year-olds also of value in pre-school age children?' or a social worker might enquire 'Would counselling techniques used successfully in Asian youths apply equally well to those from an Afro-Caribbean background?'.

Appraisal checklists

Studies vary in design, and there are key factors to look out for when appraising each type. Specific checklists have been developed for a wide range of studies and can be useful when writing or reading papers.

These checklists are all available through the EQUATOR network website where they are regularly reviewed, updated, and new ones added.[1,2] It is therefore worth checking the website for updates. As an example we have included the checklists and flow-diagrams for RCTs—the CONSORT statement later in this chapter (see 📖 pp.84–6).

Other guidelines are listed in Table 4.1, check the websites for details.

Systematic reviews and meta-analyses

Consider:
- Did the review address a clearly defined and important clinical or public health question?
- Were all relevant studies identified through a thorough search?
- Was methodological quality assessed and studies weighted accordingly?
- Was it appropriate to combine the results of the included studies?
- Was the possibility of publication bias assessed?
- Were the results interpreted appropriately and with consideration of the broader picture?

Diagnostic test accuracy studies

Consider:
- Is the study aim clearly defined? Does the study aim to estimate diagnostic accuracy or compare accuracy between tests or across patient groups?
- Has the appropriate reference test or gold standard test been chosen for comparison?
- Has the study included an appropriate spectrum of participants?
- Is the disease status of the tested participants clearly established?
- Were the methods for performing the test described in sufficient detail?
- Has work-up bias been avoided?
- Has observer bias been avoided?
- Were confidence intervals calculated for sensitivity, specificity and positive and negative predictive values of the test? (See 📖 p.16)
- Could the results for the diagnostic test of interest have been influenced by the results of the reference/gold standard test?
- Have the study findings regarding the test been placed in the wider context of other potential tests in the diagnostic process?
- Is this test relevant to my clinical practice?

Qualitative research studies

Consider:
- Was there a clearly defined question?
- Was a qualitative method appropriate for the research question?
- What was the researcher's perspective and how did this influence the methods they used for collection of data?
- Was the recruitment strategy appropriate for the aims of the research?

- Were all ethical issues duly considered?
- Were the data transcribed and analysed in a rigorous manner?
- Are the conclusions drawn justified by the findings?
- Are the findings transferable to other clinical settings?
- Do the findings provide me with useful insight for my clinical practice?

Table 4.1 Study appraisal guidelines

Acronym	Study design to be appraised	Website
CONSORT	RCTs	℘ http://www.consort-statement.org
MOOSE	Meta-analyses of observational studies	℘ http://www.equator-network.org
PRISMA	Preferred Reporting Items for Systematic Reviews and Meta-Analyses	℘ http://www.prisma-statement.org
STARD	Diagnostic test accuracy studies	℘ http://www.stard-statement.org
STREGA	Strengthening the Reporting of Genetic Associations	℘ http://www.equator-network.org
STROBE	Observational studies	℘ http://www.strobe-statement.org

References

1 EQUATOR Network website. ℘ http://www.equator-network.org
2 Simera I et al. Transparent and accurate reporting increases reliability, utility, and impact of your research: reporting guidelines and the EQUATOR Network. *BMC Med* 2010; **8**(1):24.

CONSORT statement

See Table 4.2 for the CONSORT statement, and Fig. 4.1 for flow diagram and additional recommendations.

Table 4.2 CONSORT statement[*]

Section/topic	Checklist item
Title and abstract	
	Identification as a randomized trial in the title
	Structured summary of trial design, methods, results, and conclusions (see CONSORT for abstracts)
Introduction	
Background and objectives	Scientific background and explanation of rationale
	Specific objectives or hypotheses
Methods	
Trial design	Description of trial design (such as parallel, factorial) including allocation ratio
	Important changes to methods after trial commencement (such as eligibility criteria), with reasons
Participants	Eligibility criteria for participants
	Settings and locations where the data were collected
Interventions	The interventions for each group with sufficient details to allow replication, including how and when they were actually administered
Outcomes	Completely defined pre-specified primary and secondary outcome measures, including how and when assessed
	Any changes to trial outcomes after trial commenced, with reasons
Sample size	How sample size was determined
	When applicable, explanation of any interim analyses and stopping guidelines
Randomization	
Sequence generation	Method used to generate the random allocation sequence
	Type of randomization; details of any restriction (such as blocking and block size)
Allocation concealment mechanism	Mechanism used to implement the random allocation sequence (such as sequentially numbered containers), describing any steps taken to conceal the sequence until interventions were assigned
Implementation	Who generated the random allocation sequence, who enrolled participants, and who assigned participants to interventions

Table 4.2 (*Contd.*)

Section/topic	Checklist item
Blinding	If done, who was blinded after assignment to interventions (for example, participants, care providers, those assessing outcomes) and how
	If relevant, description of the similarity of interventions
Statistical methods	Statistical methods used to compare groups for primary and secondary outcomes
	Methods for additional analyses, such as subgroup analyses and adjusted analyses
Results	
Participant flow (a diagram is strongly recommended)	For each group, the numbers of participants who were randomly assigned, received intended treatment, and were analysed for the primary outcome
	For each group, losses and exclusions after randomization, together with reasons
Recruitment	Dates defining the periods of recruitment and follow-up
	Why the trial ended or was stopped
Baseline data	A table showing baseline demographic and clinical characteristics for each group
Numbers analysed	For each group, number of participants (denominator) included in each analysis and whether the analysis was by original assigned groups
Outcomes and estimation	For each primary and secondary outcome, results for each group, and the estimated effect size and its precision (such as 95% confidence interval)
	For binary outcomes, presentation of both absolute and relative effect sizes is recommended
Ancillary analyses	Results of any other analyses performed, including subgroup analyses and adjusted analyses, distinguishing pre-specified from exploratory
Harms	All important harms or unintended effects in each group (for specific guidance see CONSORT for harms)
Discussion	
Limitations	Trial limitations, addressing sources of potential bias, imprecision, and, if relevant, multiplicity of analyses
Generalizability	Generalizability (external validity, applicability) of trial findings
Interpretation	Interpretation consistent with results, balancing benefits and harms, and considering other relevant evidence

(continued)

Table 4.2 (Contd.)

Section/topic	Checklist item
Registration	Registration number and name of trial registry
Protocol	Where the full trial protocol can be accessed, if available
Funding	Sources of funding and other support (such as supply of drugs), role of funders

*CONSORT strongly recommends reading this statement (previous pages) in conjunction with the CONSORT 2010 Explanation and Elaboration for important clarifications on all the items.

If relevant, they also recommend reading CONSORT extensions for cluster randomized trials, non-inferiority and equivalence trials, non-pharmacological treatments, herbal interventions, and pragmatic trials. Additional extensions are forthcoming: for those and for up to date references relevant to this checklist, see: ℘ http://www.consort-statement.org

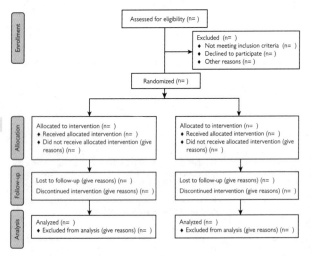

Fig. 4.1 CONSORT Statement 2010 flow diagram. From Altman DG, Moher D, for the CONSORT Group. CONSORT 2010 Statement: updated guidelines for reporting parallel group randomised trials. *BMJ* 2010; **340**:c332.

Systematic review

A systematic review is a method of providing a summary appraisal of existing evidence. Unlike traditional literature reviews, which are subjective and selective, this method is designed to be rigorous and reproducible, reducing bias.

Steps in a systematic review

- Define the question.
- Search the literature.
- Appraise the studies for relevance and quality.
- Extract the data.
- Synthesize the data.
- Report and apply the findings.

A systematic review should be based on a protocol that is produced in advance and includes the following elements:

- Clear statement of the question.
- Detailed description of the search strategy including databases to be searched and search terms to be used, and other methods for finding evidence such as use of reference lists in articles, contacting key researchers or organizations to find unpublished reports.
- Explicit inclusion and exclusion criteria for studies; e.g. define terms in advance, specify relevant populations (e.g. age range), types of study.
- Details of who will perform the search; ideally this should be done by more than one person to check that the same studies are identified.
- Methods for assessing the quality of studies: this may be through a formal scoring against pre-defined criteria, or may be a qualitative review. Again this should be done by more than one person.
- A description of data to be extracted, e.g. setting, participants, response rates, outcome.
- A method for synthesizing results; this may be a qualitative or narrative report of the findings, tables summarizing the study populations and findings, or it may lead into a quantitative synthesis through a meta-analysis (see 📖 p.90).
- A plan for reporting and applying the results.

Reporting a systematic review

Use the checklist in PRISMA (Preferred Reporting Items for Systematic Reviews and Meta-Analyses) at 🔗 http://www.prisma-statement.org. Describe the methods as in the protocol, including the details of the search. The results of the search should be presented in a standard flow-chart (Fig. 4.2). Details of the included papers should be in tables, as should key extracted data.

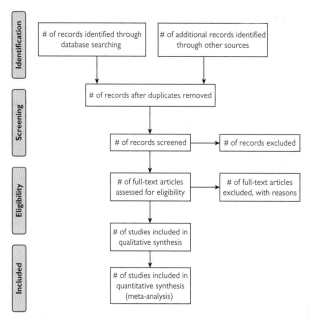

Fig. 4.2 PRISMA 2009 flow diagram. From Moher D, *et al.* Preferred Reporting Items for Systematic Reviews and Meta-Analyses: The PRISMA Statement. *PLoS Med* 2009: **6**(6):e1000097. (Reproduced under the terms of the Creative Commons Attribution Licence.)

Meta-analysis

What is a meta-analysis?

A meta-analysis is a statistical analysis of a collection of studies, often collected together through a systematic review. A systematic review provides a summary appraisal of the evidence in the systematically collected studies in a narrative form. In contrast, the statistical techniques in a meta-analysis enable a quantitative review to be undertaken by combining together the results from all the individual available studies to estimate an overall summary, or average, finding across studies. The studies themselves are the primary units of analysis and can include the range of various different epidemiological study designs that we discuss throughout this book.

Why conduct a meta-analysis?

As a result of limited study size, biases, differing definitions, or quality of exposure, disease and potential confounding data, as well as other study limitations, individual studies often have inconsistent findings. They are therefore often insufficient in themselves to definitively answer a research question or provide clear enough evidence on which to base clinical practice. A meta-analysis, however, has several advantages, including:

- Making sense of an inconsistent body of evidence by contrasting and combining results from different studies with the aim of identifying consistent patterns.
- Including more people than any single constituent study, and produce a more reliable and precise estimate of effect.
- Identifying differences (heterogeneity) between individual studies.
- Exploring whether, for the question under investigation, studies with positive findings are more likely to have been published than studies with negative findings (publication bias).
- Providing an evidence base for clinical decisions.

What are the steps in a meta-analysis?

There are 4 steps in a meta-analysis:

*1. **Extraction*** of the main result or study effect estimate from each individual study (calculation is sometimes necessary) e.g. odds ratio, relative risk etc., together with an estimate of the probability that the effect estimate is due to chance. Every study effect estimate is accompanied by the standard error, describing the variability in the study estimate due to random error. Sometimes we see this expressed as the variance, which is the standard error (SE) squared or the level of certainty we have in the estimated study result may be shown through the confidence interval (see 📖 p.229).

*2. **Checking*** whether it is appropriate to calculate a pooled summary/average result across the studies. Appropriateness depends on just how different the individual studies are that you are trying to combine. Sometimes, it is not appropriate to combine the studies at all. If it is appropriate, you must decide which method to use before you begin calculation (see 📖 p.92).

3. Calculation of the summary result as a weighted average across the studies, using either a random effects or fixed effects model (see 📖 p.93). The weight usually takes into account the variance of the study effect estimate which reflects the size of the study population of each individual study. This weighted average gives greater weight to the results from studies which provide us with more information (usually larger studies with smaller variances) as these are usually more reliable and precise and less weight to less informative studies (often smaller studies).

4. Presentation of summary results—you will often see these as forest plots (Fig. 4.3). This is a graphical representation of the results from each study included in a meta-analysis, together with the combined meta-analysis result.

In the forest plot
- The overall estimate from the meta-analysis is usually shown at the bottom, as a diamond.
- The centre of the diamond and dashed line corresponds to the summary effect estimate.
- The width of the diamond represents the confidence interval around this estimate.

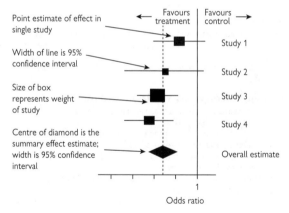

Fig. 4.3 Understanding the results of meta analysis presented in a forest plot.

Analysis and interpretation of a meta-analysis

It is not always appropriate to pool results into a statistical meta-analysis.

How do I check if it's sensible to pool results?

There are 2 elements in the decision: clinical and statistical.

Clinical

- This requires a judgement, somewhat subjective, as to whether the studies collected are addressing the same question such that calculating a summary of their results would be informative and meaningful.
- Pooling may not be appropriate if there are sufficient differences in study participants, interventions, or outcomes that suggest a different underlying research question.
- For example: if you were considering undertaking a meta-analysis of the effect of a particular treatment of depression, it would not be sensible to pool studies investigating treatment efficacy in teenagers with studies in the elderly; nor should you combine studies reporting outcomes at 6 weeks with those reporting outcomes at 12 months.
- If you have reason to believe that the studies are not estimating the same effects, do not pool the results.

Statistical

- Studies should be assessed to see if there is significant variation with respect to the populations, interventions/exposures, outcomes, clinical settings, and designs used.
- These differences or heterogeneity can be explored via Galbraith (radial) plots.

Assessing heterogeneity via Galbraith plots

Galbraith (radial) plots facilitate the examination of heterogeneity, including detection of outliers (Fig. 4.4):

- The plot is the standardized intervention/exposure effect (effect/ standard error) against the reciprocal of the SE.
- The regression line through the origin represents the pooled effect estimate; with 95% boundaries.
- Where there is little heterogeneity, the majority (95%) of studies should fall within these lines.
- The vertical spread describes the extent of heterogeneity and reveals outliers.

Calculating a pooled result

The method depends on whether there is statistical heterogeneity. If no evidence for heterogeneity is found, a fixed effects model can be used to pool the effect estimates. If some heterogeneity exists, and the underlying assumptions of a fixed effects model (i.e. that diverse studies are estimating a single effect) is too simplistic, the heterogeneity can be allowed for by using an alternative approach known as the random effects model to pool the effect estimates.

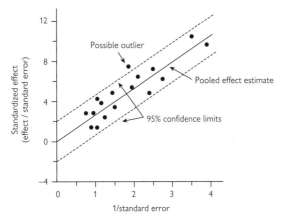

Fig. 4.4 Interpreting the Galbraith (radial) plot.

The fixed effects model
- For use where there is no evidence of heterogeneity.
- Assumes every study evaluates a common treatment/exposure effect.
- Assumes there is a single 'true' or 'fixed' underlying effect.

The random effects model
- Assumes that the true treatment/exposure effects in the individual studies may be different from each other.
- Assumes there is no single effect to estimate but a distribution of effects (due to between-study variation), from which the meta-analysis estimates the mean (and standard deviation) of the different effects.

If specific sub-groups of studies display heterogeneity, these can be pooled separately in sub-analyses, e.g. in the earlier example in this topic on the treatment of depression, pooling findings for young patients only together or pooling study findings focusing on longer-term outcomes together, etc.

Important points to remember:
- Simply adding up data from individual studies is inappropriate and is not what a meta-analysis does.
- If the studies are too heterogeneous, it may be inappropriate, even misleading, to statistically pool the results from separate studies.
- Random effects meta-analysis will tend to be more conservative than fixed effects, as it allows for an extra source of variation (between study).

Evaluating meta-analyses: what to watch out for
- Providing an overall summary measure of association/effect, can give a false impression of consistency across individual study results.
- Always look out for systematic variations in findings across studies.

- Was it appropriate to pool the studies—how well was heterogeneity explored?
- Bear in mind that no meta-analysis can compensate for the inherent limitations of the trial or observational data being combined together.*
- Consider the possibility that all studies have suffered a common systematic error, particularly before making inferences about causality.
- Publication bias—the results of a meta-analysis may be biased if the included studies are a biased sample of studies in general (this is the meta-analytic analogue of selection bias in other epidemiological study designs).

Exploring publication bias

Publication bias refers to the greater likelihood that research with statistically significant results will be published in the peer-reviewed literature in comparison to those with null or non-significant results.
When evaluating a meta-analysis, you need to consider the following:
- Failure to include all relevant data in a meta-analysis may mean the effect of an intervention/exposure is over- (or under-) estimated.
- Publication bias is caused when only a subset of the relevant data is available.
- Null or non-significant findings (especially in small studies) are less likely to be reported/published than statistically significant findings.
- Publication bias in meta-analyses can be explored using funnel plots.
- Funnel plots show whether there is a link between study size (or precision) and the effect estimate.
- A funnel plot which is symmetric about the mean effect and shaped like an upside-down funnel indicates no publication bias.
- A funnel plot with the lower right or left hand corner of the plot missing indicates that publication bias is present, as shown in Fig. 4.5.
- Detecting publication bias is not straightforward and nor is correcting for it, but the funnel plot helps us to estimate how big an impact such bias might be having on the results of the meta-analysis.

---

* Note that meta-analysis is only as good as the source data. It is no substitute for undertaking high quality original studies and trials which can then feed in to the decision-making process.

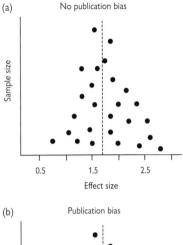

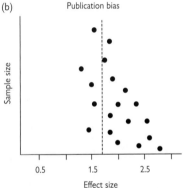

Fig. 4.5 Interpreting funnel plots: the lack of publication bias (a) and the presence of publication bias (b).

Further reading

Egger, M et al. (eds). DG. *Systematic Reviews in Health Care*. London: BMJ Publishing Group; 2001.
Greenhalgh T. How to read a paper: Papers that summarise other papers (systematic reviews and meta-analyses). *BMJ* 1997; **315**:672–75.
The Cochrane Collaboration: http://www.cochrane-net.org

Preventive medicine and screening

Prevention strategies

Most clinicians are concerned with preventing disease in individuals while public health specialists aim to prevent disease in the population. There are two broad approaches to prevention: targeting those at high risk or addressing risk across the whole population.

Population

This starts from the recognition that the occurrence of common diseases reflects the behaviour and circumstances of society as a whole. In Western societies, nearly everyone is at increased risk of many common diseases, such as heart disease, due to the widespread distribution of adverse exposures such as poor diet, lack of exercise, and smoking. If a risk factor (exposure) is widespread in the population, a prevention strategy directed at the whole population may be more effective, and cost-effective, than a high-risk approach. The population approach aims to reduce the prevalence of the risk factor in the whole population, or shift the population distribution (Fig. 5.1).

Strengths
- Equitable, targeting all those exposed even those at lower risk.
- Can get high coverage.
- Can be cost-effective.

Weaknesses
- Medicalization (e.g. widespread use of statins).
- Less acceptable to the individual (see 📖 Prevention paradox, p.98).
- Risk of over-treatment.
- Expensive.

High risk

Individuals at increased risk of disease due to established factors are targeted for interventions. If the interventions are effective then this can lead to a substantial protection for the individual.

Strengths
- Effective (high motivation).
- Efficient.
- Acceptable.
- Easy to evaluate.

Weaknesses
- Inequitable (misses a large amount of disease).
- Medicalization.
- Damage limitation as disease process already advanced.
- Can be hard to change individual behaviours.

Prevention paradox
- Many people exposed to a small risk may generate more cases of disease than the few exposed to a large risk.
- Therefore, when many people receive a small benefit the total benefit may be large.
- However, individual inconvenience may be high to the many when their individual benefit is modest.

Examples of prevention paradox

Trisomy 21: the relative risk of trisomy 21 increases steeply with maternal age. However, since there are far more births in women at younger ages the majority of Down syndrome pregnancies occur in younger women whose individual risk is low. Screening for Down syndrome has to balance detection in high-risk older women, in whom the risk of an invasive test (amniocentesis or chorionic villus sampling) may be acceptable, with detection in younger women for whom the risk of miscarriage may be too high.

Cycle helmets: cycle helmets reduce the risk of head injury in certain types of accidents. To prevent such injuries thousands of cyclists have to wear helmets on every journey, and the majority will never actually need the protection offered. It has been suggested that the wearing of helmets may have some unintended consequences including making the cyclist more reckless, drivers less cautious near cyclists, and may put some people off from cycling at all.

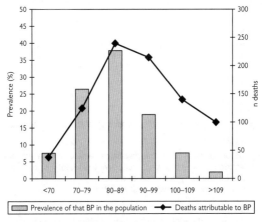

Fig. 5.1 Attributable deaths and relative risk from increased blood pressure. This shows the distribution of diastolic blood pressure (DBP) in a population (bars) together with the numbers of deaths attributable to raised BP from people with that level of DBP. Although the relative mortality is much higher for people with the highest levels of DBP (not shown), they are a small proportion of the population and therefore contribute few deaths. Though the relative mortality is lower for those with lower DBP, there is still an excess, and as they are a large part of the population they contribute more deaths than people at the top end of the BP range (after Rose).

Further reading

Rose G. Sick individuals and sick populations. *Int J Epidemiol* 1985; **14**:32–8.
Rose G. *Rose's Strategy of Preventive Medicine.* Oxford: Oxford University Press; 2008, p.2.

Levels of prevention

Clinicians have a role to play in each of the main levels of prevention as described here:

Primordial

The prevention of factors promoting the emergence of risk factors—lifestyles, behaviours, and exposure patterns—which contribute to increased risk of many diseases. For example:
- Healthy eating programmes in schools.
- Social policies to reduce poverty and inequalities.
- Healthy city programmes that promote walking, cycling, and public transport.
- The encouragement of positive health behaviour.
- The prevention of adopting risk behaviour.
- Elimination of established risk behaviour and promotion of the concept of health as a social value.

Primordial prevention applies to multiple diseases. For specific diseases, 3 levels of prevention can be described, relating to the natural history of the disease.

Primary

The prevention of the onset of disease. To limit exposure to risk factors by individual behaviour change and by actions in the community. Includes health promotion and specific protection. For example:
- Vaccination.
- Smoking cessation.
- Healthy diet.
- Condom use.
- Detection and management of hypertension and hyperlipidaemia.

Secondary

Halting the progression once the disease process is already established. Early detection followed by prompt, effective treatment. For example:
- Screening for the early detection of cancer.
- Smoking cessation after myocardial infarction.

Tertiary

The rehabilitation of people with established disease to minimize residual disability and complications:
- Rapid treatment of myocardial infarction (MI) or stroke to reduce likelihood of disability.
- Antiretroviral therapy for HIV.

One intervention, multiple levels

These levels are clearly overlapping, and interventions that are primary prevention in one situation may be secondary in another (Table 5.1). Aspirin is well established for secondary cardioprevention in people who have established cardiovascular disease, and for treatment of people who have an acute MI. It is potentially useful for the primary prevention of both cancers and cardiovascular disease although this remains under debate.[1]

Table 5.1 Levels of prevention and the example of stroke

	Primordial	Primary	Secondary	Tertiary
Disease stage	Healthy	Healthy	Early changes	Established disease
Definition	Prevent emergence of underlying determinants	Prevent the onset of disease	Early detection and treatment	Reduce disability from established disease
Types of intervention	Good health policy, health promotion	Reduce specific risk factors through health protection, health education, vaccination	Screening, case finding	Treatment and rehabilitation
Example of stroke	Smoke-free areas, reduce salt in processed food, promote sport at school	Reduce smoking, improve diet, promote exercise, identify and treat hypertension and lipid abnormalities	Detection and effective management of transient ischaemic attacks	Effective treatment, e.g. revascularization, rehabilitation, e.g. stroke unit

Reference

1 Moayyedi P, Jankowski JA. Does long term aspirin prevent cancer? *BMJ* 2010; **341**:c7326.

Preventing communicable disease

Infectious diseases remain a major cause of mortality globally despite major advances in prevention and control (see 📖 p.285). New and re-emerging infections threaten to undermine improvements in health in many parts of the world, and create specific challenges even for the most developed healthcare systems (see 📖 p.328).

Prevention can be broken down into primordial, primary, secondary, and tertiary as described earlier in this chapter (see 📖 p.100). The most important health gains have been attributed to primordial prevention through improved sanitation, housing, diet, and environmental conditions. Additional gains have been achieved through specific primary prevention programmes (vaccination, hygiene) and treatments.

Elements of communicable disease prevention

- Health protection.
- Health promotion.
- Medical interventions—vaccination, pre- or postexposure prophylaxis.
- Breaking the chain of transmission—case finding, contact management, outbreak investigation.

Health protection

This includes public health activities intended to protect individuals, groups, and populations from infectious diseases, environmental hazards such as chemical contamination, and from radiation. It is a broad concept that can include legal measures, health and social policy, health and safety at work, and the organization of diagnostic and healthcare infrastructures. Clinicians play a key role in health protection through providing information for surveillance, through notification of cases, and through alerting local public health officials to unusual cases or outbreaks.

Health promotion (see 📖 pp.52, 58)

This refers to those activities that help individual members of the public and patients to reduce their risks of infectious disease. For clinicians this may include basic advice on hygiene (to parents, for example), food handling, travel precautions, safer sex, etc.

Medical interventions

These are vaccinations or medications that are given to reduce risk of infection. This includes routine vaccinations, targeted vaccinations (for occupations, risk groups or travellers), and the use of antimicrobial agents for pre- or postexposure prophylaxis.

Breaking the chain of transmission

This includes case finding, contact tracing and management, and outbreak investigation. Unlike non-communicable disease, identifying cases can play a central role in the prevention and control of infectious disease.

This is part of the rationale for screening programmes, contact tracing and management, and trying to find the source of an outbreak (see 📖 p.68). Clinicians have a key role to play in recognizing the need for further actions such as tracing and managing contacts, e.g. in meningitis, ensuring appropriate precautions are taken to reduce onward spread (in hospital, household, or community) and in alerting the appropriate authorities to initiate further control measures.

Surveillance

Central to any organized intervention for infectious disease is accurate surveillance. In most countries surveillance is based on a number of sources of information, including compulsory notification of certain diseases, voluntary case reports, and monitoring of laboratory confirmed cases.

Notification

Responsibility for notification lies with the clinician who attends the patient and who makes, or suspects, a diagnosis of a notifiable disease. When a clinician sees a patient with a notifiable disease they should:
- Complete a notification form.
- Contact the appropriate authorities in person (e.g. in England the Consultant in Communicable Disease Control at the local Health Protection Unit) to report cases needing urgent investigation.

Which diseases are notifiable (see Box 8.2)
- Those that are relatively rare but serious, requiring rapid intervention.
- Those subject to vaccination programmes.
- Conditions requiring environmental health action such as food poisoning.

Preventing non-communicable disease: example of cardiovascular disease

In Chapter 3 we examined lifestyle changes for promotion of good health including healthy diet, smoking cessation/avoiding smoking and sensible drinking. These changes are broadly applicable to prevention of many of the common non-communicable diseases including cardiovascular disease (CVD), obesity, diabetes, and several common cancers. The epidemiology of the common non-communicable diseases is summarized in Chapter 11 including a brief discussion of preventive approaches for each disease.

Here we look in more detail at the prevention and clinical management of CVD and apply the concepts of primary and secondary prevention (see 📖 p.100) as they relate to CVD. As noted, vascular disease shares many risk factors with other chronic conditions and cancer, so the concepts, if not the detail, are applicable to other common diseases such as diabetes. Prevention, early detection, and effective management are important to reduce morbidity and mortality.

It is beyond the scope of this book to provide detailed guidance on clinical management, and since the detail changes frequently it is important to consult recommendations of appropriate local and national organizations.

CVD risk assessment

Risk assessment packages and guidelines are being produced by a number of organizations, many including software packages with calculators to estimate risk.

- A risk assessment should be carried out on all adults >40 years, and younger adults (<40 years) with a relevant family history.
- Risk assessment should include ethnicity, smoking habit history, family history of CVD, and measurements of weight, waist circumference, BP, non-fasting lipids (total cholesterol and HDL cholesterol), and non-fasting glucose.
- The results can then be fed into CVD risk prediction calculators to estimate total risk of developing CVD (coronary heart disease (CHD) and stroke) over 10 years.
- A total CVD risk of ≥20% over 10 years is defined as 'high risk' and requires professional lifestyle intervention and, where appropriate, drug therapies to achieve the lifestyle and risk factor targets.

Reducing risk

Primary prevention

Basic lifestyle and risk factor modification interventions should be provided to all, regardless of risk (see 📖 pp.58–63).

Secondary prevention

Lifestyle advice and appropriate medication (antithrombotic; BP lowering; lipid modification; diabetes control). Specific management depends on type of CVD and presence or absence of diabetes etc.

Cardiovascular protective drug therapy

Cardiovascular protective drug therapy should be considered in all high-risk people and those with established CVD to reduce risks of cardiovascular events. Detailed recommendations and doses are beyond the remit of this book and can be found in national and local guidelines, but approaches include:

Antithrombotic therapy

- Low-dose aspirin for people with established coronary or peripheral atherosclerotic disease, and for selected groups at high risk of CVD.
- Aspirin and dipyridamole for those with a history of cerebral infarction or transient ischaemic attack (if they are in sinus rhythm).
- Anticoagulation should be considered for selected people at risk of systemic embolization from large MIs, heart failure, left ventricular aneurysm, paroxysmal tachyarrhythmias, and for high-risk patients with atrial fibrillation.

Blood pressure-lowering therapy

- β-blockers are recommended for all people following MI unless there are contraindications.
- ACEi, calcium channel blockers, and diuretics should be used as necessary.

Lipid lowering therapy

A statin is recommended for:
- All high-risk people with established atherosclerotic disease.
- Most people with diabetes.
- Others at high total risk of developing CVD.
- Asymptomatic people who are at high total risk of developing CVD.

Other classes of lipid lowering drugs (fibrates, bile acid sequestrants, cholesterol absorption inhibitors, nicotinic acid, omega-3 (n-3) fatty acids) can be considered in addition to a statin if targets are not achieved.

Common protocols

Care of people with CVD should be integrated between hospital and general practice through the use of agreed protocols designed to ensure optimal long-term lifestyle, risk factor, and therapeutic management. Similarly, the care of high-risk people treated in specialist hospital clinics should be integrated with general practice to ensure, through agreed protocols, optimal long-term management.

Further reading

British Cardiac Society et al. JBS 2: Joint British Societies' guidelines on prevention of cardiovascular disease in clinical practice. *Heart* 2005; **91**(Supplement 5):v1–v52.

NICE. *Cardiovascular risk assessment and the modification of blood lipids for the primary and secondary prevention of cardiovascular disease.* London: NICE; 2008. ℘ http://www.nice.org.uk/guidance/CG67

NICE. *Hypertension: management of hypertension in adults in primary care.* London: NICE; 2011. ℘ http://www.nice.org.uk/guidance/CG127

Online resource

QRISK®2-2011 risk calculator: ℘ http://qrisk.or

Basic infectious disease epidemiology

Methods for communicable disease control vary with the epidemiology of each disease. Chapter 12 includes the epidemiology of some major infectious diseases, but here we introduce the key terms and concepts of infectious disease epidemiology. A number of key parameters influence transmission and therefore control, and basic definitions are shown in Box 5.1 and Fig. 5.2.

Basic reproductive number, R_0

This is the number of new infections caused by 1 infected individual in an entirely susceptible population. It is a useful concept that determines:
- Whether an epidemic can occur.
- The rate of growth of the epidemic.
- The size of the epidemic.
- The level of effort needed to control the infection.

For example, if 1 case of infection leads to 2 other cases (i.e. $R_0 = 2$), and each of those leads to 2 others then clearly the number of cases will increase and an epidemic will occur. If R_0 is larger than this, then the epidemic will increase more steeply and be more difficult to control.
- $R_0 > 1$ there will be an epidemic.
- $R_0 < 1$ the number of cases will decline.
- $R_0 = 1$ the disease will be endemic.

Determinants of R_0

$$R_0 = D \times c \times \beta$$

Where:
- D = mean duration of infectiousness.
- c = the rate of contact between infected and susceptive individuals.
- β = the probability of transmission on contact between an infected and susceptible individual.

Relation to control

Interventions to control infectious diseases can be analysed in relation to these determinants. For example:
- Vaccination programmes reduce c: by decreasing the numbers of susceptible people in the population there is a reduction in the probability of contact between an infected and a susceptible individual.
- Quarantine reduces c, but is only effective if the main period of infectiousness occurs after the onset of symptoms. Otherwise it is usually too late.
- Handwashing, use of protective masks, gloves, and condoms are all ways of reducing β.
- Prompt and effective treatment of infected individuals may reduce D; this can be encouraged through rapid case finding (through partner notification, for example) and good access to diagnostic services (ensuring no waiting lists for infectious disease services).

Modes of transmission
- Direct transmission:
  - Direct contact (skin-to-skin, sex).
  - Droplet spread (aerosols in close proximity).

- Indirect transmission:
  - Vehicle spread (contaminated inanimate objects, food, water, blood products, etc.).
  - Airborne (droplets over larger distance, e.g. through sneezing).
  - Vector spread (ticks, mosquitoes, etc).

Box 5.1 Glossary of terms for infectious disease epidemiology

Basic reproductive number (R_0): the number of new infections caused by 1 infection in an entirely susceptible population.

Endemic: when there is a constant presence of a disease in a particular community or geographic area.

Epidemic: when the number of cases rises above the expected level in a particular community or geographic area.

Herd (population) immunity: the immunity of a group or population. High levels of immunity in the population protect those who are not immunized.

Hyperendemic: when there is a constant presence of a high level of incidence of a disease in a particular community or geographic area.

Incubation period: the time between initial contact with an infectious agent and the first appearance of symptoms of the disease associated with that infectious agent.

Infectious period: the time during which a person is capable of transmitting the organism.

Outbreak: used interchangeably with epidemic, usually for a more localized increase in cases.

Pandemic: when an epidemic spreads over several continents.

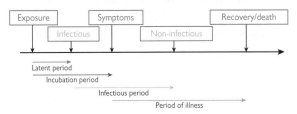

Fig. 5.2 Time periods in infectious disease.

Further reading

Hawker J et al. *Communicable Disease Control Handbook* 2nd edn. Oxford: Blackwell; 2005.
Heyman DL. *Control of Communicable Diseases Manual.* American Washington. DC: Public Works Association; 2004.

Vaccination

Vaccination is the introduction of a substance (vaccine) into the body in order to stimulate the production of antibodies against an infection without causing the active infection. Vaccination has been one of the most significant advances of medical science, saving millions of lives.

Types of immunity

Individual immunity

- Passive, short duration:
  - Maternal antibodies.
  - Passive immunization with immunoglobulin.
- Active, longer duration:
  - Following naturally acquired infection.
  - Following vaccination.

Population (herd) immunity

Population immunity is the resistance of groups of people to the spread of infection. High levels of immunity in the population protect those who are not immune, e.g. those who miss out on vaccination programmes.

Role of clinicians

Clinicians in primary care often have responsibility for the delivery of vaccinations, particularly to infants and children. Other programmes may be delivered by schools or employers. Clinicians should check that people are up to date with their vaccinations, provide a record for the individual, and complete appropriate returns to the authorities to allow coverage to be monitored.

Aim of vaccination programmes

- To provide protection to vaccinated individuals.
- To protect non-vaccinated individuals through herd immunity.

Limitations of vaccination programmes

- Partial protection (some people fail to respond).
- Waning levels of protection, for some infections need boosters or the infection may shift into an older age group.
- Some individuals (and groups of individuals) miss out on vaccination:
  - Migrants.
  - People with poor access to healthcare.
  - People with different health beliefs.

Schedules

Schedules vary by country. Standard vaccination schedules for children are shown in Table 5.2 for the UK.

Safety, ethics, and public confidence

Vaccinations are given to millions of healthy individuals and therefore any adverse effect, even if very rare, could undermine the whole programme in terms of health gain and public confidence.

Table 5.2 Standard vaccination schedule, UK, 2011

Age	Vaccine
2 months	DTaP (diphtheria, tetanus, acellular pertussis, polio)
	IPV (inactivated polio vaccine)
	Hib (*Haemophilus influenzae* type b)
	PCV (pneumococcal conjugate vaccine)
3 months	DTaP/IPV/Hib, MenC (meningitis type C vaccine)
4 months	DTaP/IPV/Hib, MenC, PCV
12–13 months	Hib, MenC, PCV, MMR (measles, mumps, rubella vaccine)
3–5 years	DTaP/IPV, MMR
12–13 years	HPV (human papillomavirus)—3 injections
13–18 years	Td/IPV(polio) booster (a combined injection of tetanus, low-dose diphtheria, and polio)
Adults	Influenza and PCV if you are aged 65 or over or in a high-risk group

Travel vaccination

Recommendations vary. Check websites for up to date information:
- The National Travel Health Network and Centre (NaTHNaC) provides advice for professionals and travellers in the UK: ℘ http://www.nathnac.org
- Fit for travel: UK, Scotland NHS website covers vaccination, malaria prophylaxis, and other advice: ℘ http://www.fitfortravel.nhs.uk

Evaluating vaccination programmes

Testing of vaccines

Vaccines are tested in the same way as drugs (see 📖 p.192) in clinical trials except that they are given to healthy individuals and therefore larger numbers are needed to demonstrate safety.
- Phase I: safety and tolerability in a small number of healthy human volunteers.
- Phase II: safe and immunogenic—dose and age range of schedules worked out.
- Phase III: vaccine tried in population intended to protect to estimate efficacy more precisely and measure common side effects.
- Phase IV: post-marketing surveillance to measure rare side effects.

Vaccine efficacy

The efficacy is a measure of how well it prevents the disease. It is estimated from clinical trails.

$$\text{Efficacy} = (I_u - I_v)/I_u$$

Where I_u is the incidence in unvaccinated, I_v is incidence in the vaccinated.

Coverage

Programmes need to meet certain coverage targets if they are to effectively control or move towards elimination. The level of coverage required for this depends on the R_0 of the infection (see 📖 p.106).

The critical proportion (p_c)

This is the proportion of the population that needs to be vaccinated to control the infection, and this is dependent on the basic reproductive number R_0:

$$p_c = 1 - (1/R_0)$$

Thus the higher the value of R_0, the greater coverage is needed to achieve control and move towards elimination. For example:

- Measles: R_0 ~16, coverage needs to be at least 94%.
- Rubella: R_0 ~4, coverage needs to be at least 80%.
- *Haemophilus influenzae* B: R_0 ~2, coverage needs to be at least 50%.

Factors influencing achievement of high immunization coverage

- Helpful government health department.
- Health professionals' acceptance and enthusiasm.
- Surveillance of adverse events.
- Continuous audit of vaccine uptake.
- Adequate supplies and high-quality vaccines.
- Adequate resources.
- Accurate confirmation of infectious disease.
- Public demand and acceptance.

Further reading

Kassianos GC. *Immunization. Childhood and travel.* Oxford: Blackwell Science; 1998.

Screening overview

Definition

Screening is the practice of investigating apparently healthy individuals with the object of detecting unrecognized disease or its precursors in order that measures can be taken to prevent or delay the development of disease or improve prognosis.

Purpose of screening

- Early detection of disease where this can lead to improved prognosis. For example, earlier detection of breast cancer allows treatment (surgery, radiotherapy, and chemotherapy) that can reduce mortality (leading to increased survival).
- Identification of people at increased risk of developing disease where interventions will reduce that risk. For example, screening for raised serum cholesterol and offering dietary advice and/or drug therapy.
- Identification of people with infectious disease where treatment or other control measures will improve the outcome for the individual (e.g. chlamydia screening), and/or prevent ongoing transmission to others (e.g. screening food handlers for salmonella, health workers for hepatitis B).

Screening tests (Table 5.3)

The *validity* of a screening test, i.e. its ability to distinguish between people with the condition and those without, is defined in the same way as for a diagnostic test (see 📖 p.16).

Table 5.3 Screening versus diagnostic tests

	Screening	Diagnostic
Population applied to	Healthy, asymptomatic	Symptomatic
Objective	To distinguish high-risk from low-risk individuals	To provide definitive diagnosis to inform management
Description	Relatively cheap, simple, and non-invasive	Can be more expensive, complex and invasive
Ideal parameters	High sensitivity to ensure no cases are missed and falsely reassured	
	High specificity to reduce number of unnecessary follow-up investigations	High sensitivity and specificity; frequently achieved through multiple investigations
	In practice may trade lower specificity for higher sensitivity to ensure no cases are missed	

Communicating results

People have different expectations from screening than from diagnostic tests, and it is important that results are carefully explained. In particular, people are likely to think that any positive screening test is indicative of certain, or almost certain, disease. In practice screening tests are often of lower specificity than diagnostic tests and therefore a positive result may still mean that the person is unlikely to have the condition. The methods described in chapter 1 for use of diagnostic tests can also be applied to screening to make communication more precise. An example is provided in Box 5.2.

Likelihood ratios are also useful in communicating the results of screening tests. The *positive likelihood ratio* is a measure of the likelihood of a positive result in a patient with the disease compared with the likelihood of a negative result in a patient without the disease (see 📖 p.22).

Box 5.2 Breast cancer screening: application of likelihood ratio[*]

A 50-year-old woman has a mammogram and the test comes back positive. She asks you whether or not she has breast cancer. How do you answer her question? You would obviously explain that she will need further investigation, but if she wants some guide you can work it out.

First establish the prevalence of breast cancer in 50-year-old women, regardless of mammogram result, let's say around 1%, and assume that mammography is 90% sensitive and 95% specific.

What is her risk? (See 📖 Likelihood ratios and post-test probabilities, p.22.)

Pre-test probability = 1% = 0.01

Pre-test odds = 0.01/(1 − 0.01) = 0.01

She has a positive test (mammogram).

$$\text{Likelihood ratio +ve test (LR+)} = \text{sensitivity}/ (1 - \text{specificity})$$
$$= 0.9/ (1 - 0.95)$$
$$= 18$$

$$\text{Post-test odds} = \text{Pre-test odds} \times \text{LR+}$$
$$= 0.01 \times 18$$
$$= 0.18$$

$$\text{Post-test probability} = \text{Post-test odds}/(\text{Post-test odds} + 1)$$
$$= 0.18/(0.18+1)$$
$$= 0.15$$

You can explain to the woman that the probability that she has breast cancer is around 15%.

[*]Numbers used are for illustration of method.

Screening programmes

Criteria for a screening programme

Before a screening programme is introduced it should meet some key criteria (see Table 5.4) in relation to the condition, the screening test, the effectiveness, and availability of treatment.

Types of screening programmes

Screening can either involve the whole population (*mass*), or selected groups who are anticipated to have an increased prevalence of the condition (*targeted*). In either of these there may be a *systematic* programme where people are called for screening (e.g. cervical cancer, breast cancer) or an *opportunistic* programme when a person presents to the doctor for some other reason and they are offered a test (e.g. chlamydia screening in young people, BP screening in older people).

First do no harm?

The concept of screening is appealing. However, by definition screening tests are carried out on apparently healthy individuals and it is always possible that screening may, inadvertently, do more harm than good. When considering the introduction of a screening programme it is essential that a careful assessment is made of the balance between benefit and harm.

Potential harm to the individual
- False alarms which induce anxiety.
- Treatment of early disease, including potential side effects, even though the disease may not have progressed.
- Unnecessary investigations, including some invasive procedures.
- False reassurance if cases are missed.

Potential harm to the population
- Waste of resources that could be used elsewhere.
- Overall could produce more harm than good through over-treatment.
- Undermine primary prevention programmes if those who test negative feel they have 'escaped' disease and can continue risky behaviours (e.g. HIV and cholesterol testing).

One study of breast cancer screening showed that for every 50,000 screens carried out, 2820 women would be found to have 'abnormal' results requiring further investigation. Only 129 of these turned out to be invasive cancer. While mortality in the population was reduced, there are also considerable costs associated with the identification of women with 'abnormal results' who face further investigation and considerable anxiety. While breast cancer screening is widely agreed to be beneficial overall, there should be continued research to reduce the harms.

Table 5.4 Criteria for a screening programme[*]

The condition	The condition should be an important health problem
	The epidemiology and natural history of the condition, including development from latent to declared disease, should be adequately understood
	There should be a detectable risk factor, disease marker, latent period or early symptomatic stage
The test	There should be a simple, safe, precise and validated screening test
	The distribution of test values in the target population should be known and a suitable cut-off level defined and agreed
	The test should be acceptable to the population
Diagnosis and treatment	There should be an agreed policy on the further diagnostic investigation of individuals with a positive test result
	There must be adequate facilities for further investigation, treatment and counseling of those who screen positive
	There should be an effective, acceptable and safe treatment

[*]Wilson and Jungner Criteria for Disease Screening. (Adopted by the World Health Organization).[1]

Reference

1 Wilson JMG, Jungner G. *Principles and Practice of Screening for Disease.* World Health Organization Public Health Papers, No. 34; 196. Geneva: WHO.

Evaluating screening programmes

Even after a disease is considered appropriate for screening and a valid test becomes available, it does not necessarily follow that a widespread screening programme should be implemented. Evaluation of a potential screening programme involves consideration of 4 main issues:

Feasibility

Feasibility will depend on how easy it is to organize the population to attend for screening, whether the screening test is acceptable, and whether facilities and resources exist to carry out the necessary diagnostic tests following screening.

Effectiveness

Effectiveness is evaluated by measuring the extent to which implementing a screening programme affects the subsequent outcomes. Does the programme reduce morbidity? Does it reduce mortality? This is difficult to measure because of a number of biases that affect most of the study designs used:

- *Selection bias* exists as people who participate in screening programmes often differ from those who do not.
- *Lead time bias:* survival appears to increase due to earlier detection. By definition, screening identifies disease at an earlier time than if there was no screening programme. Thus survival time—the time from diagnosis to death—is automatically increased even if there is no change in the outcome. This apparent improvement in the length of survival can be misleading (Fig. 5.3).
- *Length bias:* cases detected through screening may be less aggressive. Some cases may develop more slowly than others, with a longer preclinical phase, and this may be associated with a better prognosis. There is a greater probability of such 'slow' cases being picked up through screening than for more aggressive cases which may present with symptoms in between screening events. If this occurs then those detected through screening will be those with a better prognosis. Thus comparing outcomes of cases detected through screening with those presenting with symptoms will unfairly favour screening.

Cost

The cost of screening programmes is important. Resources for healthcare are limited and there are many competing demands for available money, healthcare professionals, and facilities. The relative cost-effectiveness of a screening programme compared with other forms of healthcare should therefore be carefully considered. Costs relate not just to the implementation of the screening programme but also to the further diagnostic tests and the subsequent cost of treatment. On the other hand, in the absence of screening, costs will be incurred by the treatment of patients in more advanced stages of disease.

Ethics

A screening test is a medical intervention that is done to a person who is not ill and usually to someone who has not initiated the request for the test.

For this reason the ethics of carrying out screening must be carefully considered (see 📖 p.48).

Methods for evaluating screening programmes

The gold standard is a RCT of screening compared with no screening either for individuals or in populations (see Box 5.3) There are other approaches:

- *Observational studies* in which mortality and/or morbidity are compared from before and after screening (time series), or screened individuals are compared with unscreened. These are hard to interpret (a) due to problems of bias and (b) due to confounding factors.
- *Economic analyses* are crucial to decisions about investment in screening programmes. However they are limited unless there is good evidence concerning effectiveness.
- *Mathematical modelling* can predict the impact of screening and is increasingly used, mainly in infectious disease and cancer. Again, it is only as good as the parameters entered into the model.

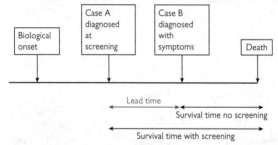

Fig. 5.3 Diagrammatic representation of lead time bias. Case A is diagnosed through screening in the pre-clinical phase and survives for twice as long as Case B who is diagnosed once she develops symptoms even though the biological course is unchanged. Hence comparing survival times of those diagnosed through screening with those diagnosed without screening will automatically favour the screening, even though there may be no true improvement in survival.

Box 5.3 Evaluating screening for colorectal cancer

A large RCT involving >170,000 men and women aged 55–64 was conducted in the UK.[1] They were randomized to either the intervention, where they were offered a single screen using flexible sigmoidoscopy, or controls who were not offered the screening. Based on an intention-to-treat analysis (see 📖 p.189) those offered screening had a 23% lower incidence of colorectal cancer and a 31% lower mortality from the disease.

Reference

1 Atkins WS *et al.* Once-only flexible sigmoidoscopy screening in prevention of colorectal cancer: A multicentre randomised controlled trial. *Lancet* 2010; **375**:1624–33.

Major UK screening programmes

(See Table 5.5.)

Table 5.5 Major UK screening programmes*

Target population	Disease	Screening test
Antenatal	Down syndrome	Serum screening, nuchal thickness in 1st or 2nd trimester
	Fetal anomalies	Ultrasound in 2nd trimester
	Sickle cell disease, thalassaemia	Blood tests for anaemia and prenatal diagnosis 1st trimester
	Syphilis HIV, hepatitis B, rubella	Blood tests
Newborn	Hearing	Oto-acoustic emissions
	Sickle cell, cystic fibrosis, phenylketonuria, hypothyroidism	Dried blood spot on Guthrie card
	Congenital anomaly	Physical examination at birth & by GP at 6–8 weeks
Children at school entry	Hearing, vision, height, weight, developmental milestones	Examination and assessment by health visitor
People <25	Chlamydia	Nucleic acid amplification test from urine or genital swab
Women aged 25–64	Cervical cancer	Cervical cytology: 3-yearly aged 25–49 then 5-yearly aged 50–64
Women aged 50–70	Breast cancer	Mammography every 3 years

*Countries in the UK and elsewhere have different standard screening programmes.

Sources of information on screening programmes

- The National Library for Health has links to all the key documents and websites on screening: ℘ http://www.screening.nhs.uk
- Healthtalkonline is a website devoted to personal experiences of health and illness, including screening, in written, audio, and video-clip format: ℘ http:// www.healthtalkonline.org
- Recommendations for screening in the USA are made by the U.S. Preventive Services Task Force: ℘ http://www.ahrq.gov/clinic/ uspstfix.htm

Evaluating clinical practice

Introduction

One of the key principles in the provision of healthcare is to provide high-quality care that is safe and effective.[1] There are 2 core activities that are necessary to achieve this:

- Clinical research to define high-quality care.
- Clinical audit to ensure that the care we provide achieves these high standards.

Clinical audit and clinical research are both fundamental to improving healthcare and delivering high-quality services. In general, they both involve the same key steps:

- Identifying an important or relevant question.
- Collecting the necessary information to answer the question.
- Analysing the information.
- Interpreting the results.
- Sharing the findings to promote change.

They are both time-consuming and challenging to do well and are subject to ethics, good practice guidelines, and data protection regulation.

It can sometimes be confusing to decide whether you need an audit or a piece of research to answer your question (see Table 6.1). As a guide, research usually involves novel data collection or analysis to answer a question about the effectiveness or safety of a clinical intervention. Audit usually looks at the clinical care being provided to see whether it meets the high standards defined by research.

Another important difference is that the findings of an audit are only applicable to the service you have studied but in research the findings can often be applied to different people or populations. This is known as generalizability—the measure of how relevant the findings of a study are to different contexts than those initially studied.

Clinical audit is usually easier to do than research, takes up less time, and uses fewer resources. Therefore it is often carried out by clinicians on top of their routine clinical responsibilities. Research is more methodologically complex and is often a full-time activity that necessitates a break from clinical practice.

These practical differences have contributed to audit becoming an integral part of clinical practice while research remains an optional activity. With this in mind, it's clear that healthcare practitioners need to understand the principles and methodology of audit well enough to participate in it. In contrast, developing practical research skills is not essential for all clinicians, although they will need to understand the principles of research in order to participate in EBM.

The following sections aim to provide an introduction to clinical audit. Rather than presenting a comprehensive review we have tried to offer practical guidance and discuss the general points you should consider if you are planning to undertake an audit.

The chapter starts by looking at the regulatory issues that underpin good audit and research and then describes a step-by-step approach to conducting your own clinical audit based on the comprehensive manual about clinical audit published by NICE in 2002, *Principles for Best Practice in Clinical Audit*.[2] Two example audits are used throughout the section to illustrate some of the practical issues. See Table 6.1 for a summary of differences between clinical audit and clinical research.

Before undertaking your own audit or research look for more detailed guidance. Further reading is suggested at the end of the chapter.

Table 6.1 Summary of differences between clinical audit and clinical research

	Audit	Research
Aim	To determine whether current practice meets best practice recommendations	To determine what best practice is
Do all clinicians need to understand it?	Yes	Yes in order to practise EBM
Do I need to carry it out?	Yes	Optional
How long does it take?	Days to few months	Months to years
Do I need ethical approval?	Often not required (but always check)	Yes
Are the findings generalizable?	No	Yes
How should I aim to share the results?	Team meetings Grand round Conference poster	Conference poster/ presentation Peer-reviewed journal

References

1 NHS. *The NHS Constitution*. London: Department of Health; 2009.
2 NICE. *Principles for Best Practice in Clinical Audit*. Oxford: Radcliffe Medical Press Ltd; 2002.

Clinical governance and ethics

Clinical governance

In the UK, clinical governance has been defined as 'the system through which National Health Service (NHS) organizations are accountable for continuously improving the quality of their services and safeguarding high standards of care, by creating an environment in which clinical excellence will flourish.'[1]

Clinical governance in the UK:
- Was introduced in 1998.
- Is central to all NHS activity.
- Made quality 'everybody's business'.
- Sets out a commitment, on behalf of NHS organizations, to constantly strive to deliver the highest quality of healthcare.
- Involves clinical audit and evidence-based practice (as defined by research).

Clinical audit

Definition

Clinical audit is 'a quality improvement process that seeks to improve patient care and outcomes through systematic review of care against explicit criteria and the implementation of change.'[2]

Purpose of audit
- To compare the care we actually provide to the care we aim to provide and checks whether care is high quality, safe, and effective.
- To identify deficiencies.
- To allow clinical teams to identify and implement change.

Audit is often represented as a circle to emphasize its continuous nature, although some argue that a spiral would be more appropriate. The key steps in an audit are illustrated in Fig. 6.1. Participation in audit is a routine part of clinical training and practice in the UK.

Steps in a clinical audit
- Planning.
- Identifying a topic.
- Choosing the standards ('explicit criteria').
- Writing a protocol.
- Choosing the sample and sample size.
- Collecting the data: what data to collect, where to find it, how to collect it, how to categorize it, how to store it.
- Analysing the data.
- Interpreting the results.
- Completing the process: changing practice, sharing findings.

The next sections in this chapter go through this process in detail, and include 2 worked examples.

Ethics

Formal ethical review and approval is required for clinical research but not necessarily for clinical audit. However, audit must be still be undertaken in line with strict ethical consideration. In the UK, formal ethical review is carried out by the National Research Ethics Services (NRES) usually via local committees. NRES produce detailed guidance on how to decide if your activity is audit or research and their website contains comprehensive advice on how to apply for ethical approval (𝄐 www.nres.npsa.nhs.uk).

For local help, there are designated teams within the Research and Development department of NHS organizations or affiliated universities that are available to provide support and advice about whether your project is audit or research and whether it needs to undergo formal ethical approval by a research ethics committee.

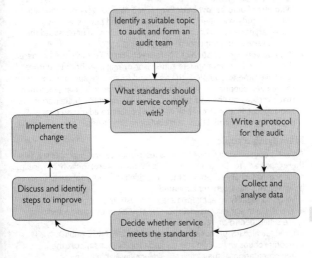

Fig. 6.1 Clinical audit cycle. Adapted from NICE. *Principles for Best Practice in Clinical Audit*. London: NICE; 2002.

References

1 Department of Health. *A first class service: Quality in the NHS*. London: DoH; 1998.
2 NICE. *Principles for Best Practice in Clinical Audit*. Oxford: Radcliffe Medical Press Ltd; 2002.

Carrying out an audit: getting started

Planning

Before you start to think about the detail of what you want to audit, there are some practical issues to consider:

- *Do you have the time?* Before you start an audit you need to make sure that you will be able to complete it (allow 2 or 3 months).
- *Who can you approach for help?* It is important to get advice and support from your seniors from the start of an audit. For people who are in training it should be a supervisor or a clinical lead within the relevant department.
- *Who else should be involved?* Even if you plan to carry out your audit independently you need to involve patients and people who work in the target service. Input from others will help you understand the clinical service and implement change.
- *Who do you need to speak to before you start?* You will need to agree the audit with an appropriate supervisor or manager both to ensure you have time to complete the audit and to arrange appropriate access to data and support. In some organizations there will be a department that oversees quality and audit and you may need to obtain permission and support from them. They will also be able to advise on data protection, data collection, and confidentiality issues.

Identifying a topic

An audit question may arise from issues in your clinical practice, e.g. when there appears to be unexplained variation in care, or when research evidence has changed good practice guidelines and you want to check how well this has been implemented.

Ways to identify an appropriate audit question:

- The department may have a shortlist of audit questions or audits that are scheduled to be repeated.
- Look for already prepared ideas e.g. in the UK, NICE publish a comprehensive list of potential audit topics that support the implementation of their clinical guidance (available online at ℘ http://www.nice.org.uk).
- Perform a literature review to find out whether there has been a significant change to the evidence base that should be reflected in your practice.
- Look for clinical guidelines or protocols in use in the department that you could audit performance against.
- Is there a part of the care pathway that might not be performing as well as it could, e.g. complication rates or complaints?
- Look at your organization's priorities.

It is advisable to choose an audit topic:

- You find interesting.
- That is an important aspect of clinical care.
- That has the potential to improve care.
- That does not duplicate recent activity in the department.

Specifying the question

Whatever topic you decide on you should try and identify a specific and answerable question from within it. Audits can be used to look at any part of clinical care, not simply whether a patient's treatment adheres to a clinical guideline. They may address:

- *Structure:* e.g. number and mix of staff, number of beds in relation to the catchment area.
- *Process:* e.g. referral, appointment booking, waiting times, the consultation, follow-up, team handovers.
- *Outcome:* e.g. re-admission rates, survival, length of hospital stay, quality of life, patient experience.

All of these dimensions can be useful targets for audit. You should also consider how you want to measure quality. Maxwell defined 6 dimensions of quality:[1]

- Effectiveness.
- Efficiency.
- Acceptability.
- Access.
- Equity.
- Relevance.

Worked examples (continued in later topics)

Management of stroke

You are working in the medical admissions unit and interested in the management of stroke. Current NICE guidance includes: 'Alteplase for the treatment of acute ischaemic stroke'.[2] To audit your unit's compliance with this guideline, start by familiarizing yourself with the guidance and identifying a specific question, '*How many people who present to your department with an acute ischaemic stroke are given alteplase within 3 hours of their symptoms starting?*' In real life, if resources allow, you would try to audit performance against all the recommendations.

Smoking cessation interventions

You are working in primary care and interested in health promotion. Current NICE guidance includes: 'Brief interventions and referral for smoking cessation in primary care and other settings'.[3] Again, you start by familiarizing yourself with the guidance and decide to ask '*how good your practice is at referring people for smoking cessation therapy*'.

References

1 Maxwell, RJ. Quality assessment in health. *BMJ* 1984; **288**:1470–2.
2 NICE. *Alteplase for treatment of acute ischaemic stroke* (TA122). London: NICE; 2007.
3 NICE. *Brief interventions and referral for smoking cessation in primary care and other settings* (PH1). London: NICE; 2006.

Choosing the standards

Audit compares clinical care to a defined set of standards or explicit criteria. Once you have identified the specific topic you wish to audit the next step is to define the standards or 'explicit criteria' for your audit.* It is important to choose or define an appropriate set of standards otherwise you risk wasting your time as the audit findings will not be meaningful or useful for service improvement.

Useful information about standards:

• They should describe 'best practice'.
• They should focus on the critical parts of the care pathway.
• They should be evidence based.
• You must be able to measure performance against the standard, i.e. be able to collect information that will tell you if your service is achieving the standard.
• You need to choose an appropriate number of standards. It can be very tempting to want to audit against everything, but be pragmatic. Define enough standards to cover the key contributors to the quality of the service but don't duplicate or collect information that isn't relevant.
• Get good coverage of the service by defining standards that look at all 3 aspects of care; structure, process and outcome.
• Choose an appropriate level of performance to achieve; do you expect your service to achieve the same as the best 5%, the same as the worst 5%, or the same as the average? This is called 'benchmarking'.

*NB: This is what differentiates an audit from a service evaluation. A service evaluation looks at the care being provided without comparing it to a defined standard.[1]

What sort of standard?

There are different approaches to finding the information/evidence on which to base your standards. Decide which example question is the most similar to your audit question:

• Is our service adhering to the local protocols/guidelines?
  • Use the protocol/guidelines to identify the key components of care.
  • NB: an assumption is made here that local protocols/guidelines will have been developed to reflect the evidence base or expert consensus where the evidence is not available.
• Is our service adhering to national protocols/guidelines?
  • Find the published national guidelines and identify the key components of care.
  • Many organizations publish national guidelines e.g. NICE or SIGN (Scottish Intercollegiate Guidelines Network) and the Royal Colleges (see 📖 pp.38–41).
  • NICE also publishes audit guides to support the implementation of their clinical guidelines, complete with pre-defined audit standards.
• Is our service adhering to evidence-based best practice or where this does not exist, expert consensus best practice?
  • This is the most challenging way of defining standards and should only be needed where local and national guidelines do not exist.
  • Start with a systematic review of the relevant literature to define quality care (see 📖 Systematic review, pp.88–9).
  • For a detailed description of how to formulate criteria from the evidence refer to NICE guidance.[1]

Once you have identified the information you will use to define your audit standards you need to begin the process of turning the document/ evidence into a set of standards. This can be a complex process get help from your seniors/colleagues and always try to use published audit standards where they exist. Further support can be found on the NICE website (http://www.nice.org.uk).

Examples of NICE guidance documents:

- *Clinical guidelines:* 'recommendations on the appropriate treatment and care of people with specific diseases and conditions within the NHS in England and Wales'.
- *Public health guidance:* 'recommendations for populations and individuals on activities, policies and strategies that can help prevent disease or improve health'.
- *Technology appraisal:* 'guidance on the use of new and existing medicines and treatments within the NHS'.
- *Interventional procedures:* 'guidance looks at whether interventional procedures are safe enough and work well enough to be used routinely or whether special arrangements are needed for patient consent'.

Worked examples (see ▭ p.125)

Management of stroke

NICE guidance on alteplase[2] defines 4 criteria, but the one you have chosen is 'The percentage of patients diagnosed with acute ischaemic stroke treated with alteplase within 3 hours of onset of the stroke symptoms.'

This criterion has defined:

- Eligible patients: people diagnosed with acute stroke.
- Timeframe for intervention: 3 hours from symptom onset.
- Treatment to receive: alteplase.

The guidance also suggested that people diagnosed with an intracranial haemorrhage are excluded from this criterion.

NICE recommends 100% attainment for this criterion (for full details please refer to the guidance document[2]).

Smoking cessation interventions

NICE guidance on smoking cessation[3] defines 5 criteria for audit, but you are planning to look at how good your practice is at referring people for smoking cessation therapy. This is the relevant criterion:

'Percentage of patients on GP lists who smoke, who have within the last 12 months:
  a) been referred to the NHS Stop Smoking Service.
  b) been offered pharmacotherapy (e.g. received a prescription for nicotine replacement therapy (NRT)).
  c) both (a) and (b).
  d) been referred to an intensive stop smoking support service other than the NHS Stop Smoking Service.
  e) none of the above.'

This criterion has defined:

- Source of the sample of patients: GP register.
- Eligible patients: people who smoke.
- Timeframe for intervention: last 12 months.
- Types of smoking cessation therapy.

The NICE guidance recommends that 'everyone who smokes should be advised to quit unless there are exceptional circumstances' and 'those who want to stop should be offered a referral to an intensive support service' or pharmacotherapy. NICE recommends 100% attainment for the criterion, i.e. everyone who smokes should be offered referral or treatment at least every 12 months.

References

1 NICE. *Principles for Best Practice in Clinical Audit*. Oxford: Radcliffe Medical Press Ltd; 2002.
2 NICE. *Alteplase for treatment of acute ischaemic stroke (TA122)*. London: NICE; 2007.
3 NICE. *Brief interventions and referral for smoking cessation in primary care and other settings (PH1)*. London: NICE; 2006.

Online resources

National Research Ethics Service: ℔ http://www.nres.npsa.nhs.uk
NICE: ℔ http://nice.org.uk
Royal College of Physicians: ℔ http://www.rcplondon.ac.uk/resources/clinical/guidelines
SIGN: ℔ http://www.sign.ac.uk

Writing your protocol

Having decided on the topic and defined the criteria it is important to prepare a protocol. If you skip this stage and go directly to pulling data it is likely that you will not collect the correct information from an appropriate sample of patients, and may have to go back and repeat the work.

The protocol:
- Should be written before you start.
- Will describe all the activity that will take place from start to finish of the audit.
- Will identify potential problems.
- Will allow you to rectify any problems before they occur.
- Will be your point of reference throughout the project.
- Can be shared with others.
- Should be referred back to at regular intervals.
- Will help to keep the project on track.

A protocol should be detailed enough to guide someone else who wishes to repeat the audit, but not so detailed that it takes longer to write than to complete the audit.

A typical audit protocol should contain the following:
- Title.
- Background (brief):
  - Why is this an important topic?
  - Description of your clinical setting, e.g. number of patients per week.
- Audit question and standards ('explicit criteria'):
  - Describe how they were obtained/developed.
- Data collection (see 📖 Data collection, pp.132–3):
  - What data will you collect and why?
  - How will you collect the data?
- Analysis plan (see 📖 Analysing data, pp.136–7).
- Plan for completing the audit cycle.
- Resources:
  - Staff: e.g. administrative staff to pull case notes, IT support for database design or data extraction.
  - Materials: e.g. computer/printer/statistical software.
- Timeline/key milestones:
  - Data collection, data analysis, draft report of results, key departmental meetings, final report, etc.
- Relevant appendices:
  - e.g. clinical guideline, previous audit results.

Once you have drafted your protocol you should circulate it, initially to those directly involved in the audit. Collect any feedback or comments and revise it as needed. You should then share this completed protocol with any other relevant staff in your department.

It is worth taking the time to discuss the audit with your colleagues from an early stage as their support will make it much easier to complete the audit and implement any change to the service.

Choosing the sample

Your sample should be defined in terms of:
- Time:
  - This can be prospective or retrospective (see Table 6.2).
  - The duration will be influenced by the volume of activity in the service and your resources.
  - For example, if only 1 patient is admitted per week, then you may need to collect information for at least 6 months, whereas if you admit 100 patients per week you may only need to look at a period of a few weeks.
  - Be explicit in the definition, i.e. state a time and date for the start and finish.
- Person:
  - Sex.
  - Age range.
  - Diagnosis or presenting complaint or intervention.
- Place:
  - Health authority or local geographical area.
  - Primary care surgery.
  - Community or hospital clinic.
  - Hospital ward or department.
- Sampling method:
  - Consecutive patients.
  - Random sample of patients.
- Decide whether the sample should be prospective or retrospective:

Table 6.2 Prospective or retrospective sample

Prospective	Retrospective
Period from the start of the audit.	Previous period of time.
Example: form completed by clinician or patient at time of consultation.	Example: from medical records.
Can collect additional information to that routinely collected.	Have to use what is usually collected.
People are aware of the data collection and may change practice.	Study cannot affect the content of information already collected.
More resource intensive.	Less resource intensive.

NB: audit samples tend to be chosen in a pragmatic way, known as a convenience sample, i.e. chosen because of the ease of availability. However, you still need to make sure that the choice of sample is appropriate to the question and avoids bias. You are trying to build a fair picture of how the clinical area is performing against certain standards.

Examples of a sampling frame:
- 100 consecutive patients aged 18 years or over, presenting to Accident and Emergency in Trust A with back pain from 0900 on 1 February 2010.
- Consecutive patients aged 75 years and over attending the anticoagulation clinic at Trust B between 0900 on 1 February 2010 until 0900 on 7 February 2010.

Sample size (see 📖 p.240)

A sample size calculation determines the number of patients you need:
- To detect an effect/change of a defined size.
- With a defined level of statistical certainty.
- And with a defined probability of detecting this change.

Unlike in research you *do not need* to calculate a sample size for an audit if your results are not intended to be generalizable beyond your clinical environment. However, it is good practice to calculate a sample size before you start. By doing this you will be able to compare the results of this audit to future or previous audits.

In practice, the sample size is often a pragmatic decision guided by:
- How much information there is, e.g. patients or procedures.
- How long you have to conduct the audit.
- How many hours you have to collect the data.

Data collection

What to collect?

Research often involves collecting new data but there are usually fewer resources available for audits so you will need to rely on existing information or that which can be collected quickly and easily. The data you decide to collect will be informed by the audit standards, but on a practical note, the availability of data may actually influence the standards that you are able to audit against.

Only collect information that is relevant to the standards. This will save time and help when it comes to interpreting the findings:

• List the information needed to compare your performance to these standards.
• List additional information that may help interpret the findings, e.g. patient characteristics (e.g. age, gender, ethnicity), provider characteristics (e.g. clinician, time of day, type of clinic).

Where to find the information? (See Chapter 8)

Is the information you need already recorded somewhere? Example sources of information include medical case notes (paper or electronic), a register (e.g. cancer registries), a surveillance system (e.g. infectious disease notification data), or management and activity data (e.g. prescribing data, hospital episode statistics).

If the information you need is stored in some electronic form then you need to list the exact data that you want extracted. If it is paper form you will need to design a simple form or template that includes all the variables that you need when you go through the records to extract the data.

If the information does not already exist then you will need to collect it yourself. Identify the best setting to collect the information and design a form or template. This may involve clinicians or patients completing a form during the clinical consultation. This may be on paper or, increasingly, it will be an electronic form which will reduce errors introduced during data entry.

Categorizing data

If you are using a form to extract data from records or to collect new data from clinicians or patients it is essential to carry out a pilot. This will ensure that whoever is collecting the data is clear about what is required. This is particularly important when it comes to categorizing data. Define the information you want to collect precisely so that:

• Data collection is consistent.
• The information from each case is comparable.
• You can repeat the process.
• You collect the right information at the start.
• You can limit the amount of information you collect.

The importance of a clear definition can be seen from the relatively simple example of age. Do you want:

• Age at time of event (e.g. admission, discharge)? If so, what other dates do you need to collect (e.g. date of event)?
• Age in years, years and months, or in 5-year bands?
• Date of birth so you can calculate exact ages?

If you are unsure, it is best to collect raw data and group into categories when you analyse the data. However, this adds to the work and may be unnecessary if you are sure that you are only going to analyse by 5-year age bands.

You may also want to analyse people by clinical categories, e.g. *type of operation* if you want to audit against a standard on postoperative wound infection rates. In this situation defining the categories before you start data collection may improve coding accuracy as information from the medical notes can be used if there is ambiguity.

Storing the data

Paper based or electronic: this will depend on how much information you are collecting and what analysis you intend to do. More information is available from the Caldicott Guardian at your Practice/Trust.[1]

General principles for storing information:

- Information should be stored for the duration of the audit and for an agreed time after (until the audit is going to be repeated, for example).
- Paper forms should be kept in a locked drawer in an appropriate office.
- Electronic information should be stored on your organization's computer server (ideally password protected, encrypted and with restricted access according to local regulations).

Reference

1 Department of Health. *NHS Caldicott Guardians* [online] 2011. http://www.dh.gov.uk/en/ Managingyourorganisation/Informationpolicy/Patientconfidentialityandcaldicottguardians/ DH_4100563

Online resources

Cancer registries: http://www.statistics.gov.uk
Hospital Episode Statistics: http://www.hesonline.nhs.uk
Infectious disease notifications: http://www.hpa.org.uk

Data collection: examples

Management of stroke (see 📖 p.127)

The information you need for this audit criterion can be found in the patient's medical notes and the hospital admission system. NICE suggest that the audit is conducted retrospectively and define the sample as:
- Time: all presentations in the previous 6 months.
- Person: people diagnosed with acute ischaemic stroke.
- Place: hospital.
- Sampling method: consecutive sample of all patients presenting over the previous 6 months.

Data to be collected
- Age at presentation, recorded in 5-year age band (50–≤54; 55–≤59; 60–≤64, etc.).
- Time* and date of onset of stroke symptoms.
- Time and date of presentation.
- Initial diagnosis:
  - Stroke Yes/No
  - Other ....
- Time of request for brain imaging.
- Time of CT head (or other imaging).
- Diagnosis from report of CT head (or other imaging):
  - Acute ischaemic
  - Haemorrhagic
  - Other..............................
- Definitive diagnosis:
  - Acute ischaemic stroke: Yes/No
  - Other ....
- Name of treating clinician: recognized initials
- Alteplase given Yes/No with time and date:

*All times in 24-hour clock format.

You may also decide to collect gender, ethnicity, past medical history, medication, etc.

These data can be collected simply onto a paper form. You can calculate the duration after the onset of symptoms that each stage of care occurred. This will allow you to identify any potential delays in the care pathway.

Smoking cessation interventions

The information you need for this audit criterion can all be found in the patient's electronic record at the GP surgery.

NICE suggest that the audit is conducted retrospectively and define the sample in terms of:
- Time: all consultations over the previous month.
- Person: people who smoke.

- Place: GP surgery.
- Sampling method: consecutive sample of all patients from the start of the previous month to the end of the month.
- Sample size: ideally the complete sample of 1 month's patients will be used, but if resources do not allow or there is a particularly high prevalence of smoking in your practice, consider truncating the sample to 1/2/3 weeks. But remember, this will reduce the representativeness of the sample.

To measure your practice's performance against the audit criterion, you will need to go through each patient's record and collect the following information: if they smoke, and if so were they referred to a smoking cessation service and/or prescribed pharmacotherapy.

Suggested data to collect:
- Age: based on date of birth, recorded in five year age band (15–≤19; 20–≤24; 25–≤29, etc.).
- Referral in last 12 months: Yes/No.
- Type of referral: NHS Stop smoking service/other.
- Pharmacotherapy prescription given: Yes/No.
- Reason given for lack of referral/prescription: Yes/No.
- Detail of reason.

These data can be collected simply onto a paper form and aggregated into a simple database for analysis and presentation.

Analysing data

The aim of the analysis is to determine whether your service has achieved the standards set out in the audit. If you have used well-defined measurable standards then this process should be straightforward.

Steps in data analysis:
- Collate the information or 'raw data'.
- Save a copy of the raw data for reference.
- Look through for any errors, often called a 'sense check'. This is a way of saying look for any obvious mistakes in the data, e.g. date of birth that is incompatible with the recorded age or the wrong sex of a patient (e.g. male hysterectomy patient).
- If you find any errors it may be possible to go back to the original source and re-extract the information.
- Where possible anonymize the data by removing any patient-identifiable details.
- The specific analysis will depend on your question and the chapters on statistics (see Chapters 9 and 10) will be able to provide you with more guidance about this.
- The commonest statistic you are likely to need is a simple proportion, e.g. what percentage of patients received treatment X for condition Y?
- Consider a rough 'sub-group analysis' to see if the overall figure of performance varies when you look at smaller groups of patients, e.g. grouped by age, sex, ethnicity, or time of presentation (out of hours/daytime), consultant, or clinic. This will not always be appropriate and you need to be careful not to assign too much importance to the findings, but they could point to areas where your service is performing well or less well.
- Summarize the performance of your service against every audit standard.

Worked examples (see 📖 p.134)

Stroke management

Calculate the denominator, i.e. the total number of patients presenting with a diagnosis of acute ischaemic stroke within the last 6 months, and the numerator, i.e. the number of those who were given alteplase within 3 hours of the onset of symptoms.

Remember to exclude people from both the numerator and denominator if there is insufficient information to know whether the alteplase was given in time.

You may also wish to do some subgroup analyses to see if performance varies by age or gender of the patient, or by clinician grade.

Smoking cessation

From the data you should be able to show the numbers of patients in each of the categories defined by NICE:
a) referred to the NHS Stop Smoking Service.
b) offered pharmacotherapy (e.g. received a prescription for NRT).
c) both (a) and (b).
d) referred to an intensive stop smoking support service other than the NHS Stop Smoking Service.
e) none of the above.

Percentage of patient's referred to smoking cessation therapy or prescribed pharmacotherapy, let's call this n%, is equal to all those who received a referral (a+d) plus all those who received a prescription (b) minus those who received both (c) divided by the total number of people who smoke in the sample (a+b+d+e–c):

$$n\% = \frac{(a+b+d)-(c)}{(a+b+d+e-c)} \times 100$$

Again, you may want to see if this outcome varies by patient or clinician characteristics.

Interpreting findings

You need to make an informed decision about the clinical relevance and importance of the findings. This requires consideration of the findings in context, i.e. with an understanding of your local population/services/resources.

If your service has achieved the standard:

- This may indicate that your service is performing well.
- Consider everything you learnt about the service and whether you can identify any potential improvements not specifically related to the standards.
- If the audit did not identify any areas for improvement it may be appropriate to focus resources on other clinical areas that may not be performing as well.
- Plan to repeat the audit at a suitable interval.

If your service has not achieved the standard:

- You need to decide how significant this is for patient care.
- Remember that you have not collected a random sample of cases so it is not appropriate to calculate significance in the statistical sense; you need to make a judgement about the clinical relevance of this finding.
- Use any additional information you collected to help interpret the findings, e.g. you may have collected reasons for any deviation from the standard.
- As you become more experienced or familiar with a particular field, judging the clinical significance will become easier—don't be afraid to ask for the input and experience of senior colleagues.
- Prioritize the ways in which your service did not meet the standards in terms of their clinical significance.
- Address the issues raised in the order of their clinical significance.

Potential factors contributing to clinical significance:

- Severity of condition.
- Number of patients affected.
- Urgency of need for care.
- Potential harm from poor-quality care.

Worked examples (see 📖 p.136)

Stroke management

Let's say that your audit found that only 75% of appropriately diagnosed patients received alteplase within 3 hours of the onset of stroke symptoms. You did not achieve the 100% target—what does this mean about the quality of your service and what will you do to rectify the situation?

To answer this question you would probably like to know some additional information. For example, the time the patient presented to healthcare (whether this was within the 3-hour window); the grade of the treating physician (whether they are appropriately experienced); the report from CT head (or other imaging) (whether a haemorrhagic stroke has been ruled out).

Collecting this information could show that 15% of patients presented to hospital too late and that 10% were not able to undergo imaging within the timescale.

This additional information will change how you interpret the quality of your service and provide further information needed to plan improvements.

Results
- 75% of eligible patients received the recommended treatment.
- 15% presented to hospital too late.
- 10% were not able to undergo imaging within the timescale.

Suggested actions
- Review the time at which a decision was taken to request brain imaging.
- Look at the time and date of admission of patients who did and did not receive brain imaging within the designated time window.
- Look at the systems in place for arranging emergency CT head scans.
- Consider the need for health promotion to raise awareness of the symptoms of stroke and promote early presentation.

Smoking cessation interventions
Let's say that your audit found that only 25% of patients were referred or given a prescription for pharmacotherapy. You did not achieve the 100% target—what does this mean about the quality of your service and what will you do to rectify the situation?

To answer this question you would probably like to know some additional information. For example, whether the patient refused the offer of referral or treatment; whether there were 'exceptional circumstances' to explain why a referral was not made.

Collecting this information could show that 65% of the patients were offered a referral or treatment and declined, 5% had a documented reason to explain the lack of referral or treatment ('exceptional circumstances') and the remaining 5% were not offered intervention with no reason given.

This additional information will change how you interpret the quality of your service.

Suggested actions
- Speak to practitioners involved in specific cases where no intervention was offered and no reason given to find out why this occurred—identify steps to improve the offer of intervention.
- Speak to a group of patients to find out why they refused intervention—identify steps to improve uptake of intervention.

Changing practice

The previous steps should have produced a list, in order of priority, of the areas where your service has not achieved the audit standards. This list tells you where changes need to be made. But the step from knowing what you have to change to deciding how to change can be difficult.

This is an example of a step-wise approach to identifying what changes to make:

- Work independently at first to think about possible solutions.
- Conduct a search of the literature looking for case studies or related examples and compile a list of ideas from their results.
- Informally discuss with other members of the department.
- Hold a meeting with key people in the department (e.g. clinician, patient, nurse, ward clerk, physiotherapist, porter, etc.), present the findings from the audit and use your initial work to stimulate the discussion. NB: be careful not to steer the conversation too closely in the direction of your ideas!
- End the meeting with a list of possible actions.
- Work through these ideas to determine their likely impact. For example, will they require additional resources, e.g. extra equipment, more staff, more time, or will they require less resources, e.g. potential staff redundancies?
- From this investigation identify a list of potential actions or recommendations that will improve the service within the available resources.
- Discuss these recommendations at a team meeting and make a consensus decision about what action to take given your local context and wider resource limitations.

Once you have agreed on an appropriate change you need to write an action plan that describes the steps you will need to take to implement it. You should also plan for a system to monitor the impact of this change. This will save time in the future and make the process of repeating the audit much simpler.

Implementing change

- The most challenging part of an audit.
- The area where junior staff often have least experience.
- Easier with a detailed action plan.
- Easier if you have strong senior support and the support of your team/department.
- Often a gradual process.

A senior champion, e.g. the clinical lead in the department can:
- Use their role to promote the change.
- Use their leadership skills to encourage others to adopt the change.
- Assist in finding any resources needed to support the change.

Implementing a change successfully can take longer than you think. Be realistic and give yourself plenty of time to put everything in place before you 'launch' the change as people can get disheartened when they are expecting something great and it doesn't deliver quickly.

After the change is implemented:
- Don't assume that everyone will find it easy to change their practice.
- Continue to make people aware of the change to practice.
- Look for opportunities to keep people interested/motivated, e.g. present a brief progress update at team meetings.
- Give people a chance to feedback their ideas and adapt things if needed. This should improve the change process and increase the chance of people being supportive.

Worked examples (see 📖 p.138)

Stroke management

The department agrees:
- To recruit an extra member of staff to undertake the transport of patients to and from the radiology department after 8pm and on the weekends.
- To repeat the audit after 6 months, to allow time to fill the new post.

Smoking cessation interventions

The practice decides:
- To run training on brief interventions for smoking cessation and provide information about the services and interventions available.
- All clinical areas should have a poster clearly displayed with a summary of how to refer patients to smoking cessation services and the doses for pharmacotherapy.
- The audit should be repeated at 12 months to allow all staff to participate in the training.

Completing the process

Once the audit has been completed you should write a final report. Keep it brief and cover the following sections:
- Context to the audit.
- Methods of data collection.
- Methods and results of data analysis.
- Interpretation of results.
- Recommendations.
- Chosen action and justification.
- Action plan for change (including milestones and timeline).
- Suggested date for repeat audit.

Audit is a continuous process. It is useful to plan for the re-audit before the first audit is completed. The timing of the repeat audit will depend on what your audit identified and what changes were made to the service.

You need to allow enough time to incorporate the new change into practice, but you don't want to leave it too long—consider the potential implications if the novel approach turns out to be less effective than the original.

Depending on your specific circumstances, you should plan to repeat the audit anywhere between 6 months to 3 years.

Remember that you may have left your current post before it is time to repeat the audit. Therefore it is important to plan for someone to take over responsibility when you leave. This could be the lead clinician involved in the audit but check if there are other systems within your institution.

If you move on from the post, you should be able to hand over:
- Audit protocol.
- Data collected.
- Final audit report.
- Proposed date for the repeat audit.

Sharing your findings

Sharing findings of audits can be very important in helping others to improve quality. Publishing in academic journals is one important avenue, but there are many others that are often forgotten, e.g. presenting to local audit networks, patient panels and relevant professional groups.

Consider the following to decide whether your work will be interesting or relevant to others:
- Novel approach to audit methodology, e.g. data collection or analysis.
- Audit of a novel service.
- Identified an innovative solution to meet the standards.
- Successful implementation of change.
- Good example of multidisciplinary working.

Possible avenues for sharing your work include:
- Team meeting.
- Lunchtime meeting of other specialties in your hospital.
- Grand round.
- Poster presentation at a relevant conference.
- Short report for a relevant journal.

Epidemiological methods

Introduction

The previous sections outlined how epidemiological methods and knowledge are used in the clinic and in the practice of evidence-based care. We now move on to the methods that are central to epidemiology but also applicable to many parts of clinical research and practice. Clinicians need to be aware of the ways that evidence and knowledge are generated, whether from empirical research or through analysis of existing routine data sets. With the rapid growth in the amount of information and the ease with which it can be obtained by doctors and patients alike, it is essential that clinicians be armed with the knowledge and skills to find, evaluate, and apply evidence appropriately. This involves appreciating how research is carried out, understanding where data come from and how valid they are, different techniques for presenting and analysing data, and, crucially, the ability to distinguish strong from weak or even incorrect evidence. While most clinicians will not have a career in full-time research, familiarity with the principles of good scientific method are invaluable for any branch of medicine.

Chapter 7 describes the different types of studies that produce epidemiological and clinical knowledge, starting with the basics that distinguish quantitative and qualitative, observational, and experimental forms of evidence. We outline the major study designs and include a guide as to when they are appropriate, how they are analysed, and what limitations to look out for.

Chapter 8 provides a brief overview of sources of routine data, such as hospital and mortality statistics, again with a pointer to how these may be used and interpreted but also how to treat them with caution. We also indicate the important role of clinicians in providing the raw data for many of these systems, with a plea to pay attention to the quality of coding and reporting in order to avoid the pitfall of 'rubbish in, rubbish out'.

Chapter 9 outlines the concepts used in statistics that are relevant to clinical medicine. It covers basics such as the ways that data are categorized, described, and presented, explains how sampling variability underpins statistical methods, and introduces different distributions, hypothesis tests, and sample size calculations. It also distinguishes statistical and clinical significance, and provides guidance on what resources you might use, such as statistical packages, and when you should consider consulting a statistician.

Chapter 10 concludes this section with a description of the main statistical techniques that you will come across in reports of clinical research. Each topic covers a type of statistical test and describes what it is for, when it is used, what it does, the output produced and how to interpret it, and any limitations on its use. These descriptions are not intended to be a complete guide to doing your own statistical analysis, but more as a way of helping you understand research papers and know what tests are appropriate. More detail is available in the excellent *Oxford Handbook of Medical Statistics*.[1]

Reference

1 Peacock A, Peacock P. *Oxford Handbook of Medical Statistics*. Oxford: Oxford University Press; 2010.

Types of study

Types of evidence and study designs

Clinical medicine is based on a wide range of disciplines, and scientific methods should underpin them all. Epidemiology is the study of the distribution and determinants of health and illness in populations and its scientific methods are relevant to much clinical research which is based on observation and enquiry relating to groups of people.

The best type of evidence depends on the question. For treatment decisions randomized controlled trials (RCTs) provide the strongest evidence of effectiveness, while informing people about prognosis after a cancer diagnosis should be based on evidence from large follow-up studies. Understanding the factors leading to a positive experience of care may best be achieved through a qualitative study.

Observational research

Epidemiological research is mostly observational. That means the investigator uses naturally occurring variation in the population to identify patterns and associations. Clinical research is also often observational, studying the natural history of disease or comparing outcomes in people who present in different ways. Good observational research requires close attention to the design, selection of participants, inclusion of controls, careful measurement of exposures, outcomes and potential confounders, and robust data analysis.

Types of observational study include:
- Case series.
- Time trend and geographical studies (ecological).
- Surveys and cross sectional studies.
- Case–control studies.
- Prospective (cohort) studies.
- Qualitative studies.

Experimental research

Much science is based on experiments in which the investigator controls some factor and then measures the variation in outcome. In clinical medicine, experimental methods underpin clinical trials that compare treatments. In epidemiology trials are used to measure the impact of preventive interventions such as vaccines or behaviour change programmes. As with observational studies, it is essential that trials are well designed, carried out and analysed.

Types include:
- RCTs.
- Cluster (community) RCTs.
- Cross-over trials.
- Factorial trials.

Modelling and simulation research

Observational and experimental studies are both forms of empirical research. A growing field of biomedical and epidemiological research is based on the development of complex models and simulations that are then used to test hypotheses. Such research is strongly linked to the development of theories to explain systems, and the validity of the research depends on the strength of these theories and of the data that are used to set model parameters. Mathematical modelling is commonly used to study infectious disease transmission, and statistical models are widely used to help interpret empirical data.

A hierarchy of evidence?

Although the best type of study depends on the question being asked, there is a general acceptance in medical research of a 'hierarchy' of evidence, with some providing stronger proof than others. The suggested hierarchy is, from highest to lowest:

- Systematic review and meta-analysis of trials.
- RCTs.
- Cohort studies.
- Case–control studies.
- Ecological studies.
- Cross-sectional studies.
- Case reports and case series.
- Expert opinion.

Animal-based, *in vitro*, and qualitative research are relevant to different questions and do not fit well in this concept of a hierarchy of research.

This hierarchy has been developed in relation to standardizing evidence for the effectiveness of treatments and is used by organizations making policy recommendations and developing guidelines. It therefore places greatest weight on results of trials. While trials avoid many of the limitations of observational studies, including confounding and bias in allocation, their results should be subject to the same careful appraisal as any other study. Trials and systematic reviews can be excellent, but they may also be wrong if poorly conducted. Forms of evidence lower down the hierarchy are critical in the research process and should not be dismissed, and may be the only source of evidence available.

Further reading

Glasziou P, Vandenbroucke JP, Chalmers I. Assessing the quality of research. *BMJ* 2004; **328**:39–41.

Basic concepts in epidemiological research

An important aspect of epidemiology is to identify, describe, and quantify factors that increase or decrease the risk of disease or death. If we find out that a particular factor or exposure, e.g. smoking or taking a drug, is associated with the risk of a particular health outcome, we can then assess if the association is likely to be causal or not, and postulate causal mechanisms. Even in the absence of established causal mechanisms, evidence of association can guide public health policy and action, and clinical practice, to reduce the risk of disease or death and protect, restore, and promote health.

Exposure

This is used to describe something that might affect an outcome. In statistical analysis exposures are *explanatory* or *independent variables* (see 📖 p.221). It may refer to an environmental hazard or infectious agent, but is also used in epidemiology to describe other factors such as a genetic factor e.g. human leukocyte antigen (HLA) type, or demographic characteristic such as ethnicity. The exposure of primary interest is the one which is included in the hypothesis under investigation, e.g. if the hypothesis is that aflatoxin causes liver cancer, then aflatoxin is the primary exposure of interest. In contrast, if the hypothesis is that the individual's ability to metabolize aflatoxin determines their risk of liver cancer, then the metabolic enzyme phenotype or genotype is the exposure.

Outcome

This is also used in a broad sense, and may be disease, death, or recovery. Some studies, particularly cohorts, can look at multiple outcomes in relation to one or more exposures. In statistical analysis outcomes are *response* or *dependent variables* (see 📖 p.221).

Confounder

This refers to any factor that is independently associated with *both* the exposure and the outcome under study. Confounding can lead to bias and wrong conclusions, and therefore care needs to be taken to measure confounders in any study in order to control for them in the analysis. For example, there is an association between playing football and going bald. Before concluding that football makes you go bald, it would be important to control for gender, which is associated with the exposure (football) and the outcome (baldness). Common confounders in epidemiological studies would include age, sex, socioeconomic status, smoking, etc. Confounders are also *explanatory* or *independent variables*.

Bias

Bias is a deviation from the truth that can occur in studies. When present it means that the results of the study are wrong. For example, if a study aims to estimate the prevalence of HIV in the whole population, and the sample used is people attending sexual health clinics, the result will be an overestimate of the true population prevalence. Those who are recruited are selected in a way that is likely to relate to their HIV risk, i.e. they are more likely to be engaging in high-risk sexual behaviour than the rest of the population who do not attend clinics.

Systematic error (bias) is different from random error. The latter occurs because of random variation in observation or measurement. Increasing the sample size of a study can reduce random error, but cannot reduce bias.

There are 2 main types of bias in studies: selection bias and measurement (or information) bias:

Selection bias refers to errors introduced by recruiting participants based on some characteristic that is likely to be linked to the exposure and/or the outcome. For example, in estimating the case fatality rate for pandemic influenza you need to measure the deaths (numerator) and total cases. If you conduct the study in a hospital, than you will only record the most serious cases, missing all those who are asymptomatic or treated for milder symptoms at home. The result will be an overestimate of the case fatality rate. Selection bias is also likely to occur in allocation of participants to intervention in non-randomized studies (see 📖 p.187). Non-responders in a study are likely to introduce selection bias, as those who take part are likely to differ in many ways from those who prefer not to. Indeed there is a specific type of bias called the *healthy participant effect*, in which those who volunteer to take part in studies tend to be healthier than those who don't.

Measurement bias refers to systematic errors in measurement including errors in the allocation of participants to the appropriate groups for exposures, outcomes, or confounders. For bias to be introduced, the measurement has to be systematically wrong, e.g. in the measurement of a physiological or lifestyle variable of interest (e.g. mean BP or prevalence of hypertension) or in quantifying the relationship between the exposure and outcome. One example is recall bias which is a common limitation in case–control studies (see 📖 p.174). This is when people with a disease (cases) recall past exposures differently from controls who do not have the disease, in part because the cases are seeking explanations for their condition. Other examples are when researchers are inadvertently influenced by knowledge of the disease or exposure status of the participant when taking clinical measurements; e.g. in a study of the association between lifestyle and BP, a research nurse may tend to record a lower BP in those who report regular exercise. Minimizing bias is at the heart of good study design, good epidemiology and good science.

Interpreting associations

An association is the statistical dependence between 2 variables, and indicates the degree to which an outcome is higher or lower in those with or without the exposure. An association can also be referred to as a link, relationship or correlation.

When 2 things are found to be associated in a study, it is essential to explore whether this can be explained by factors other than a causal link, in other words look for all possible alternative explanations before concluding that it might be causal.

There are 3 important alternative explanations for an observed association:

- Chance.
- Bias.
- Confounding (see 📖 Confounding, p.154).

Role of chance

- Chance may lead to a false association between exposure and disease under investigation.
- Epidemiological studies make inferences from samples of individuals as studying whole populations is often impractical.
- For example, to assess MMR immunization coverage in a district, epidemiologists may study the immunization status of a random sample of children in the district and extrapolate the observed coverage in their sample to all children.
- However, if they were to repeat the study in different random samples of children, the observed immunization coverage would be different.
- We, therefore, use statistical methods producing a p-value and confidence intervals to assess the probability of obtaining an observed estimate by chance alone, and also to assess the range of values within which the true underlying estimate (if the whole population were studied rather than a sample) is likely to fall (see 📖 p.232).

Using confidence intervals to examine the role of chance

- A study of men in the USA measured the relative risk of dying from lung cancer in smokers compared to non-smokers. The study included 1.2 million people.
- The authors reported a relative risk (RR) and 95% confidence intervals (CIs) for this relative risk: RR = 27, (95% CI 19, 38).
- This *relative risk* can be interpreted to mean that, as a best estimate, an American male is 27× more likely to die from lung cancer if he smokes than if he has never smoked.
- The *confidence intervals* quoted give an idea of how certain we are of the estimate of *risk* reported. In this case, the results indicate that we are 95% confident that a male is between 19–38× more likely to die from lung cancer if he smokes than if he doesn't smoke.
- If the *confidence interval* had spanned 1 (a *risk* of 1 would mean that smokers are just as likely as non-smokers to die from lung cancer) e.g. had ranged from 0.2 to 38, (1 lying being between 0.2 and 38), then we are not able to say that the risk of dying from lung cancer is statistically different in smokers and non-smokers.
- Or, in other words, we would not be able to exclude chance as an explanation for our finding of a greater lung cancer risk amongst smokers than non-smokers, without more evidence of a smoking effect.

Bias

- Bias is a systematic error in the design, the conduct, or the analysis (or a combination of these factors) of a study that can give rise to a false association. In some instances, bias may lead to a false lack of association.
- There are many different types of bias, the main ones are:
  - *Selection bias:* this is where there are systematic differences (related to exposure or disease under investigation) in the characteristics of cases and controls in a case–control study.
  - *Recall bias:* this is where there are systematic differences in the recall of exposure information related to case–control status.
  - *Observer bias:* this is usually more relevant in RCTs, and occurs where the researcher is aware of which treatment the participant is being given and the awareness biases their interpretation of symptoms/outcomes.
  - *Information/measurement bias:* this is where there are systematic differences in the way information on exposure and disease are collected so that there is a difference in the quality of the information between the groups being compared in the study.

Understanding the affect of information/measurement bias in more detail

- Information (or measurement) bias occurs if an inaccurate measurement, or misclassification, is made of an exposure or outcome.
- Individuals are then assigned to the wrong exposure or outcome category and this will result in an inaccurate or distorted estimation of the association between exposure and disease.
- The size and the direction of the distortion of an observed association due to such misclassification depend on which type of misclassification has occurred. There are 2 types:
  - Non-differential misclassification.
  - Differential misclassification.

What is non-differential misclassification?

- This occurs when the probability of exposure being misclassified is the same regardless of disease status, or when the probability of disease status being misclassified is the same regardless of exposure status.
- This form of misclassification is sometimes referred to as random misclassification.
- This form of misclassification usually biases estimates of association towards the null, i.e. no association because it reduces the true differences between the groups being compared.

Example:

- In a cohort study of birth weight and consumption of fish oil during pregnancy, women estimated their own consumption according to frequency.
- Non-differential misclassification is likely as women may not recall accurately and even if they do, frequency of eating does not indicate actual quantity eaten, etc.
- This misclassification would not depend on birth weight as consumption was determined prior to delivery.

What is differential misclassification?

- This occurs when the probability of exposure being misclassified depends upon disease status, or when the probability of disease status being misclassified depends upon exposure status.
- This form of misclassification can bias estimates of association in either direction, i.e. higher or lower than the true magnitude of association between the exposure and disease under investigation.

Example:

- Women with newly diagnosed breast cancer were found to be more likely to give an accurate account of the number of abortions they had had, compared to healthy controls who tended to underestimate their number of abortions.
- In a case–control study, this would lead to an overestimate of the strength of the association between breast cancer and a history of abortions.

Confounding

- Confounding gives rise to a false association between an exposure and disease under investigation because it distorts the observed association through a third factor known as the confounder.
- Confounding is therefore also thought of as a mixing of effects and reflects the fact that epidemiology is an observational science, observing human behaviour in its free-living environment.
- In order for a variable to be a confounder, it must be independently associated with both the exposure and the disease under investigation.

Understanding confounding (Fig. 7.1)

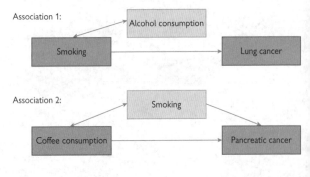

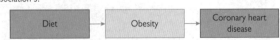

Fig. 7.1 Understanding confounding in more detail.

Association 1:

- Smoking is observed to be associated with lung cancer.
- Alcohol consumption is related to smoking but not with lung cancer.
- Alcohol does not confound the association between smoking and lung cancer.

Association 2:

- Coffee consumption is observed to be associated with pancreatic cancer.
- Smoking is related to both coffee drinking and pancreatic cancer.
- Smoking confounds the association between coffee drinking and pancreatic cancer.

Association 3:

- Diet is observed to be associated with coronary heart disease.
- Obesity is found to be related to diet and to coronary heart disease but not independently.
- Obesity is a factor on the causal pathway between diet and heart disease but is not a confounder of the association.

How do we take into account, or adjust for, confounding?

- At the design stage of a study, confounding can be dealt with by:
  - Randomization (in RCTs, randomly allocating participants to treatment and placebo groups which should mean that the distribution of confounding factors is the same in both groups; see ▢ p.187).
  - Matching (in a case–control study, we can select cases and controls to ensure they match on essential characteristics e.g. age and sex).
- Alternatively, confounding variables can be controlled or adjusted for at the analysis stage by:
  - Stratification.
  - Standardization.
  - Multiple regression.

Worked example of adjustment for confounding

- In a study investigating the effect of occupational exposure on lung cancer risk, the odds ratio for lung cancer was 1.5 (95% CI 1.1–2.1) for those working as dockers or freight handlers, compared with those working in other occupations.
- If we want to establish the impact of occupation on lung cancer risk, we need to take the effect of smoking on lung cancer risk into account in some way.
- In this case–control study, multiple regression was used to control/ adjust for the effect of smoking on lung cancer risk.
- The lung cancer risk associated with working as a docker or freight handler after controlling for the effect of smoking was reduced to 1.3 (95% CI 0.9–1.9).
- Although the odds ratio for lung cancer is still higher (by 30%) for dockers or freight handlers, after adjustment for confounding by smoking, the CI now spans 1 and so we cannot reject the null hypothesis that working as a docker or freight handler has no independent effect on lung cancer risk because the higher odds ratio for lung cancer reported for dockers could just have been found by chance.

Reference

1 Richiardi L et al. Effect of different approaches to treatment of smoking as a potential confounder in a case-control study on occupational exposures. Occup Environ Med 2005; 62(2):101–4.

Association or causation?

If you can exclude chance, bias, and confounding (see 📖 pp.150, 151, 154) as the likely explanations for your finding, then you can conclude that there is a true association between the risk factor/drug and disease under investigation. Association, however, does not mean the same as causation. Two things can be statistically associated without being causally associated, e.g. when analysing data country by country on an international scale, there is a positive association between increasing prevalence of car ownership and higher rates of certain types of cancer. This is not because car ownership causes cancer but because cars are a reflection of a country's development and some cancers are more prevalent in developed countries.

Assessing causality

The concept of cause can be considered at many levels, and has deep philosophical implications. Modern science is predicated upon a system of cause-and-effect relationships. Within the epidemiological framework, however, unravelling an observed relationship requires distinguishing between association (statistical measure) and causation (necessary or sufficient or contributory). Further assessment is, therefore, required for a cause–effect relationship to be considered likely. This judgment is based on a chain of logic that addresses 2 main areas:

• The observed association between an exposure and a disease is considered to be valid.
• The totality of evidence taken from a number of sources supports a judgement of causality.

A checklist of criteria to consider when assessing whether an association is likely to be causal was originally proposed by Bradford Hill in 1965 (Table 7.1). These criteria serve as a guide but not all criteria must be fulfilled to establish scientific causation.

Table 7.1 Bradford Hill criteria for assessing causation

Criteria	How do I assess this?	Example	Don't forget!
1. Strength of association	This is measured by the magnitude of the relative risk The stronger the association the less likely the relationship is due to confounding or bias	Oesophageal cancer in smokers might be 10 × higher than in non-smokers. To account for such a high risk by a second factor associated with oesophageal cancer, the second risk factor would have to be present in smokers at a very much higher rate than in non-smokers and this becomes very unlikely	A weak (small magnitude) association does not rule out a causal connection, only that in such cases it is more difficult to exclude alternative explanations

Table 7.1 (Cont'd)

Criteria	How do I assess this?	Example	Don't forget!
2. Consistency of association	Repeated demonstration in different populations and with different study designs	The assessment of causality in the association between cigarette smoking and coronary heart disease is enhanced by the fact that similar results have been found in numerous studies, over a long period of time, using case–control and cohort designs.	A lack of consistency does not exclude a causal association since different exposure levels and other conditions may reduce the impact of the causal factor in certain studies
3. Specificity of association	One-to-one relationship between cause and outcome	The rabies virus that leads to only one disease outcome	One-to-one relationships between exposures and disease are rare. Most exposures e.g. poor diet, lead to many possible outcomes, e.g. cancer, heart disease, therefore, this is one of the weakest criteria in the checklist and the lack of specificity should not be used to refute a causal relationship
4. Temporal sequence of association	The suspected risk factor must have occurred, or be present, before the outcome developed		This is an essential criterion for causality and probably the most important of all in the checklist. It is easier to establish temporality in cohort studies than in cross-sectional or case control studies when measurements of the possible cause and the effect are made at the same time

(Continued)

Table 7.1 (Cont'd)

Criteria	How do I assess this?	Example	Don't forget!
5. Dose–response relationship (biological gradient)	Monotonic relationship (gradient of risk) between exposure to, or dose of, risk factor and risk of disease	Those who smoke a moderate number of cigarettes have a risk of lung cancer that is higher than that of non-smokers but lower than that of those who are heavy smokers. This adds credibility to the hypothesis that smoking increases the risk of lung cancer	Some causal associations show a single jump (threshold effect) rather than a monotonic trend
6. Biological plausibility of association	Is there a known or postulated biological mechanism by which the exposure might reasonably alter the risk of disease?	The association between consumption of moderate amounts of alcohol and decreased risk of coronary heart disease is enhanced by the fact that alcohol is associated with higher levels of high density lipoprotein which is associated with a decreased risk of coronary heart disease	Lack of a known mechanism should not rule out causality because this may simply reflect lack of scientific knowledge at any given time
7. Coherence of association	Absence of conflict with other knowledge about the natural history and biology of the disease		Absence of coherent information as distinguished from the presence of conflicting information, should not be taken as evidence against an association being causal

Table 7.1 (Cont'd)

Criteria	How do I assess this?	Example	Don't forget!
8. Experimental evidence (reversibility)	Does removal of the risk factor decrease or prevent the disease outcome?		This is a very powerful criterion. If reduction in a particular exposure is followed by a reduction in risk of a particular disease, this strengthens the conclusion of a real cause–effect relationship
9. Analogy	Are there analogies with other similar, well established, causal associations?		Absence of such analogies only reflects lack of imagination or experience, not falsity of the hypothesis

The nature of causality

The provisional nature of 'causal' understanding

- Causation in epidemiology is something we think about, but cannot see.
- Causality, as pointed out by David Hume long ago, is always an inference from the observed conjunction of events; the causal 'process' itself cannot be observed.
- A causal interpretation is our best attempt to identify the specific antecedent events/circumstances that alter the probability of disease occurrence. That interpretation is limited by the body of available knowledge at any time in history and its associated prevailing scientific paradigm.
- In retrospect, we often get 'the cause' wrong or at least incomplete. Therefore we should always be circumspect when discussing causality.
- We should never assume that there are absolute truths to be discovered or that causal factors are universal in their importance and impact.

An example: coronary heart disease (CHD)

- About 50 years ago, American epidemiologists began explaining the modern epidemic of CHD in terms of lifelong cholesterol accumulation in the inner lining of the coronary arteries, assisted by the damaging effects of high BP and smoking upon the vessel walls.
- Since then, other theories about CHD aetiology have emerged, reflecting the advent of new types of observations, ideas, and new levels of measurement/techniques. These include:
  - The importance of antioxidant micronutrients.
  - The role of certain vitamins in reducing tendency of blood to clot.
  - The beneficial effects of fish oils.
  - The protective effect of moderate alcohol consumption.
  - The possible role of long term infection with *Helicobacter pylori*.
  - The possibility that part of the risk of late-life CHD is 'set' by birth.
  - The role of common genetic variants in influencing risk of disease.
- Did early epidemiologists get CHD causation 'wrong'?
- Are some, none, or all of the listed factors involved in the causation of CHD?
- It is essential we understand that CHD, like most diseases, has multiple and complex aetiologies and that our understanding of aetiology today is merely 'knowledge-in-transition'.

How relevant is causality to public health?

- Absolute proof is rarely attainable in the empirical sciences.
- Critics often point out that epidemiology whilst identifying statistical associations is unable to specify the actual causal mechanisms for associations.

But how important are causal mechanisms?

Much of our experience in the public health domain indicates that knowledge of the causal mechanism is not essential for effective preventive strategies.

Examples to prove the point!

- In Biblical times, 2 millennia before Germ Theory, it was known that avoidance of contact with people who had leprosy would reduce the risk of transmission of the disease (lepers were kept outside of the city/camp).
- In the British Navy, Captain James Lind found that shipboard diets supplemented with limes reduced the occurrence of scurvy in the crews, despite vitamin C not being discovered for a further 2 centuries.
- John Snow, in 1854, identified that contaminated drinking water was the source of cholera epidemics in London which was sufficient for effective public health intervention, long before the identification of the cholera bacterium.
- Today, we know that smoking is associated with lung cancer and that smoking reduces that risk, but we still have not identified all the carcinogenic chemical constituents or the mechanisms by which they act.

Time trend and geographical (ecological) studies

Overview

Ecological studies examine the association between exposures and outcomes by using aggregate data. Data are analysed at a group rather than individual level. For example, the study might explore whether changes in cardiovascular disease over time correlate with changes in diet over time. The grouping may be by time, also known as trend studies, or place (geographical studies). They can be used to:

- Explore quality of care, e.g. in comparing mortality ratios over time or between hospitals or countries.
- Explore inequalities in care, e.g. whether mortality is higher in hospitals with higher proportions of people from deprived areas.
- Generate hypotheses about variations in illness, diagnosis, and response to treatments.
- Examine possible correlations between changes in disease rates and changes in risk factors or the introduction of an intervention over time.
- Study exposures that are measured over groups/areas, e.g. diet, temperature, and climate variation, air pollution, water supply.

Ecological studies require data on exposure and outcome at the same level of aggregation (e.g. town, country, period of time). They often use routine data collected for other purposes, so are efficient but rely on availability of the necessary data.

Analysis and interpretation

Analysis includes charts of trends, scatterplots of exposure and outcome. A simple linear regression may be used to show the relationship between an exposure variable, such as average salt excretion in a population, and the outcome variable, average systolic blood pressure. The strength of the association will be given by the correlation coefficient, r:

$r = 1$ indicates a perfect positive correlation (i.e. straight line).

$r = -1$ a perfect negative correlation.

r^2 = the proportion of the total variation that can be explained by the regression line.

e.g. if $r = 0.7$, $r^2 = 0.49$ meaning that approximately half of the variation in the outcome variable is 'explained' by variation in the exposure variable (although this association does not mean the exposure caused the outcome) (see 📖 p.262).

When looking at the results check for:

- Changes in case definitions, disease coding, diagnostic methods, or data collection over time or between places: this is a major potential weakness and can lead to artefactual errors. For example, a more sensitive test that detects more cases will lead to an increase in observed rates; a revision of the International Classification of Diseases used to clinically code diseases may make it difficult to compare rates before and after the change.
- Confounding—although disease rates can be standardized to take into account age and sex differences within and between populations, data on other potential confounders are often unavailable.

Strengths

- Can look for associations in large populations.
- Used to initiate further research by hypothesis-generation.
- Use existing data therefore may be efficient and relatively quick.

Limitations

- Cannot confirm association at the individual level.
- Can be surprisingly difficult or costly when exposure data, e.g. to environmental toxins, are not readily available.
- Potential of an 'ecological fallacy' (see Box 7.1).

Box 7.1 The ecological fallacy

Durkheim on suicide

- In 1897 Durkheim (Fig. 7.2) published a work on suicide rates in provinces across Bavaria. He found relatively high rates of suicide in provinces with high proportions of Protestants and low rates of suicide in provinces with many Catholics.
- He concluded that Protestants are more likely to commit suicide than Catholics.
- Subsequent in-depth investigation of his work showed that most of the suicides that had taken place in the Protestant provinces were actually by Catholics.
- Catholics living in predominantly Protestant provinces were a minority group and due to the social isolation they felt, some had committed suicide.
- Durkheim inappropriately inferred group level information to individuals giving rise to the ecological fallacy. His mistake is often quoted as a classic example of ecological bias.

How do we interpret these findings?

- What happened to minority Protestant groups living in predominantly Catholic provinces—were they also more likely to commit suicide due to social isolation?
- It seems like there is an interaction of effects between religion at *individual* level and religious composition of *area*.
- Ultimately, group level data are unlikely to provide us with a definitive interpretation but can be an important source of evidence and generate hypotheses that could be examined further with individual level data.

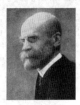

Fig. 7.2 Émile Durkheim, 1858–1917.

Reference

1 Durkheim É, *Suicide* (Spaulding JA, Simpson G (trans)). Glencoe, IL: Free Press; 1951.

Ecological studies: examples

Carrying out a simple ecological study

We want to know whether coverage of a screening programme varies according to social deprivation at a local level.

Data needed

- A deprivation measure (e.g. Carstairs index) at a small area level.
- Proportion of people covered by the screening programme at same small area level.

Analysis

- Plot a chart with deprivation (exposure or independent variable) on the × axis, and screening coverage (outcome or dependent variable) on the y axis.
- The association is then presented as a scatter plot and strength of association assessed by the correlation coefficient.
- Consider confounding (results would need to be standardized for age, for example).

Interpretation

Consider the ecological fallacy (see Box 7.1)—people living in deprived areas are not all poor, particularly in places like London. It is possible (unlikely) that it is the wealthier people living in deprived areas who do not go for screening.

Are mobile phones associated with acoustic neuroma?

An ecological study was carried out to look at trends in mobile phone use, based on numbers of subscriptions, together with rates of acoustic neuroma in England and Wales. Fig. 7.3 shows that rates of neuroma rose before the widespread use of mobile phones, and then began to decline. This does not disprove an association, but suggests that detailed work needs to be done to understand changes in diagnosis and reporting to understand the fluctuations, and better exposure data and longer follow-up are needed.

The relationship between wealth and health?

Fig. 7.4 shows the relationship between wealth in a country (gross domestic product per capita) and the average life expectancy at birth. It appears that survival increases with GDP up to a point when the curve evens out. Although there is a general trend, at the lowest average incomes there is a huge variation in life expectancy, suggesting that poverty is only one of the factors involved. Further exploration of the data has been carried out to try and identify interventions that can improve survival with limited resources. At the other end of the distribution, there is quite large variation in life expectancy between relatively wealthy countries.

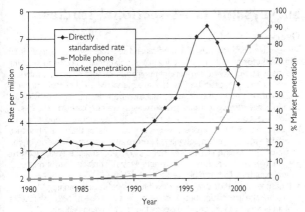

Fig. 7.3 UK mobile phone market penetration, 1980–2004 (right scale) and age-standardized rate of acoustic neuroma and other benign cranial nerve neoplasms among people of all ages in England and Wales, 1980–2000 (left scale). Reproduced from Nelson PD *et al.* Trends in acoustic neuroma and cellular phones: Is there a link? *Neurology* 2006; **66**:284–5, with permission from Wolters Kluwer Health.

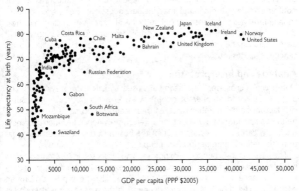

Fig. 7.4 Life expectancy at birth vs average annual income. Source: Gapminder ℗ http://www.gapminder.org

Surveys and cross-sectional studies

Overview

Surveys are commonly used in medical and social research. A survey is an instrument for measuring something in a population, usually through asking questions and/or taking measurements from a sample of that population. These studies are described as cross-sectional when they collect information at one point in time. They can also be referred to as prevalence studies, since they collect data on existing (prevalent) cases of diseases.

Cross-sectional studies may be primarily descriptive, reporting the frequency and distribution of exposures or outcomes, or analytical when they investigate the association between exposure and outcome. The distribution of factors or disease can be described in relation to time (year, season), person (gender, age, race, occupation, lifestyle), place (neighbourhood, region, country). They can be used to:

- Measure population prevalence to inform healthcare planning.
- Explore the association between risk factors and disease, e.g. risk factors in an emerging infectious disease, or the link between diet and BP.
- Describe the experience of patients using a service.
- Explore the knowledge, attitudes and beliefs of patients and relate this to adherence to treatment regimens.

In a cross-sectional study, data are collected on each individual study participant. Data collection methods depend on the exposures and/or outcomes being studied, and may include questionnaires (through face-to-face interviews, by post, or online), clinical examination, and investigation. Additional information may be obtained from routine sources, e.g. if linked data on the individual are being recorded through medical records, cancer registries, etc.

Analysis and interpretation

Data from a cross-sectional study are used to calculate prevalence. The prevalence is the number of people who report a particular exposure/risk factor, or the number of cases of a health outcome of interest, in a defined population at a point of time. Period prevalence includes both new (incident) cases and existing cases of the health outcome under investigation in a defined time period (see 📖 p.6).

The association between exposure and disease is presented as a prevalence ratio, which is the prevalence in exposed individuals divided by the prevalence in the unexposed. Studies may also be reported using an odds ratio. The choice of measure depends on the nature of the data and in particular the prevalence of disease and/or exposure in the study population.

A cross-sectional study will produce basic data that can be tabulated (Table 7.2).

Table 7.2 Cross-sectional study data

	Disease	No disease
Exposed	a	b
Unexposed	c	d

$$\text{Prevalence of disease} = (a+c)/(a+b+c+d)$$

$$\text{Prevalence of exposure} = (a+b)/(a+b+c+d)$$

$$\text{Prevalence of disease in exposed} = a/(a+b)$$

$$\text{Prevalence of disease in unexposed} = c/(c+d)$$

$$\text{Prevalence ratio} = \frac{\text{prevalence in the exposed}}{\text{prevalence in the unexposed}}$$

$$\text{Odds ratio} = (a/c)/(b/d) = ad/bc$$

Cross-sectional data may also be explored to look at the correlation between continuous measures of exposure and continuous outcome measures, e.g. relationship between dietary variables and BMI or BP. These basic measures will usually be followed by more complex analyses to control for possible confounding, e.g. using logistic regression (see 🕮 p.272).

When looking at the results check:
- Was a clear definition of a case and/or an exposure identified before the collection of data?
- Was there a reasonable response rate from eligible participants? A low response rate may introduce selection bias where those who agree to take part differ from those who decline in relation to prevalence of exposure and/or outcome.
- Were validated questionnaires used? If not, were they thoroughly piloted and tested? This is important to ensure that they elicit valid responses and avoid measurement errors and bias.
- If data were collected indirectly using routine sources, what was the quality of the data and how valid were they for measuring the objectives of the research study?
- Were outcome measurements similarly validated and applied in a consistent way?
- Were known confounders measured and then controlled for in the analysis?

When interpreting findings, always consider 'reverse causality' as a possible explanation. For example, in a cross sectional study, CHD mortality risk was found to be 50% lower in those claiming high orgasmic frequency. It appears as if lots of sex is good for your health! However, as temporality cannot be determined when risk factor and disease status are determined at the same time, we need to consider the possibility that those with early CHD symptoms, actually slow down and lower their frequency of energetic activities like sex.

Strengths
- Relatively easy and quick to conduct providing timely insights particularly in emerging conditions.
- Often relatively cheap.
- Can provide information on a wide range of exposures and outcomes at the same time.
- Regular surveys of random samples of the population (e.g. family health surveys) provide valuable snapshots of exposures and outcomes.

Limitations
- They are biased towards inclusion of people with chronic illness rather than acute illness because only prevalent cases are included.
- As data on exposure and disease are collected simultaneously it can be difficult to assess the temporal relationship between the exposure and the outcome.

Cross-sectional studies: examples

Impact of bed nets on malaria in children

In areas where malaria is common it causes considerable illness in children, including anaemia. In the 1990s controlled trials showed that the use of bed nets could reduce malaria substantially, and so they started to be widely distributed.

This study[1] looked at the impact of bed net use on malaria and on anaemia in children <2 years. A random sample of children in Tanzania was recruited at their homes; a questionnaire was used with parents to record use of bed nets, and samples were taken to test for malaria parasitaemia and anaemia.

Findings (Table 7.3)

Table 7.3[1] Use of bed nets and prevalence of malaria parasitaemia and anaemia in children < 2yrs

	Parasitaemia n (%)	Odds ratio (95% CI)	Anaemia N (%)	Odds ratio (95% CI)
No net (n=198)	132 (70)	Reference group	103 (54)	Reference group
Untreated net (n=233)	115 (49)	0.49 (0.24, 1.00)	90 (39)	0.63 (0.27, 1.46)
Treated net (n=326)	120 (37)	0.38 (0.23, 0.62)	70 (21)	0.37 (0.19, 0.73)

The results showed that only treated nets had a substantial impact on the health of children with an odds ratio for malaria parasitaemia of 0.38 and 95% CI that does not span 1. Although this was a cross-sectional study and could not prove causation, the findings strongly supported other evidence of the effectiveness of this cheap and simple intervention.

Worked example: mobile phones and headaches

Question: are mobile phone users more likely to suffer headaches than non-mobile phone users?

Study: a hypothetical cross-sectional study asking 50 mobile phone users and 50 non-mobile phone users in a high school to report whether they had headaches or not during a one week period. The results are shown in Table 7.4.

Table 7.4[2] Results from a hypothetical cross-sectional study on mobile phone use and prevalence of headaches

	Headache	No headache
Mobile phone	18	32
No mobile phone	7	43

Period prevalence in exposed = 18/50 = 36%

i.e. the prevalence of headaches amongst mobile phone users was 36%

Period prevalence in unexposed = 7/50 = 14%

i.e. the prevalence of headaches in non-mobile phone users was 14%

Prevalence ratio = 36%/14% = 2.57

To see if this result could be explained by chance, a statistical test is needed. In this case a chi-squared test shows that the difference is statistically significant, $p=0.0198$ (Fisher's exact test, two-tailed p value, see 📖 p.254), meaning that the difference in headache prevalence between the 2 groups was unlikely to have occurred by chance.

In this hypothetical example, the prevalence of headaches in mobile phone users was $2.57\times$ higher than the prevalence of headaches amongst non-mobile phone users. Of course, this does not mean that the mobile phones caused the increase in headaches as mobile phone users might differ from non-users in other ways.

Sex work and HIV

In the 1980s it was unclear whether HIV would spread among heterosexuals in the UK. We carried out a cross-sectional survey to measure HIV prevalence in women sex workers in London.[2] Between 1989 and 1991, 280 women were recruited from a sexual health clinic and during outreach.

The prevalence of HIV was 0.9%, with 2 of 228 women testing positive for HIV. HIV was strongly associated with drug use, with an odds ratio of 20.6. Results were interpreted with caution as findings might be biased in relation to participation and particularly agreement to HIV testing (were they more health conscious than non-participants and those who declined?).

References

1 Abdulla S et al. Impact on malaria morbidity of a programme supplying insecticide treated nets in children aged under 2 years in Tanzania: community cross sectional study. *BMJ* 2001; **322**: 270.
2 Ward H et al. Prostitution and risk of HIV: male partners of female prostitutes. *BMJ* 1993; **307**(6900):359–61.

Case–control studies

Overview

A case–control study is where people with a condition (cases) are compared with those who do not have the condition (controls) with respect to one or more exposures of interest.

If the exposure is higher in cases than controls, it may be a risk factor for the disease; if it is lower then it may be a protective factor. For example, a study may look at whether children with leukaemia are more likely to have been exposed to radiation while *in utero*. Affected children will be recruited and their mothers asked about exposures in pregnancy; a similar group of children without leukaemia will be recruited and their mothers asked the same questions.

In case–control studies information on exposures is retrospective. As participants are defined by disease (or absence of disease) then the exposure of interest will be in the past (e.g. previous smoking). This can make measurement of exposure difficult unless the exposure is a persistent trait, such as a genetic factor, or there are records of past exposure, e.g. birth records in a study looking at birth weight and adult risk of diabetes.

Since the definition of the study groups is by disease, you can assess the relationship of the disease with any number of exposures (see Fig. 7.5). Case–control studies can be used to:

- Identify potential causal factors for disease.
- Explore the association between risk factors to help identify causal pathways.
- In clinical research case–control studies are widely used to identify different clinical patterns, presentations and associations.

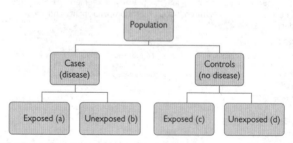

Fig. 7.5 Overview of case–control studies.

Selection and recruitment of cases

Cases must be clearly defined with inclusion criteria and a recruitment framework. The study protocol needs to specify whether cases can be anyone with a condition (prevalent cases) or only new (incident) cases. Usually incident cases are preferred. The protocol should also include how cases will be identified—through a disease register, a clinical service, a primary care practice, a patient support group. Each of these has potential advantages and disadvantages. Ideally cases should be as representative as possible of all cases in a defined population group unless otherwise defined (some studies may focus on part of the spectrum of a disease).

Selection and recruitment of controls

Selection of appropriate controls is often the most difficult and critical part of the study.

- Controls should be representative of people without the disease, and should come from the same population as the cases, in other words if they were cases they would be eligible for the study.
- Controls may be randomly selected from the population, using primary care records for example, may be patients with other conditions, or may be 'matched' to the cases in some way such as a friend or neighbour. Each approach has strengths and weaknesses. The most important principle is that controls should not be selected in a way that could alter their risk of the exposure of interest.
- There may be 1 or more controls for each case. More controls per case increases the statistical ability (power) of the study to exclude chance as an explanation for any association of exposure with the disease. Obtaining >1 control per case is particularly useful when cases are rare or difficult to recruit (e.g., rapidly fatal conditions).

Measurement of exposures

Collecting information on the exposures may be done using a participant questionnaire or through looking up past records. If questionnaires are used they must be carefully tested and validated. The same method should be used for collecting exposure data in cases and controls.

Analysis and interpretation

A case–control study will produce data like those shown in Table 7.5.

Table 7.5 Case–control study data

	Case	Control
Exposed	a	b
Unexposed	c	d

The primary comparison is between the prevalence of exposure in the cases and in the controls.

Incidence is not measured in case–control studies so relative risk (incidence in the exposed divided by incidence in the unexposed) cannot be directly calculated. Instead we use odds ratio (OR) which is the odds[*] of exposure amongst the cases divided by the odds of exposure amongst the controls:

$$\text{Odds} = \text{prevalence}/(1 - \text{prevalence}).$$

$$\text{Odds ratio} = (a/c)/(b/d) = ad/bc$$

Interpreting an odds ratio:

- OR = 1: no association between the exposure and the disease.
- OR > 1: the exposure is a potential risk factor for the disease.
- OR < 1: the exposure is potentially protective for the disease.

If the study uses matched cases and controls then a more complex analysis is necessary using conditional logistic regression models.

When looking at results look out for:

- Selection of cases and controls. Could there have been any bias in relation to the exposure of interest? If controls were other patients, could their disease be linked to the same exposure (see 📖 p.176).
- Measurement of exposure: is there likely to be recall bias, with cases having different recall than controls?
- Were confounders measured and adequately controlled for in the analysis?

Strengths

- Can be relatively quick and cheap.
- Much quicker than cohort studies for investigating diseases with long latent periods between exposure and onset.
- Efficient way of studying rare diseases.
- Can look at several different possible risk factors for single disease.

Limitations

- Unable to measure incidence, therefore can't calculate attributable risk (see 📖 p.180).
- Susceptible to recall and selection bias if not well designed.
- Inefficient for rare exposures.
- As with many epidemiological studies, it may be difficult to be sure about the temporal relationship between exposure and disease.

Case–control studies: examples

Example 1 (Fig. 7.6)

One of the most famous case–control studies was carried out by epidemiologists Richard Doll and Bradford Hill in the 1940s. They were investigating the huge increase in lung cancer over previous decades. Two main causes had been suggested: pollution linked to the increase in cars, or smoking.

BRITISH MEDICAL JOURNAL

LONDON SATURDAY SEPTEMBER 30 1950

SMOKING AND CARCINOMA OF THE LUNG

PRELIMINARY REPORT

BY

RICHARD DOLL, M.D., M.R.C.P.

Member of the Statistical Research Unit of the Medical Research Council

AND

A. BRADFORD HILL, Ph.D., D.Sc.

Professor of Medical Statistics, London School of Hygiene and Tropical Medicine; Honorary Director of the Statistical Research Unit of the Medical Research Council

In England and Wales the phenomenal increase in the number of deaths attributed to cancer of the lung provides one of the most striking changes in the pattern of mortality recorded by the Registrar-General. For example, in the quarter of a century between 1922 and 1947 the annual number of deaths recorded increased from 612 to

whole explanation, although no one would deny that it may well have been contributory. As a corollary, it is right and proper to seek for other causes.

Possible Causes of the Increase

Two main causes have from time to time been put for-

Fig. 7.6 Front page of Doll and Hill's paper. Reproduced with permission from Doll R, Hill AB. Smoking and carcinoma of the lung. *BMJ* 1950; **ii**(4682):739–48.

The study was carried out in 20 London hospitals; cases were patients diagnosed with lung cancer, controls were patients in the same hospital, same gender and age group, but who did not have cancer (lung or other). Results for men and women are shown in Table 7.6.

Table 7.6 Doll and Hill's case–control study on lung cancer

	Men		Women	
	Case	Control	Case	Control
Smoker	647	622	41	28
Non-smoker	2	27	19	32

One of the most striking things about the results was that almost all men smoked, cases and controls!

Analysis

For men, OR (ad/bc) = $(647 \times 27)/(622 \times 2) = 14.04$ ($p<0.00001$)

For women, OR = $(41 \times 32)/28 \times 19) = 2.47$ ($p=0.016$)

The p values are from significance tests using a chi-squared statistic.

Comment

The strong association did not prove that smoking caused lung cancer, but was very strong evidence, followed up with even more definitive cohort studies. The odds ratio they found was actually an underestimate of the effect of smoking, in part due to the fact that controls were also ill and may well have had one of the many other conditions that we now know are also caused by smoking.

Example 2: use of sun-beds and risk of melanoma

The incidence of invasive melanoma has been increasing in many Caucasian populations. The link with sunlight is well established, but this has not deterred a huge growth in the tanning industry. In the USA in many cities there are more tanning salons than there are branches of McDonalds.

The authors of a study in Minnesota recruited 1167 cases of invasive cutaneous melanoma and compared them to 1101 age and gender-matched controls from the population.[1] Cases and controls were asked in detail about their sun-bed use.

Findings

They found that 62.9% of cases and 51.1% of controls had tanned indoors, OR 1.74 (95% CI 1.42, 2.14); the OR increased with years of use, hours of use and numbers of sessions and use of high intensity machines.

Discussion

The evidence for the association includes a strong dose response, and the results fit with other studies. In this kind of study bias is possible if cases were more likely to recall use of sun-beds than controls. The authors attempted to measure this and found that there was probably over-reporting of sun-bed use in both cases and controls.

References

1 Lazovich D *et al.* Indoor tanning and risk of melanoma: a case-control study in a highly exposed population. *Cancer Epidemiol Biomarkers Prev* 2010; **19**:1557–68.

Cohort studies

Overview

In a cohort study, a group of people are followed over time to measure the incidence of a disease, comparing incidence rates among those who are exposed to 1 or more factors to those who are unexposed. For example, a study may look at whether eating fruit and vegetables reduces the risk of stroke. A cohort of healthy people would be recruited and asked about their diet, and categorized according to their fruit and vegetable intake (the 'exposure'). They would be followed for many years, and any episodes of stroke noted from medical records. At the end of the study the incidence of stroke in those with high intake would be compared with the incidence in those with low intake, producing a relative risk. Cohort studies can also be useful in clinical medicine to follow up people with a particular condition or disease to look at natural history, survival rates, etc. (see Fig. 7.7).

Cohort studies are used to:
- Identify potential causal factors for disease (see 📖 p.156).
- Explore the association between factors to identify causal pathways.
- Identify biomarkers for disease.
- Evaluate outcomes in people with different diseases.

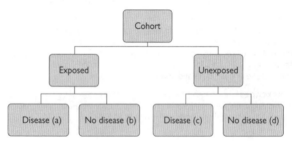

Fig. 7.7 Overview of cohort studies.

Selection and recruitment of cohort

This depends on the aim of the study. Cohorts may be:
- A random selection of the population.
- Defined by a life event, e.g. a birth cohort (e.g. all babies born in a particular week) or a pregnancy cohort.
- An occupational group or groups.
- People with specific exposures, e.g. people known to have worked with asbestos and a comparison group with no known exposure to asbestos to estimate risk of mesothelioma and other cancers.
- Defined by one disease to measure the incidence of others or of complications; e.g. people who have HIV and a comparison group without HIV to estimate the increased risk of coronary heart disease.

Cohorts are generally *prospective*—participants are recruited and then followed over time. They can be *retrospective*, meaning that the disease has already occurred by the time the study starts, but the cohort is still defined by exposure, e.g. looking back to occupational records to identify all workers in a factory at a point in time, or medical records to identify women who gave birth in a particular year.

Key point: both prospective and retrospective cohorts are longitudinal, and participants are selected by exposure not outcome.

Measurement of exposure
Participants are categorized by exposure and the measurement of this may be through questionnaires, records (e.g. occupational exposure such as radiation) or baseline tests (e.g. blood biomarkers, BP, or anthropometry). Since people may change their behaviours such as smoking or diet over time, cohort studies often need to collect repeated measurements of exposures to correctly categorize participants.

Measurement of outcome
Assessment of outcome may be through record linkage, where the participants' details are tagged, e.g. in cancer registries, and if they are diagnosed then the research team will receive a notification. Other outcomes can be obtained through links to medical records or regular re-interview and examination.

Analysis and interpretation
Data from a cohort study are used to calculate the incidence in the exposed and unexposed. The incidence (sometimes called cumulative incidence) is the number of new cases of a disease in a group or population over time. The incidence rate (sometimes called the cumulative incidence rate) is the number of new cases of a disease in a defined period divided by the size of the population. (Note this is actually a proportion rather than a true rate.)

A cohort study will produce basic data that can be tabulated (Table 7.7).

Table 7.7 Cohort study data

	Disease	**No disease**
Exposed	a	b
Unexposed	c	d

From this the following measures can be calculated

Overall incidence rate of disease $= (a+c)/(a+b+c+d)$

Incidence rate of disease in exposed $I_e = a/(a+b)$

Incidence rate of disease in unexposed $I_o = c/(c+d)$

$$\text{Relative risk} = \frac{\text{incidence rate in the exposed}}{\text{incidence rate in the unexposed}}$$

Attributable risk $= I_e - I_o$

Interpreting a relative risk (see 📖 p.179)
- RR = 1: no association between the exposure and the disease.
- RR > 1: the exposure is a potential risk factor for the disease.
- RR < 1: the exposure is potentially protective for the disease.

A relative risk of 2 means that people who are exposed are twice as likely to get the disease as those who are unexposed. A relative risk of 0.6 means those with the exposure are 40% less likely to get the disease, i.e. it is a protective factor.

Interpreting attributable risk (see 📖 p.179)
The attributable risk is an absolute measure with the same units as the incidence rate, e.g. per person per year. It indicates the number of cases of the disease among the exposed group that could theoretically be prevented if the exposure were completely eliminated (assuming the risk is causal). See Chapter 3 for examples.

Fixed and dynamic cohorts
Table 7.7 assumes that all participants are followed for the same length of time, a *fixed cohort*, and reports incidence rate as a proportion (see Box 7.2).

Box 7.2 Key outputs from a static cohort

$$\text{(Cumulative) incidence} = \frac{\text{New cases of disease in time period}}{\substack{\text{number of disease-free} \\ \text{people in population at start of time period}}}$$

$$\text{Relative risk} = \frac{\text{incidence rate}^* \text{ in the exposed}}{\text{incidence rate}^* \text{ in the unexposed}}$$

$$\text{Attributable risk} = \text{incidence rate}^* \text{ in the exposed} - \text{incidence rate}^* \text{ in the unexposed}$$

*While the term rate is used it actually refers to a proportion.

Key outputs from a dynamic cohort

$$\text{Incidence rate} = \frac{\text{number of new cases of disease in period}}{\text{person-years at risk during period}}$$

$$\text{Rate ratio} = \frac{\text{incidence rate in the exposed}}{\text{incidence rate in the unexposed}}$$

$$\text{Attributable rate} = \text{incidence rate in the exposed} - \text{incidence rate in the unexposed}$$

In a *dynamic cohort* the variation in follow-up time is accounted for: people can be recruited at different times, and are followed to the point where they leave the cohort when:

- They acquire the disease and are no longer part of the disease-free denominator.
- They are lost to follow-up (e.g. if they die, leave the area, decide they don't want to take further part in the study).
- The study ends.

Each person will have contributed a certain amount of time to the cohort, and these are summed to make a total time, usually 'person years at risk'. This is then used as the denominator for incidence, which is then a 'true' rate (rather than a proportion), and the association is described as the rate ratio.

Things to look out for

The cohort study is generally considered the 'gold standard' of observational study designs, although it is not always applicable or possible.

But like any other study, a cohort study can be excellent or poor. Things you should watch out for include:

- Selection bias: if a high proportion of eligible people refuse to participate then this may bias results (if non-participation is associated with exposure and outcome risks) though this is much less of a problem than in case–control studies; more commonly, it may reduce the extent to which results can be generalized to the wider population.
- Was exposure measurement accurate, unbiased, sufficiently detailed, and of comparable quality in both the exposed and unexposed groups? Cohort studies are not vulnerable to recall bias since exposure is measured before the outcome has occurred.
- Could there have been misclassification of outcome status leading to bias? Could knowledge of exposure status have influenced outcome measurement?
- How long was the follow-up? Was it long enough for the outcome to occur? And how complete was it (were there considerable numbers lost during the follow-up period)?
- Loss to follow-up—people may be lost for various reasons. This could bias the study if the loss is linked to the exposure and outcome. Otherwise it could reduce the power of the study to find associations.
- Was sufficient adjustment made for potential confounding factors?
- What is the magnitude of the association between exposure and disease and could the reported association be due to chance?
- Is there a dose-response gradient e.g. increasing exposure is associated with increasing disease?

Strengths

- Temporal sequence between exposure and disease can be established—essential criteria for assessing a causal association.
- Measurement of incidence rate of disease in exposed and non-exposed.
- Examination of multiple outcomes (diseases, mortality) for any 1 exposure.
- Suitable for the study of rare exposures by focusing on particular groups, e.g. asbestos exposure amongst factory employees.
- Minimize biases associated with case–control studies, e.g. selection bias and recall bias.

Weaknesses

These include:
- Long time until completion meaning results and conclusions may be delayed.
- Non-participation in cohort studies may be high if they require repeated surveys and measurements.
- Losses to follow-up possibly leading to bias and making interpretation more difficult.
- Expensive to carry out.
- Not suitable (inefficient) for the study of rare diseases unless cohorts are very large (e.g. UK Biobank).

Cohort studies: examples

British Physicians Study

Perhaps the most famous cohort study is the British Physicians Study initiated by Sir Richard Doll and Sir Austin Bradford Hill in the 1950s. Rates of lung cancer in the UK had increased markedly in the early 1900s but nobody knew why. Evidence from case–control studies (see 📖 p.172) suggested that patients with lung cancer were more likely to smoke than those without but this may have been partly due to bias.

The British Physicians Study followed up 40,000 doctors split into groups of non-smokers, light, moderate, and heavy smokers. After more than 40 years of follow-up, the study has consistently shown a substantial excess risk of lung cancer and all-cause mortality amongst smokers compared to non-smokers. The strength of the evidence from this cohort study is such that it is universally accepted that there is a causal association between smoking and lung cancer despite the fact that we still do not have complete understanding of the exact mechanistic pathways by which tobacco smoke causes mutagenic changes at the cellular level. And we don't have randomized trial evidence in support of this conclusion—the epidemiological (observational) data were strong enough to infer causality in the absence of trial data.

The Million Women Study

This UK study enrolled 1.3 million women with a median age of 56 who are being followed up to look at a wide range of outcomes linked to various baseline measures and exposures. The study has produced major insights into cancer and cardiovascular disease risk.

The study also provides a rich source of data for other analyses. For example, using records of the women for 7.8 million years of follow-up, they looked at the relationship of BMI to gallbladder disease.[1] Women with higher BMI were more likely to be admitted and to spend more time in hospital for gallbladder disease (Table 7.8).

The authors estimated that a quarter of all hospital bed-days for gall bladder disease in middle aged women were attributable to obesity.[1]

Table 7.8 Relationship of BMI to gallbladder disease in the Million Women Study[1]

BMI	Days in hospital for gallbladder disease (per 1000 py)
18.5–24.9	16.5
25–29.9	28.6
30–39.9	44.0
40	49.4

Does *Chlamydia trachomatis* cause reproductive tract infection?

A cohort study was carried out in Uppsala, Sweden using routinely collected data on *Chlamydia* screening in women and was able to link these to hospital records of admissions for pelvic inflammatory disease (PID), ectopic pregnancy (EP), and tubal infertility.[2] Women aged 15–24 in the 1980s were followed until 1999. Using Cox proportional hazards regression models (see ▢ p.279), the authors estimated the increased risk associated with having had any positive *Chlamydia* test compared with those who only tested negative. They used survival analysis to produce hazard ratios, (similar to relative risk but taking into account the speed at which the events happen). Increased risks associated with a positive *Chlamydia* test ranged from 38% for infertility to 52% for pelvic inflammatory disease (Table 7.9).

Table 7.9 Chlamydia screening and incidence of reproductive tract complications

	Incidence per 100 person years		
	PID	Ectopic	Infertility
Chlamydia positive	5.6	2.7	6.7
Chlamydia negative	4.0	2.0	4.7
Hazard ratio (95% CI)	1.52 (1.25, 1.84)	1.42 (1.06, 1.88)	1.38 (1.15, 1.66)

References

1 Liu B *et al.* Relationship between body mass index and length of hospital stay for gallbladder disease. *J Public Health* 2008; **30**:161–6.

2 Low N. *et al.* Incidence of severe reproductive tract complications associated with diagnosed genital chlamydial infection: the Uppsala Women's Cohort Study. *Sex Transm Infect* 2006; **82**:212–18.

Intervention studies and clinical trials

Overview

A clinical trial is a planned *experiment* in humans, designed to measure the efficacy or effectiveness of an intervention. The intervention is usually a new drug, but the method can equally be applied to the assessment of a surgical procedure, a vaccine, complementary therapy, etc.

Experimental studies like trials are different from most epidemiological studies (surveys, cross-sectional, cohort, case–control, ecological) which are observational. In observational studies the investigator measures what happens but does not control it. For example, an investigator may record a person's serum cholesterol level and relate this to whether or not they develop heart disease. In contrast, in a clinical trial, the investigator would allocate 1 group to an intervention such as a drug or dietary or lifestyle change, and the others to some sort of 'control' intervention or placebo, and then measure the effect on some outcome, such as changes in serum cholesterol or incidence of heart disease. Trials can also be done where the person acts as their own control, e.g. cross-over trials. It is useful to distinguish trials that study *efficacy* (the true biological effect of a treatment) from those designed to measure *effectiveness* (effect of a treatment when actually used in practice). The important thing about well-designed and conducted trials is that because they are experiments, they are not subject to problems such as confounding and bias which are a feature complicating the interpretation of many observational studies.

Features of clinical trials

- Must contain a control group or the person acts as their own control.
- Prospective: participants are followed though time.
- Participants should be randomized to intervention or control groups or to intervention/control periods in cross-over trials.
- Intervention and control groups enrolled, treated, and followed over same period of time.
- Ideally the participants and the researcher are unaware as to whether a person has been assigned to the intervention or control group or period. This is known as (double) blinding.

Types of clinical trials

- Parallel, where individuals are assigned to different interventions (usually 2, the intervention and control arm, but there may be >2 arms).
- Cross-over trials, where each participant acts as their own control, taking the intervention and the control treatment in random order, with a wash-out period in between.
- Cluster trials, where groups of patients, clinics, or even geographic areas form the basis of the intervention, and the outcome is compared between these groups rather than between individuals. This is appropriate if an intervention is likely to have a group or population effect (e.g. testing a vaccine or other preventive intervention) or if interventions aimed at some people are likely to spill over to others in the community, e.g. a dietary trial.

Why a control group?

The control group is composed of those study participants who do not receive the intervention under assessment. They may instead receive placebo or standard clinical practice. A control group must be included otherwise you cannot be sure why the outcome happened; it may be due to the new treatment or it may have happened anyway.

Why randomize?

Randomization is done to remove *bias* in treatment allocation. Without randomization it is possible (indeed likely) that the investigator will choose different patients for each group.

In a famous early study of the BCG vaccine for TB in children, deaths from TB were 5x higher in the control group than the vaccinated children.[1] Further investigation showed that doctors had tended to offer the new vaccine to children whose parents were more 'cooperative', and left the rest as controls. These cooperative parents were likely to have been more educated, health conscious, and therefore to have a lower mortality from TB regardless of the vaccination (see Fig 7.8).

Why blind or double-blind?

Blinding means that the patient does not know whether they are getting the new treatment or not. In a double-blind trial neither the patient nor the investigator knows which treatment they are getting. This is to prevent bias in measurement or reporting of the outcome, *measurement* or *ascertainment bias*. People who are getting a new treatment (or treatment compared with no treatment) often report improvement in subjective symptoms because they are enthusiastic and hopeful. Similarly if a researcher knows that a patient is on the new or active drug they may look for better outcomes.

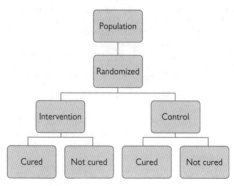

Fig. 7.8 Overview of randomized trials.

Open-label studies

Sometimes it is not possible to conduct a blind or double-blind trial, e.g. when a surgical intervention is compared with a medical treatment. However, it is still important to include randomization and controls and, where possible, to ensure that people doing outcome measurements are blinded to which treatment the participant received.

Ethics and consent

Clinical trials are strictly regulated to ensure that patients are protected. All clinical trials have to be registered, reviewed by an independent scientific committee, be approved by a Research Ethics Committee, and adhere to government and international guidelines. Trials will have an independent data monitoring committee—a group of independent researchers who can check progress during the trial; they will usually unblind the results to see if there is any major difference in outcome (improvement or side effects) between the intervention and control groups. If there is a large difference they have the power to stop the trial.

All participants in a trial must provide informed consent, and be free to withdraw at any time without affecting their care.

Analysis and interpretation

The analysis and presentation of results of a clinical trial varies according to the exact nature of the trial. Since they are prospective, analysis is often done using similar methods as cohort studies such as survival analysis (see 📖 p.274).

A trial will usually produce:
• Experimental event rate (EER), the incidence in the intervention arm. The 'event' might be progression, cure, death, or side effect.
• Control event rate (CER) the incidence in the control arm.
These can then be used to estimate:
• Relative risk (or hazard ratio, odds ratio): this is a ratio of the event rate in the experimental group and in the control group.
• Absolute risk reduction (ARR): this is the difference between the experimental and the control groups presented as a rate.
• Number needed to treat (NNT): this is the number of people who need to receive the experimental treatment to prevent one adverse outcome. It is the reciprocal of the absolute risk reduction (NNT = 1/ ARR).

See Chapter 2 for examples (see 📖 pp.42–5).

Things to look out for

Clinical trials should be reported according to the CONSORT (Consolidated Standards of Reporting Trials) guidelines (see 📖 p.84) These ensure that papers about trials include all the relevant information for readers to critically appraise the paper. Briefly, check:
• Is it a high-quality trial addressing an important question?
• Was randomization adequately done?
• How complete was follow-up and was it similar in both arms of the study?
• Did they look for negative as well as positive outcomes and were these measured blind?
• Does it apply to my practice—were patients adequately described?

- Was the intervention adequately described? This is very important in trials of behavioural or complex interventions.
- Was the analysis based on intention to treat or per-protocol?

Intention-to-treat or per protocol analysis

In many trials there will be some deviation from the trial design. For example, some people who are randomized to a treatment will stop taking it because of side effects. Others will shift to another treatment for clinical reasons. A decision then has to be made about what to do with people who deviate from protocol. This depends on the aim of the study. Usually the trial investigators should report intention to treat analysis as only this maintains the original randomization and therefore differences between the groups should reflect the treatment and not other (confounding) factors. If the aim is to assess efficacy of the treatment then it may be appropriate to analyse those who stuck to the protocol. However, this will give less idea of how the treatment will work in practice (effectiveness). If, for example, one-third of people stop taking the treatment because of side effects then this will affect the effectiveness of a strategy that makes it a first-line treatment (see ⬛ Clinical trials: examples, pp.190–1).

Reference

1 Levine MI, Sackett MF. Results of BCG immunization in New. York City. *Am Rev Tuberculosis* 1946; **53**:517–32.

Clinical trials: examples

Cross-over trial

In a randomized, double-blind, placebo-controlled cross-over trial, patients with migraine received 12 weeks of tonabersat and 12 weeks of placebo with a washout period of 4 weeks in between. The order of treatment was randomly allocated (see Fig. 7.9).[1]

Overall 31 patients completed the trial and could be analysed for efficacy. There were fewer aura attacks in the tonabersat than the placebo group: median 3.2 (IQR 1.0–5.0) over 12 weeks on placebo compared with 1.0 (0–3.0) in the tonabersat group (p = 0.01). There was no significant difference in other outcomes (including headache), and side effects were more common with tonabersat.

The data show:
- Relative reduction in aura = (3.2 − 1.0)/3.2 = 69%.
- ARR = 3.2 − 1.0 = 2.2.
- NNT = 1/ARR = 1 / 2.2 = 0.45 (i.e. 0.45 people treated for 12 weeks to produce 1 fewer episode of aura).

European Coronary Surgery Trial: coping with deviation from protocol

This trial from the 1970s asked whether men with significant coronary artery disease should have a trial of medical management or go straight to surgery. 768 men were enrolled and randomized: 373 to medical management and 394 to surgical. However, during the study some of the men randomized to medical management ended up having surgery because of clinical indication, and a few of those randomized to surgery did not have it in the end. This makes analysis and interpretation complicated. The flow chart shows what actually happened, giving mortality for each group (Fig. 7.10).

Analysis could be done in 1 of 3 ways, according to the initial randomization (intention to treat), according to randomization but excluding people who didn't stick to protocol (per-protocol), or according to actual treatment (comparing medical with surgical care). Each gives different results:

The appropriate analysis depends on the aim of the study, though in most (or all) cases intention to treat (ITT) is the preferred analysis as this retains the original randomization and (if follow up is complete) is not affected by selective deviation from protocol or withdrawal.

- The ITT approach measures the effectiveness of the policy of advocating surgical or medical intervention, and shows it to be better than trying medical management first.
- The per-protocol analysis, i.e. excluding people who deviate from protocol, shows the efficacy of the approach by including only those who were managed according to protocol, but this would not be replicated in a real-world setting where not everyone will be fit for surgery, for example. Although it retains the original randomization for those left in the trial, people may have selectively deviated from protocol or dropped out of the trial in the 2 treatment arms for a variety of reasons that may be related to survival, so it is possible that the results could be biased.
- Basing analysis on actual treatment regardless of randomization will re-introduce the selection bias that a trial is designed to overcome, and therefore is not a valid method.

Intention-to-treat (i.e. all those randomized)
- Mortality in those randomized to medical management = 69/373 = 18.5%.
- Mortality in those randomized to surgery = 41/394 = 10.4%.
- Relative reduction in mortality = (18.5 − 10.4)/18.5 = 43.8%.

Per-protocol (excluding people who deviated from protocol)
- Mortality in those randomized to medical management = 60/273 = 22.0%.
- Mortality in those randomized to surgery = 33/368 = 9.0%.
- Relative reduction in mortality = (22.0 − 9.0)/22.0 = 59.1%.

Actual treatment (ignoring randomization)
- Mortality in those managed medically management = 68/299 = 22.7%.
- Mortality in those managed surgery = 42/468 = 9.0%.
- Relative reduction in mortality = (22.7 − 9.0)/22.7 = 60.4%.

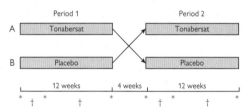

Fig. 7.9 Design of a cross-over trial of patients with migraine.

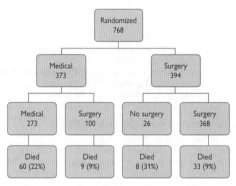

Fig. 7.10 Results of the European Coronary Surgery Trial.

References
1 Hauge AW *et al.* Effects of tonabersat on migraine with aura: a randomised, double-blind, placebo-controlled crossover study. *Lancet Neurol* 2009; **8**:718–23.
2 European Coronary Surgery Study Group. Long-term results of prospective randomised study of coronary artery bypass surgery in stable angina pectoris. *Lancet* 1982; **2**:1174–80.

Clinical trial phases

In the development of a new drug or treatment, there are several stages which must be followed to ensure that it is safe and effective.

Phase I

Phase I trials aim to test the safety of a new treatment. This will include looking at side effects of a treatment, e.g. does it make people sick, raise their BP, etc? Phase I trials involve only a small number of people, who may be healthy volunteers.

Phase II

Phase II trials test the new treatment in a larger group of people who usually have the disease for which the treatment is to be used, to see whether the treatment is effective, at least in the short term. Usually a few hundred people are involved at this stage. Phase II trials also look at safety.

Phase III

Phase III trials test the new treatment in a larger group of people. Phase III trials compare the new treatment with the treatment currently in use, or with a placebo. These trials look at how well the new treatment works, and at any side effects it may cause. Often several thousand patients will be involved in a phase III trial. They may use different hospitals and live in different countries. For example, the MRC Clinical Trials Unit runs phase III trials across Europe, parts of Africa, and the USA. The smaller the expected advantage of one treatment over another, the more people will be needed to take part in a trial.

Phase IV

Phase IV studies are done after the drug or treatment has been marketed to gather information on the drug's effects in various populations and any side effects associated with long-term use, or use in much larger populations than was possible in Phase III. These studies are observational and therefore subject to the same potential problems of confounding and bias as other observational studies, but they do provide essential 'real world' information about the use of the drug or treatment in actual clinical practice.

Classic randomized controlled trials (RCTs)

Streptomycin trial, 1948[1]

One of the classic trials that helped develop the clinical trial methodology was of the use of streptomycin in patients with pulmonary TB. Patients were randomized to receive streptomycin or control (bed rest alone) and outcomes documented at 6 months (Table 7.10).

Table 7.10 Results of the streptomycin trial (1948)

Treatment	Died	Survived	Mortality
Streptomycin	4	51	7.3%
Bed-rest	15	37	35.7%

- Relative reduction in mortality = 28.4/35.7 = 79.6%.
- Number needed to treat (to save one life) = 100/28.4= 3.5.
- Absolute reduction in mortality = 35.7% − 7.3% = 28.4%.

Unfortunately there were a large number of side effects, resistance developed rapidly, and the relative improvement was not sustained. However, this was a landmark trial in terms of both the treatment of TB and the use of randomization in clinical trials.

Salk Polio vaccine

An RCT was carried out on the new Salk vaccine for polio in 1954. The study involved hundreds of thousands of children who were then followed up to see if they developed polio. There are many aspects to the trial, but the basic results are shown in Table 7.11.

Table 7.11 Results of the Salk vaccine trial (1954)

Group	Number	Cases of polio	Rate per 100,000
Vaccinated	200 745	33	16
Control	210 229	115	57

- The relative risk of polio in the unvaccinated group was 57/16 = 3.6.
- The vaccine efficacy (see 📖 p.109) is then (57 − 16)/57 × 100 = 72%, i.e. the trial showed a 72% reduction in polio cases.

Reference

1 Medical Research Council. Streptomycin treatment of pulmonary tuberculosis. *BMJ* 1948; **2**:769–82.

Further reading

MRC Clinical Trials Unit: ♒ http://www.ctu.mrc.ac.uk/TrialInfo.asp

Choosing the right type of study

The types of study described in this chapter can all measure associations, e.g. between a risk factor and a disease, an exposure and an outcome. So how do you know which design is the most appropriate to investigate your particular research question? With information on the strengths and weaknesses provided in this chapter, you can start to weigh up which design might be the best fit.

In reality, you will find that the most appropriate design will also be dictated by resources available, e.g. time/money, and the importance of the research question.

Considerations include:

• What is your exact question?
• What is already known? If there is already a lot of research on the question but no clear answers it may be appropriate to do a systematic review and meta-analysis. If there have been observational studies showing an association it may be appropriate to move onto a clinical trial.
• If you find that other researchers have already conducted ecological or case–control studies on your research question and there is evidence suggestive of an association, a cohort study might be appropriate, especially if the exposure is rare so case–control studies may not be efficient (but beware, given the large size, long-term nature, and cost of many cohort studies this might not be a feasible option for you).
• On the other hand, if there are only a handful of case-reports available that hint to 2 things being associated, it would not be sensible to jump straight into carrying out an expensive, long-term cohort study. You might first conduct a cheaper and quicker study, e.g. a cross-sectional or ecological study, to further assess the evidence.
• If the outcome is rare it may make sense to do a case–control study, e.g. where you can recruit all known cases, whereas a cohort study would be highly inefficient as not many cases would accrue in the cohort.
• What is the likely time between the exposure and outcome? If there is a 30-year lag then a cohort study would not be the first choice, since you would have a long time to wait for any results. A retrospective study, such as a case–control or a retrospective cohort, would be preferable.

Table 7.12 gives a summary of the main features, applications, advantages and disadvantages of each study design and will act as a checklist to help you further evaluate when and where each design is most appropriate.

Example: HIV and circumcision[1,2]

In the 1980s clinicians and epidemiologists noticed that that HIV appeared to be less common in men who were circumcised. Evidence came from a number of studies:

• Ecological studies: populations with high levels of circumcision had a lower prevalence of HIV. However, this could be due to confounding, e.g. if circumcised men had less risky sexual behaviour.
• Case–control studies of men with and without HIV supported the association, but they too could be subject to confounding by sexual behaviour which might be poorly recalled.

- Cohort studies also showed an association, and were better able to control for sexual behaviour.
- Finally the evidence was felt strong enough to conduct trials which have proved that circumcision is protective against the acquisition of HIV.

Table 7.12 Summary of features of different types of study

	Ecological	Case–control	Cohort	RCT
Features				
Study population	Group (geographic, time)	Defined by outcome/ disease status	Defined by exposure	Randomly allocated to exposure
Applications				
Rare disease/outcome	Possibly	Yes	No	No
Rare exposure	Possibly	No	Yes	Yes
Studying multiple outcomes		No	Yes	Yes
Assessing temporal sequence	No	No	Yes	Yes
Direct measure of incidence	No	No	Yes	Yes
Studying long latency	Maybe	Maybe	Usually only in retrospective cohort	No
Advantages and disadvantages				
Time required	Short	Medium	Long	Variable
Cost	Low	Medium	High	High
Risk of selection bias	n/a	High	Low	Low
Recall bias	n/a	High	Low	Low
Loss to follow-up	n/a	n/a	High	Variable
Confounding	High	Medium	Medium	Low

References

1 Johnson KE, Quinn TC. Update on male circumcision: prevention success and challenges ahead. *Curr Infect Dis Rep* 2008; **10**(3):243–51.
2 Moses, S *et al.* The association between lack of male circumcision and risk for HIV infection: a review of the epidemiological data. *Sex Transm Dis* 1994; **21**(4):201–10.

Sources of data

Introduction: good quality data

The focus of this book is on the ways epidemiology can help clinicians in their everyday practice. In this chapter we approach the relationship from the other side and ask how clinicians can help epidemiologists. Epidemiological knowledge derives from research studies and routine data about health, exposures, illness, and outcomes. Routine data come from many sources such as the population census, population health surveys, birth and death certification, patient data, and registries. Clinicians have a direct role in recording much of the information that forms routine data.

Rubbish in, rubbish out?

The provision of data, through death certification, disease notification, or coding of visits to hospital or the GP, is often fairly low on the priority list for clinicians. The consequence is often poor data which can lead to inadequate or incorrect conclusions about individuals and about population trends, the impact of interventions, and health service activity. An incorrectly completed death certificate may cause delay and distress to relatives, and may lead to incorrect national data about trends in causes of death.

Increasingly, routine data from clinical settings—including diagnoses, prescribing, and other activity—are being used for monitoring performance, safety, efficiency, and health outcomes. Poor quality data could therefore also have far-reaching consequences for the individual clinician, the organization where he or she works, and the health of the population.

Clinicians are most likely to care about data quality when the data are useful to them. This in turn depends on the information cycle being completed through the production of reports which are fed back to those who provide the data in the first place (Fig. 8.1). Turning data into useful reports is not necessarily simple, and requires linking with denominator (usually population) data, stratification (by sex, age, ethnicity, etc.), analysis, and interpretation.

Quality of data depends on:

- *Coverage:* the proportion of eligible cases that are included.
- *Completeness:* for all required fields including dates, diagnoses, demographic information, personal identifiers.
- *Validity:* is the diagnosis (or code or category) based on a good interpretation of available information? Have responses been checked, e.g. with validation rules that make sure responses are within certain ranges?
- *Consistency:* have diagnostic codes changed, are they being used in the same way by different clinicians, hospitals, etc. and over time?
- *Timeliness:* if data are returned late then they cannot be incorporated into routine analyses and reports, and may delay recognition of important new trends.
- *Relevance:* the data must be collected, collated, analysed, and reported in a way that is relevant to the needs of the clinician, public health specialist, policy maker, and other users, including the patient.
- *Accuracy:* the data must closely represent the 'real' situation.
- *Precision:* if the data collection is repeated, e.g. recoding medical notes, it should result in the same information being collected.

If these criteria are met, then quality is more likely to be achieved at each step in the process, and the data are more likely to be useful and used.

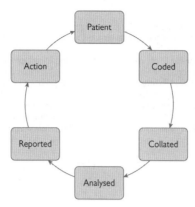

Fig. 8.1 The data cycle.

Places to look for relevant data
UK
- Association of Public Health Observatories: 🖰 http://www.apho.org.uk
- British Heart Foundation: 🖰 http://www.bhf.org.uk
- Cancer Research UK: 🖰 http://info.cancerresearchuk.org/cancerstats
- Department of Health: 🖰 http://www.dh.gov.uk
- Dr Foster Intelligence: 🖰 http://www.drfoster.co.uk
- Health of Wales Information Service: 🖰 http://www.wales.nhs.uk
- Health Protection Agency: 🖰 http://www.hpa.org.uk
- Health Protection Scotland: 🖰 http://www.hps.scot.nhs.uk
- Information Services Division, Scotland: 🖰 http://www.isdscotland.org
- Ireland and Northern Ireland's Population Health Observatory
  (INIsPHO): 🖰 http://www.inispho.org
- National Cancer Intelligence Network: 🖰 http://www.ncic.org.uk
- National Data Archive: 🖰 http://www.ndad.nationalarchives.gov.uk
- National Primary Care Trust Database: 🖰 http://www.primary-care-db.
  org.uk
- NHS Information Centre: 🖰 http://www.ic.nhs.uk
- Scottish Public Health Observatory: 🖰 http://www.scotpho.org.uk
- UK Statistics Authority/Office for National Statistics (ONS):
  🖰 http://www.statistics.gov.uk

USA
- American Heart Association (AHA): 🖰 http://www.americanheart.org
- Center for Disease Control and Prevention (CDC): 🖰 http://www.cdc.gov
- National Cancer Institute (NCI): 🖰 http://www.cancer.gov
- National Center for Health Statistics (NCHS): 🖰 http://www.cdc.gov/nchs
- National Heart, Lung, and Blood Institute (NHLBI): 🖰 http://www.nhlbi.
  nih.gov

International
- Global Health Council ⌗ http://www.globalhealth.org
- International Agency for Research on Cancer (IARC): ⌗ http://www.iarc.fr
- Organization for Economic Co-operation and Development: ⌗ http://www.oecd.org
- United Nations: ⌗ http://www.unstats.un.org
- World Bank: ⌗ http://www.worldbank.org
- World Health Organization: ⌗ http://www.who.int, including:
  - WHO Global Health Observatory: ⌗ http://www.who.int/gho/en
  - WHO Regional Office for Europe: ⌗ http://www.euro.who.int

Routine data

Routine health data* are sources of information relating to the health of the population that are collected in an ongoing way rather than for any specific research project.

They include:

- Broad population data such as vital statistics (including registrations of births and deaths).
- Detailed mortality data, such as numbers and causes of death.
- Morbidity data such as diagnoses of cancer or infectious diseases.
- Health service activity data such as hospital episodes, prescribing, vaccination coverage.
- Limited data on determinants of health such as smoking, physical activity, and occupation.
- Limited data on environmental exposures such as air and drinking water quality.

Routine data are often collected for statutory purposes, e.g. information about terminations of pregnancy is required by law, but the data are then used for a variety of health and social analyses.

*Note that the word 'data' is plural, the singular being datum and relates to a single item only.

Vital statistics

One of the most important sources of routine data derives from vital statistics based on universal registrations of births and deaths. These data—counts of the number of births and deaths—are combined with information from a periodic population census and migration statistics to produce estimates of population size and make-up. Universal registration and therefore vital data are not available in some less developed countries, and therefore population estimates have to be based on surveys.

Mortality data

Mortality data are more detailed than the death count included in the vital statistics. They include numbers and causes of death together with limited demographic information about the deceased. In the UK, they are obtained from death certificates and are important for monitoring trends in disease (see 📖 p.210). The different indices are shown in Box 8.1.

Box 8.1 Mortality definitions

- Maternal mortality rate: the number of maternal deaths per 100,000 births.
- Infant mortality rate: the number of deaths of infants aged <1 year per 1000 live births in a given year.
- Neonatal mortality rate: the number of deaths of infants aged <28 days per 1000 live births in a given year.
- Under 5 mortality rate: the probability that a newborn baby will die before reaching age 5, as a number per 1000 live births.

Morbidity data

In addition to mortality, we also need data on morbidity and risk factors for planning healthcare, informing prevention programmes and studying variations in the incidence of diseases and their underlying causes. Morbidity data can be disease-specific (e.g. cancer registries, infectious disease notifications, congenital anomalies registers) or relate to healthcare activity (e.g. prescribing data, hospital episode statistics). More detailed data on determinants, and experience of ill health and disability, can be obtained from periodic surveys. Most of these are based on interviewing a representative sample of the population (see 📖 p.162). For example, the Health Survey for England (HSE)[1] is an annual survey of 20,000 individuals who are intended to be representative of the whole population. This survey includes data on self-reported health, disease, and risk factors. The National Health And Nutrition Examination Survey (NHANES)[2] collects similar data from an age/sex/ethnicity weighted sample chosen to be representative of the overall population in the USA. These data can be used to describe the distribution of disease and its determinants in the population, and to make estimates of future trends.

Advantages of routine data

- Relatively cheap to use.
- Already collected and available, accessible from ONS (UK), NCHS (USA) etc.
- Regularly updated.
- Standardized collection procedures.
- Relatively comprehensive—population coverage, large numbers.
- Wide range of recorded items.
- Available for past years.
- Experience in use and interpretation.

Limitations of routine data

- May not answer the question (no information or not enough detail).
- Incomplete ascertainment for morbid events (not every case captured).
- Need careful interpretation.
- Often used regardless of lack of completeness, inaccuracies etc.
- Diagnostic codes change, geographical boundaries change.
- Accurate population data may be limited, e.g. decennial census.
- Often out of date due to lack of timely returns.

Examples of routine sources of data

Demographic and vital statistics

- Births.
- Deaths.
- Migration.
- Marriage.
- Census (includes socioeconomic data and ethnicity).

Health care activity data
- Hospital episode data.
- Prescribing data (PACT).
- GP data on consultations and prescriptions.
- Vaccination records.
- Screening records.

Health data
- Cancer registrations.
- Notification of infectious diseases.
- Terminations of pregnancy.
- Congenital anomalies.
- Road traffic accidents.
- Child health.

Health determinants
- Lifestyle: General Lifestyle Survey (GLF) (Great Britain).
- National Survey of Sexual Attitudes and Lifestyles (NATSAL) (Britain).
- Health surveys, e.g. HSE, NHANES, National Food Survey (Great Britain).
- Environmental exposures e.g. air pollution.
- Employment.

References
1 Health Survey for England (HSE): Ӎ http://www.ic.nhs.uk/statistics-and-data-collections/health-and-lifestyles-related-surveys/health-survey-for-england
2 The National Health And Nutrition Examination Survey (NHANES): Ӎ http://www.cdc.gov/nchs/nhanes.htm

Clinical uses of routine data

Clinicians provide many of the routine data used by epidemiologists and public health specialists. Many of the data sources can also be useful to clinicians, e.g. in planning services, anticipating or understanding changes in demand, clinical governance (see 🕮 p.122), quality and safety monitoring, and audit.

Planning services

The demand for clinical services, e.g. for obesity and related conditions such as diabetes, depends on long-term trends in the health status of the population. The Health Survey for England (HSE) collects information on height and weight in a representative sample of the population each year. The data can be used to measure the levels of overweight and obesity in the population today, and to estimate levels in the future. The data can also be analysed to show the distribution of overweight and obesity by gender, age, ethnicity, and region of the country.

Quality and safety monitoring

Routine data are becoming increasingly important in monitoring of outcomes of healthcare. For example in the UK, hospital episode statistics (HES) are used and published by organizations like the Care Quality Commission (🕾 http://www.cqc.org.uk), the Department of Health, and commercial organizations like Dr Foster Intelligence.

League tables

Fig. 8.2 shows the potential use of mortality data from HES to monitor performance of different clinical centres. These kinds of data are used to produce reports of outcome for centres and by individual consultants or teams. Outcomes include mortality, infection rates, other complications, lengths of stay, and re-admission rates. These kinds of reports, sometimes brought together in 'league tables' of performance, are difficult to interpret. Inevitably, even if the underlying mortality of all units (be they hospitals or surgeons) were the same, because of random variation, there will always be someone at the top of the league table and someone at the bottom. In addition, around 50% of units will be below average. This means that league tables are less than perfect for comparing outcomes between units. Using the data presented in the figure, hospitals can be ranked in a league table (Table 8.1). However, presented in this way the data suggest major differences between the units while Fig. 8.2, which includes confidence intervals, shows that all but 3 of the units had performance that was not significantly different from the average performance.

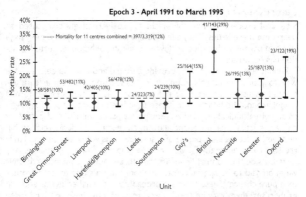

Fig. 8.2 Paediatric surgical mortality, using hospital episode statistics. This figure plots paediatric cardiac surgery mortality rate in 11 English hospitals in the early 1990s based on routine hospital data (HES). The red diamonds show the mortality and the bars show the 95% confidence intervals. The Bristol centre has a significantly higher mortality than the average. This analysis was done in the aftermath of a scandal alleging medical negligence in paediatric cardiac surgery in Bristol. Although HES data are incomplete, routine analysis could have identified the problem earlier. Figure adapted from Aylin P et al. BMJ 2004; **329**:825–7. Reproduced with permission from BMJ Publishing Group Ltd.

Table 8.1 Example league table using information presented in Fig. 8.2

Rank	Hospital	Risk of mortality
1	Leeds	7%
=2	Birmingham	10%
=2	Liverpool	10%
=2	Southampton	10%
5	GOSH	11%
6	Harefield/Brompton	12%
=7	Leicester	13%
=7	Newcastle	13%
9	Guy's	15%
10	Oxford	19%
11	Bristol	29%

Statistical process control charts

Statistical process control (SPC) charts are increasingly being used to overcome these issues. They allow you to monitor activity (e.g. mortality) and compare it with expected levels to identify when unexpected variation has occurred.

Funnel plots, a type of SPC, provide a simple and easily understandable way to plot institutional or unit level comparisons. Outcome data are plotted against a measure of its precision, so that the control limits form a funnel around the benchmark. These have been promoted as providing a strong visual indication of divergent performance with the advantage of displaying actual event rates and allowing an informal check of a relationship between outcome and volume of cases. Any units within the control limits are said to be 'in-control', with their variation explained by chance. Any units outside the control limits are said to be 'out of control', with their variation said to be special cause variation, and thus due to factors other than pure chance. These units are probably worth further investigation. In many cases, there may be good clinical reasons why these units appear to be 'out of control' due to complexity of cases, case-mix, etc.

Cumulative sum charts

Although funnel plots are generally used to compare outcomes at a particular point in time, they are looking back in time to discover problems that have already occurred and are not ideally suited to detecting a problem as soon as possible. A prospective monitoring system accumulates data continuously over time and the analysis is repeated at every time point. The cumulative sum chart (CUSUM) is one such method, derived from the monitoring of laboratory performance. A number of different CUSUM charts have been used in applications of routine health surveillance, such as the exponentially weighted moving average chart (EWMA), the log-likelihood CUSUM chart, and the sequential probability ratio test (SPRT). What distinguishes the various methods is the way in which the test statistic is derived. Each test statistic is added to the previous value, and plotted on a chart. When the cumulative sum of this value exceeds a predefined threshold, the chart signals, and can serve as a prompt for further investigation.

Case mix

Presented as crude rates (e.g. deaths per 100 operations), outcomes may be very misleading as they do not take into account differences in case mix. Florence Nightingale recognized the limitations of naïve calculations of surgical mortality rates 'without reference to age, sex or cause of operation'. Case mix can be adjusted for using indirect or direct standardization, or through statistical risk prediction models derived from regression analysis. Examples of common surgical risk prediction models include POSSUM (Physiological and Operative Severity Score for the Enumeration of Mortality and Morbidity), EuroScore, and ASA (American Society of Anesthesiologists). These scores take into account the poorer outcomes expected in more complex, or older cases.

Further reading

Association of Public Health Observatories (APHO). Statistical process control methods in public health intelligence. York: APHO; 2009.

Death certification

The system of monitoring deaths is based on the issuing of Medical Certificates of Cause of Death, more commonly known as death certificates. In this section we specifically refer to the legal processes in England and Wales, but many of the principles will apply elsewhere. It is essential that death certification is as accurate and timely as possible in order to minimize the chance of the relatives having problems with the burial and funeral arrangements, to ensure that anything suspicious is appropriately referred, and to provide reasonable information for health surveillance purposes.

The process of death certification in England and Wales is currently being improved and new regulation is expected to come into force by April 2012.

Purposes of death certification

- To provide a permanent legal record of the fact of death and the cause of death. This allows the relatives to arrange the funeral and the deceased's estate to be settled.
- To ensure that anything suspicious is appropriately referred for investigation.
- To provide a record that can be used for public health purposes including monitoring health of populations, planning healthcare, and prioritizing resources.

Who issues the death certificate?

- If you are the attending physician you are required under the Births and Deaths Registration Act 1953 to certify the cause of death and issue a certificate.
- Who is the attending physician?
  - A registered medical practitioner who attended the deceased during their last illness.
  - In hospital this will be one of the team caring for the patient, from junior to consultant medical staff. Ultimately however, it is the responsibility of the consultant in charge of the patient's care to ensure that the death is properly certified.
  - In the community this will be the GP.
  - In future, the role may be extended to include other members of the multidisciplinary team such as nurse practitioners.
- When can you not issue a certificate?
  - If you have not been directly involved in the patient's care at any time during the illness from which they died.
  - If you have not seen the patient either after death or within 14 days of death.
  - If there are any other indications for referral to the coroner (see 📖 p.214).
  - In these situations, or if you are in any doubt, you must refer the death to the coroner before it can be registered. If the coroner decides to take on the case, then they must investigate before they issue a death certificate. They may, however, choose simply to instruct the registrar to accept the doctor's medical certificate of cause of death.

Importance of death certification

- Relatives will be spared the distress of delay in funeral arrangements caused by unexpected referral of the death to the coroner.
- Doctors will avoid being asked to clarify their certificate by the Registrar of Birth and Deaths or by the Coroner.
- Everyone will benefit from more reliable information on mortality.

The death certificate

In addition to the cause of death statement, the certificate includes sections covering the personal details about the deceased, the circumstances of certification, and whether or not there was a referral to coroner or whether a hospital postmortem was carried out. The following should be carefully completed:

- Name of deceased, age, date of death, place of death.
- Date last seen by the doctor issuing the certificate for registration.
- The doctor should circle 1 or more of the following:
  - This certificate takes account of information obtained from a postmortem examination.
  - Information from the postmortem examination may be available later.
  - A postmortem examination not being held.
  - I have reported this death to the coroner for further action.
- There is also an option for 1 of the following statements:
  - Seen after death by me.
  - Seen after death by another medical practitioner but not by me.
  - Not seen after death by a medical practitioner.
- The death might have been due to or contributed to by the employment followed at some time by the deceased. It is important to consider this and to discuss with the relatives as this may affect pensions or other claims from employers.

Cause of Death Statement

This is in 2 parts (Table 8.2).

Table 8.2 Cause of Death Statement

CAUSE OF DEATH The condition thought to be the 'Underlying Cause of Death' should appear in the lowest completed line of Part I		Approximate interval between onset and death
I	(a) Disease or condition directly leading to death	
	(b) Other disease of condition, if any, leading to I(a)	
	(c) Other disease of condition, if any, leading to I(b)	
II	Other significant conditions CONTRIBUTING TO THE DEATH but not relating to the disease or condition causing it	

Part I

This should show the immediate cause of death, and then work back in time to the disease or condition that started the process.

The top line (1a) should therefore identify the disease or condition that led directly to the death, moving down to any antecedent or intermediate causes of that event or disease or condition in the lines below until the 'Underlying cause of death' is given in the lowest completed line of Part 1.

If only providing a single cause of death, then this should be placed in Part 1(a). The underlying cause of death is the disease or injury which initiated the chain of morbid events leading directly to death. It is not the mode of dying, such as heart failure or asphyxia.

Part II

This should include other significant conditions contributing to the death but not related to the disease or condition causing it.

There are detailed instructions on how to complete a certificate in the front of the book of medical certificates of cause of death which you should refer to.

In completing the certificate, the attending physician should write clearly, check information including correct spelling of names, dates, etc., and not use abbreviations. All parts of the form should be completed.

Medical certificates of cause of death

There are 3 types of medical certificates of cause of death:
• Medical Certificate of Cause of Death: any death after 28 days of life.
• Neonatal Death Certificate: within 28 days if child breathed regardless of gestation.
• Certificate of Still-birth: if child born dead after 24 weeks' gestation.

Ascertaining the fact of death

Before issuing a death certificate, clearly the doctor has to ensure that the person is dead. This requires an examination to check for pulse, breath sounds, and heartbeat. These should be checked for at least 2min. In addition, corneal and/or light reflexes should be checked. Doctors should clearly record the time of death and time of examination in the notes.

In the case of someone with hypothermia, death should not be pronounced until the body has warmed sufficiently.

Criteria for ascertaining brainstem death can be found in Wijdicks (2001).[1]

Example of completing the medical certificate of the cause of death

An 84-year-old retired midwife was admitted to hospital with a community-acquired pneumonia. She improved but a suspicious shadow was reported on her chest X-ray. The bronchial biopsy showed an inoperable squamous cell bronchial carcinoma. She was discharged home despite her limited mobility. 1 week later she was readmitted with a deep vein thrombosis. She declined further investigation or treatment. The following day she became acutely short of breath and died the next night.

Certificate:
- Part I(a): Pulmonary embolism.
- Part I(b): Deep vein thrombosis due to immobility.
- Part I(c): Squamous cell carcinoma of bronchus.
- Part 2: empty, no relevant information given.

Reference

1 Wijdicks EFM. The diagnosis of brain death. *NEJM* 2001; **344**:1215–21.

Referral to the coroner

The coroner (or procurator fiscal in Scotland) must be informed about any death where there is uncertainty about the cause of death or where further investigation may be required. The coroner is part of the criminal justice system, and has the power to issue a death certificate following investigation which may include a postmortem. Once a death has been referred to the coroner it cannot be registered until the ensuing investigation has been completed. A death should be referred to the coroner if:

* The cause of death is unknown.
* The deceased was not seen by the certifying doctor either after death or within 14 days of death.
* The death was violent, unnatural, or suspicious.
* The death may be due to an accident (whenever it occurred).
* The death may be due to self-neglect or neglect by others.
* The death may be due to an industrial disease or related to the deceased employment.
* The death may be due to an abortion.
* The death occurred during an operation or before recovery from the effects of an anaesthetic.
* The death may be due to suicide.
* The death occurred during or shortly after detention in police or prison custody.

In the event of uncertainty, the coroner's office can provide advice on whether a death should be formally reported to them.

Resources

Death certification in England and Wales

The General Register Office provides updated guidance on many of the issues doctors often ask about, and clarifies best practice under current legislation. The guidance will be updated to reflect any new legislation. Available online at: ℘ http://www.gro.gov.uk/medcert

Scotland and Northern Ireland

Deaths are registered in a similar way to in England and Wales. In Scotland the role of the Coroner is played by the Procurator Fiscal.

Death certification in the USA

Department of Health and Human Services' Centers for Disease Control and Prevention's National Center for Health Statistics (NCHS) Physician's handbook on medical certification of death, 2003 revision. Available online at: ℘ http://www.cdc.gov/nchs/data/misc/hb_cod.pdf

Infectious disease notification

Doctors in England and Wales have a statutory duty to notify a 'Proper Officer' of the Local Authority of suspected cases of certain infectious diseases. The Proper Officers are required every week to inform the Centre for Infections (CfI) currently at the Health Protection Agency (HPA), details of each case of each disease that has been notified. The Information Management & Technology Department within the CfI has responsibility for collating these weekly returns and publishing analyses of local and national trends.

Which diseases are notifiable (Box 8.2)?

- Those that are relatively rare but serious, requiring rapid intervention.
- Those subject of vaccination programmes.
- Conditions requiring environmental health action such as food poisoning.

Box 8.2 Notifiable diseases in England[1]

- Acute encephalitis
- Acute meningitis
- Acute poliomyelitis
- Acute infectious hepatitis
- Anthrax
- Botulism
- Brucellosis
- Cholera
- Diphtheria
- Enteric fever (typhoid or paratyphoid fever)
- Food poisoning
- Haemolytic uraemic syndrome (HUS)
- Infectious bloody diarrhoea
- Invasive group A streptococcal disease and scarlet fever
- Legionnaires' Disease
- Leprosy
- Malaria
- Measles
- Meningococcal septicaemia
- Mumps
- Plague
- Rabies
- Rubella
- SARS
- Smallpox
- Tetanus
- Tuberculosis
- Typhus
- Viral haemorrhagic fever (VHF)
- Whooping cough
- Yellow fever.

Reference

1 HPA. *Health Protection (Notification) Regulations*, 2010. ℘ http://www.legislation.gov.uk/uksi/2010/659/contents/made

Cancer registration

Cancer registries provide important information on the incidence and survival rates of cancers. In the UK, cancer registries have been collecting data for the last 40 years. There are 8 regional cancer registries in England. The National Assembly for Wales is responsible for cancer registration in Wales, the registration system in Scotland is coordinated by the information and statistics division (ISD) of the NHS in Scotland, and cancer registration in Northern Ireland is carried out by the Department of Health and Social Services and Queen's University, Belfast. The national cancer intelligence centre (NCIC) at the Office for National Statistics (ONS) coordinates the national collection of cancer registration data.

Cancer registries collate data on individual patients from multiple sources and over long time periods. In the UK, these sources include both NHS and private institutions, private hospitals, cancer screening programmes, primary care, nursing homes, and death certificates.

Use of cancer data
- The evaluation of the effectiveness of cancer screening programmes.
- Cancer survival rates.
- Trends in incidence.
- Inequalities in cancer treatment.
- International comparisons.
- The study of environmental effects on cancer incidence.
- Investigating the presence and causes of cancer clusters.

Online resources
Cancer Research UK. ✍ http://www.cancerresearchuk.org
National Assembly for Wales. Available online at ✍ http://www.wcisu.wales.nhs.uk
National Cancer Intelligence. Available online at ✍ http://www.ncri.org.uk
United Kingdom Association of Cancer Registries. Available online at ✍ http://www.ukacr.org

Statistical concepts

Introduction

Statistics is the science that helps us to make sense of data. It can be as simple as summarizing a distribution ('the children were aged between 5 and 14, the mean age was 8') or identifying whether 2 variables are correlated. Statistics is crucial for biomedical science as it enables us to make sense of data that have been collected in an experiment or survey and to assess whether the observed results may just have arisen by chance.

Statistics contributes to robust research by improving the design of studies and suggesting ways to analyse the data once they are collected. It is important for those doing the research to do it well, and for those keeping up to date with current research to be able to distinguish between strong and weak studies.

Populations and samples

Research is almost always carried out with samples from a population with the aim of drawing some conclusions about the whole population. For example, during election campaigns there are many opinion polls which survey a proportion of potential voters and ask about their voting intentions. Understanding the relationship between the sample and the population is a key function of statistics, and helps us to understand the results.

If the poll shows that Party A has 60% of the preferences, Party B 30% and Party C 10%, we would like to know if Party A is going to win come election day. In other words we want to know if our sample is providing a good estimate of the true voting preferences in the population as a whole.

To answer that we need to know:
• How big was the sample?
• Was it representative of the population or were there possible biases?

Assuming that the poll was based on a representative sample of potential voters, then the key factor here would be the size of the sample. If the poll was based on asking 10 people, then we would be less confident about predicting victory for Party A than if we had asked 10,000 people.

Statistics provides us with methods for showing how confident we are in such estimates.

Biological variability

Consider the measurement of the heart rate of a person at various times of day. In this case, heart rate is a *variable* that will vary throughout the day and will take on one of a set of allowed values each time it is observed. Multiple measurements of a variable form a *sample*. We would not expect each measurement to be the same, but together they can tell us something about the underlying process. The use of samples to make inference about an underlying process, or population, is at the heart of statistics.

In this chapter we provide an overview of the basic concepts and tools relevant to clinical practice, and also introduce some of the more complex statistics that are reported in studies. Reading and understanding research requires a familiarity with the use, outputs, and limitations of statistical tests. We provide examples to demonstrate the use of different methods.

Data and variables

Types of variables

Variables may be qualitative (having distinct values or classes) or quantitative (having a numeric value).

Qualitative variables

These take on distinct values or classes. They may be:

- Categorical: e.g. whether someone travels to work by car/bus/train/foot/bicycle/motor cycle. These are called nominal data.
- Ordered categorical: e.g. whether someone is a non-smoker/light/moderate/heavy smoker or has low/medium/high BP. These are called ordinal data as there is an order to the classes.
- Binary: a special case of variables which take on 1 of 2 possible values, e.g. true/false, male/female, survived/died.

Collecting and recording qualitative data

If you are setting up a data collection system from scratch, think carefully about the categories in advance. For example, if you want to analyse ethnicity, you should ask people to self-define from a pre-set list (preferably using a standard census list). Otherwise you may get a number of categories that do not map to each other. When you record data for analysis, make sure you record them in the form they were obtained rather than collapsing them. You will then be able to collapse categories later.

For example, if you ask people whether they travelled to work by car, bus, train, foot, bicycle, motor cycle, record them in this form. If some groups are very small, you may decide to collapse the groups into high emission/private vehicle (car, motor cycle), medium emission/public transport (bus train), and low emission (foot, bicycle). For another analysis you may be interested in car or other.

Quantitative variables

These take on numeric values and can be:

- Discrete: e.g. number of patients in a study, number of cases of disease; or
- Continuous: e.g. temperature, BP.

Categorizing continuous variables

Continuous quantitative variables can have their values grouped into classes and presented as discrete or ordered categorical variables. For example, Table 9.1 groups measurements of the systolic blood pressure (SBP) in a sample of 648 men suffering from self-reported fatigue. These data can then be grouped further into an ordered categorical classification e.g. low, medium, and high BP.

Recording continuous data

If you are collecting data for research or audit, you need to decide in advance how you are going to record them. In the BP example, you may decide to record the categories, low, medium, or high. However, if you subsequently decided to re-analyse the data you would be limited to those broad groups. In general it is better to record as continuous data (actual SBP reading) and categorize later.

Explanatory and response variables

Variables are often distinguished as being either *explanatory* or *response* variables (see 📖 p.149). The purpose of a study is frequently to assess the dependence of the response variables (e.g. disease outcome) on explanatory variables (e.g. exposure). For example, in a study of the effect of a whooping cough vaccination in young children the explanatory variable would be whether a child has been vaccinated or not and the response, the occurrence or absence of whooping cough.

Table 9.1 Continuous data from measurements of the blood pressure of 648 men grouped in 2 ways (based on results from Wessley et al. 1990[1])

SBP (mmHg)	Group	Number of men	Percentage
<100	'Low'	12	1.9%
100–119.9	'Low'	209	32.3%
120–129.9	'Medium'	286	44.1%
140–159.9	'Medium'	111	17.1%
≥160	'High'	30	4.6%
Total		648	100.0%

Reference

1 Wessley S et al. Symptoms of low blood pressure: A population study. *BMJ* 1990; **301**:362–5.

Summarizing sample data

Various statistics are routinely used to describe samples. These split into two broad groups:
- Those that aim to give a summary of location of the central value of the data, e.g. the mean, median, or mode.
- Those that give an idea of the spread of the data around this central point, e.g. the interquartile range or standard deviation.

Example

The data in Table 9.2 shows a selection of waist girths (in cm) for a sample of 180 women.[1]

Table 9.2 Example data

60.7	61.4	61.5	61.7	62.4	62.5
62.7	62.7	62.9	63.5	63.7	63.8
...	...	...	...	...	...
78	78	78	78.3	78.5	78.7
79.2	79.4	79.6	80	88.2	90.1
90.5	93.4	94.2	96.2	96.3	101.5

Presented in this way it is difficult to interpret, and would certainly be difficult to compare with a table from a different set of health centres or at a different point in time. We therefore present the data in a more accessible way using a graphical format (e.g. histogram) or through the use of statistics to summarize the data.

Histograms

The distribution of e.g. the cost of the drugs can be presented graphically using a *histogram*, which shows the relative frequencies of a quantitative variable. The area of each bar has a natural interpretation as a proportion of the total area of all the bars displayed. Fig. 9.1 shows a histogram of the waist girths.

Summary statistics

Many statistics can be calculated from these data and a selection of them are shown in Table 9.3.

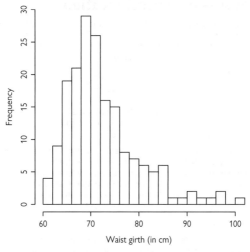

Fig. 9.1 A histogram of the waist girth of a sample of 180 women.

Table 9.3 Summary statistics for the waist girths (cm) of a sample of 180 women

Statistic	Symbol	Value
Sample size	N	180
Mean	$\bar{x}$	72.4
Median		70.5
Mode		68.3
Variance	s^2	55.0
Standard deviation	s	7.4
Minimum	x_{min}	60.7
Maximum	x_{max}	101.5
Range	$x_{max} - x_{min}$	40.8
Lower quartile	Q_l	67.5
Upper quartile	Q_u	75.5
Interquartile range	IQR	8
Standard error of the mean	SE	0.55

Reference

1 Heinz G et al. Exploring relationships in body dimensions. *J Stat Educ* 2003;**11**(2).

Measures of central location

The commonly used term 'average' can actually refer to 3 different measures which aim to summarize data in terms of its central value.

- Mean: an arithmetic calculation which is the sum of the observations divided by the number of observations.

$$\text{mean} = \overline{x} = \frac{1}{N} \sum_{i=1}^{N} x_i$$

- Mode: the most frequent value that is observed.
- Median: the value that splits the distribution in half, i.e. 50% of the values lie below this value and 50% above.

If the data are roughly symmetrical, the value of the mean will generally be close to of the mode and median. If there are extreme values, however, then the mean and the median can be very different. Under these circumstances, usual practice would be to use the median as it is far more robust to extreme values. The mean, however is the basis of the majority of formal statistical analyses and is widely used.

Non-symmetrical data

In cases where the distribution of the data is not symmetric, it may be possible to transform the data to introduce symmetry and then use the mean. In addition, many statistical tests rely on the underlying assumption that the data can be represented by the Normal distribution, which is symmetrical.

There are different types of transformation that can be applied to enable standard statistical tests to be performed.

Types of transformation you will see:

- Logarithmic (using $\log_{10}$ or $\log_e$): used where continuous data are non-normally distributed and have a skew to the right.
- Square transformation: used where continuous data are non-normally distributed and have a skew to the left.
- Logit (logistic): used for data where each observation is a proportion.

Example

Returning to the example given in Table 9.2, the distribution of waist girths is asymmetric, i.e. there is an extended tail of higher girths to the right. It is this asymmetry, or *skewness*, that is causing the mean, median, and mode to have different values.

One way to make a distribution more symmetric is to transform the values of the observations, e.g. by taking the logarithm of the data prior to calculating the sample statistics. Fig. 9.2 shows the distribution of the log values of the girths.

The distribution is now more symmetrical, with the mean now being closer to the median and mode (Table 9.4), although there is still some evidence of right-skewness.

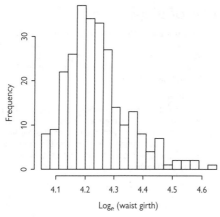

Fig. 9.2 Distribution of the log values of the waist girth data from Table 9.2.

Table 9.4 Summary statistics for the log values of waist girth data from Table 9.2

Statistic	Symbol	Waist	Log$_e$ (waist)
Sample size	N	180	180
Mean	$\bar{x}$	72.4	4.3
Median		70.5	4.3
Mode		68.3	4.2

Measures of dispersion

In addition to measuring the centre of a distribution we generally want to describe the spread around this value. The most appropriate measure of dispersion relates to the measure of centrality. For example, when using the median we usually quote the interquartile range, while when using the mean we use the standard deviation.

Interquartile range

This is used to describe dispersion when the median is the central measure. The median is the 50th percentile, i.e. 50% of the distribution lies above it and 50% below. Together with the median, 2 other values can be found that will cut the distribution into quarters, the lower quartile (or 25th percentile) and the upper quartile (75th percentile). An idea of the spread of the data can then be given by calculating the *interquartile range*:

$$IQR = Qu - Ql$$

(Where Qu and Ql are the upper and lower quartiles, respectively.)

Standard deviation

When using the mean, the associated measure of the spread of the data is referred to as the standard deviation (SD) which is commonly denoted by the Greek letter sigma, σ.

The standard deviation is the square root of the *variance*, which is based on the squared differences or deviances of the individual observations from the mean.

$$\text{variance} = \sigma^2 = \frac{1}{N} \sum_{i=1}^{N} (x_i - \bar{x})^2$$

The standard deviation is then equal to the square root of the variance

$$SD = \sigma = \sqrt{\sigma^2}$$

Provided that the data are roughly symmetrical, we would expect the mean to be roughly equal to the mode and the median and an interval of 1 SD either side of the mean to contain roughly 70% of the data and an interval of 2 SDs either side to contain approximately 95% of the distribution, that is roughly 2.5% at either end of the distribution. Fig. 9.3 shows examples of the proportions contained within 1, 1.5, 1.96, and 2 SDs either side of the mean.

Sample standard deviation

In the expression for the variance given, the sum of squared deviations is divided by N (the number of observations). This is used when we have data for the entire population. In the common case where we have data from a sample the divisor is (N − 1) rather than N. Mathematically, this adjusts for the bias which would be present when we don't have data for the entire population. A variance calculated using sample data is commonly denoted by s^2, in order to distinguish it from σ^2 and the corresponding standard deviation by s.

$$\text{sample variance} = s^2 = \frac{1}{N-1}\sum_{i=1}^{N}\left(x_i - \bar{x}\right)^2$$

The sample standard deviation is then equal to the square root of the sample variance

$$\text{Sample standard deviation} = s = \sqrt{s^2}.$$

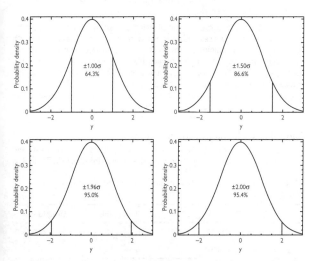

Fig. 9.3 Examples of the proportions of the data contained within 1, 1.5, 1.96, and 2 standard deviations either side of the mean of a normal distribution.

Sampling variability

Sample statistics can be used to estimate the characteristics of the underlying population or process from which the sample is drawn (Fig. 9.4). We must be aware of 2 factors when attempting to make generalizations from a sample to a population of interest:

- *Bias:* the sample may be biased, i.e. it may not representative of the population as a whole. This may be due to way the study was designed or carried out.
- *Chance:* the sample may differ to a greater or lesser extent from the population by chance alone.

The first factor is important in the planning of a study, where we must be clear about any possible selection effects that may bias a sample (see 📖 p.34). For example, public opinion surveys on the street on weekdays will miss out many different types of people, in particular the working population, who may have strongly differing views on various issues. If we have a well-designed and carefully executed study bias should not pose a major problem.

The second factor is unavoidable. Where variability is present, the sample statistics calculated from any particular sample will be different to those calculated from another independent sample.

Sampling variability of the mean

A random sample of size N is taken from a population, the mean and standard deviation of the population and the sample are shown in Table 9.5.

Table 9.5 Measures of central location and dispersion for populations and samples

	Population	Sample
Mean	μ	$\bar{x}$
Standard deviation (SD)	σ	s

Example

The packed cell volume (PCV) was measured in 302 children aged 1–3 years in Western Kenya:[1]

Mean $(\bar{x})$ = 24.9, standard deviation (s) = 3.5

Note that the symbols used here refer to values calculated from the sample. The sample mean, $\bar{x}$, is an estimate of the true population mean, μ, of all 1–3-year-olds and the sample standard deviation, s, is an estimate of the true population standard deviation, σ.

What can we say about the true mean of PCV in this population of children?

If we repeatedly take random samples from the overall population and each time record the mean and the standard deviation of their PCV values we would find:

- The values of $\bar{x}$ and s would vary from sample to sample.
- The values of $\bar{x}$ would be distributed symmetrically around the true population mean, μ, the value we are interested in.
- Values near μ would occur more frequently than those far from μ.

Statistical theory tells us that no matter what the original distribution of the data, the distribution of sample means will follow the Normal distribution. The standard deviation of this distribution of sample means is known as the standard error (SE).

Standard error

The SE is the standard deviation of the distribution of sample means. It is equal to the population standard deviation divided by the square root of the sample size.

$$SE = \sigma / \sqrt{N}$$

When the true population standard deviation is unknown, as is generally the case, the sample standard deviation may be used in place of σ.

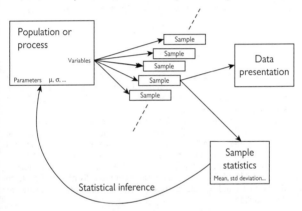

Fig. 9.4 Schematic of the sampling process to enable inference about populations.

Reference

1 Nabakwe EC, Ngare DK. Health and nutritional status of children in Western Kenya in relation to vitamin A deficiency. *East Afr J Public Health* 2004; **1**(1):1–5.

Probability distributions

Probability distributions come in a variety of shapes and sizes depending on the type of variable they represent. They may be expressed in tables, bar charts, histograms, or as mathematical formulae. They share out probabilities among a set of possible outcomes and those probabilities always sum up to 1.

The Normal distribution

The Normal distribution is the most commonly used mathematical distribution in statistics. It is also referred to as the Gaussian distribution or as a bell-shaped curve.

It is defined for quantitative variables that can take any value from minus infinity to plus infinity, and is characterized by 2 parameters, its mean μ and standard deviation σ. Thus a Normal distribution is described by

$$N\left(\mu, \sigma^2\right)$$

Fig. 9.5 shows a Normal distribution with mean 0 and standard deviation 1, N(0,1), known as the unit Normal distribution.

Whenever a probability distribution is expressed as a curve on a graph as discussed, or as a histogram, then the proportion of the area underneath the curve between any pair of values is the probability of observing a value in that range.

In the case of the Normal distribution the chances of a value lying between, say, the mean and 1 standard deviation above the mean are always the same no matter what the value of the mean and standard deviation. Additionally, a Normal distribution with any mean and standard deviation can be transformed or *standardized* to make a unit Normal distribution, N(0,1). This allows us to easily compare distributions, perform statistical tests, and use standardized tables, or computer programs, to find probabilities.

Other probability distributions

Probability distributions are at the heart of statistical tests used to estimate if observations or groups differ from each other. The Normal distribution is not always the most appropriate one to use. A detailed description of the theory behind the different distributions is beyond the scope of this text, but for information the other commonly used distributions are:

- The t-distribution is used under similar circumstances to the Normal but where the variance is unknown, as is often the case, and has to be estimated from a sample along with the mean. The t-distribution allows for the additional uncertainty that is introduced. For large enough samples (N >30) the t-distribution is approximated by the Normal distribution.
- The binomial distribution where there are only 2 outcomes (e.g. diseased or non-diseased).
- The Poisson distribution where the outcome is a count, e.g. the number of new cases of a disease in a population.
- The Chi-squared distribution used for analysing categorical data.
- The F-distribution used when comparing the variance of samples.

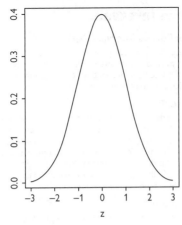

Fig. 9.5 The unit normal distribution, with mean equal to 0 and standard deviation of 1.

Confidence intervals

What is a confidence interval (CI)?

Given a sample of data, the sample mean will be the best estimate of the true population mean although there will be some uncertainty associated with this. A confidence interval quantifies this uncertainty and gives a range of values in which we are confident the true population value will lie.

When is it used?

It is used to indicate the level of precision associated with an estimate from a sample. Estimates calculated from large samples will be more precise than those arising from small samples. Often they are used to assess whether a particular value is likely or not, a specific case being when estimating the difference in means between 2 groups in which case the interest is in whether zero is a reasonable estimate for the difference, i.e. is zero included in the confidence interval?

What is the output?

A symmetrical interval centred around the sample mean. It is usually given as a 95% interval either side of the sample mean, e.g.:

$$mean = 24.9 \left(95\% \; CI \; 24.5, \; 25.3\right)$$

Note the 95% CI might not be symmetrical if there has been a transformation of the data before taking the mean (e.g. log) and then a back-transformation (e.g. exp) to put back into the original units.

How do we interpret it?

The CI will be calculated based on a pre-specified level of significance, commonly 95%, in which case we are 95% 'confident' that the true population value will lie within the given interval.

A wider interval means that there is more uncertainty. If 2 CIs overlap, then we cannot say that the 2 means are significantly different (at the pre-specified level of significance).

Are there any restrictions on its use?

The calculation relies on normality and crucially symmetry. In certain cases this will not be a tenable assumption, e.g. when dealing with proportions that are close to 0 or 1 or with very low counts of disease where negative values are prohibited. In such cases, exact methods based on the true underlying probability distributions should be used.

We can use CIs to make certain inferences about population means using the observed values from a sample. For example, we might ask: are the (unknown) means of 2 populations different?

The procedure is to construct CIs and then to see whether or not the values of interest lie in those intervals.

From properties of the Normal distribution, 95% of the distribution will fall between 1.96 SEs either side of the sample mean. Hence a 95% CI is given by:

$$\bar{x} \pm 1.96 \frac{s}{\sqrt{N}}$$

It is important not to confuse the 2 different standard deviations here, there is the standard deviation of the population σ (estimated by s) and there is the standard deviation of the sample means, SE, denoted by $\frac{s}{\sqrt{N}}$.

Example
In the PCV example (see 📖 p.228):

$$\text{Mean} = \bar{x} = 24.9$$

$$s = 3.5$$

$$N = 302$$

$$\text{standard error} = s/\sqrt{N} = 3.5/17.4 = 0.20$$

Thus the 95% CI for the population mean:

$$95\% \text{ CI} = \bar{x} \pm 1.96 \text{ SE} = 24.9 \pm (1.96 \times 0.20) = (24.5, 25.3)$$

What does this mean? We are 95% 'confident' that the true mean lies between 24.5 and 25.3.

  NB: when we say we are 95% 'confident', it is not same as saying that there is a 95% probability that the true population mean is within this interval. The true population mean is fixed (and is thus either inside the interval with probability 1 or 0) and it is the CIs themselves that are variable as they are based on sample statistics which will vary from sample to sample. Under repeated sampling, we expect 95% of the calculated intervals to contain the population mean.

Hypothesis tests

Research involves the development and testing of hypotheses. These may concern estimates of a particular measurement or association. Statistical tests help us to evaluate these hypotheses.

To do this, two alternative conclusions (hypotheses) are set up, and on the basis of the experiment one is accepted and the other rejected. This acceptance and rejection is always on the basis of some pre-specified levels of confidence.

The 2 hypotheses are:
- The null hypothesis, H_0: we hypothesize that *there is no difference* between e.g. the mean of 2 groups, or no association between an exposure and an outcome.
- The alternative hypothesis, H_A: we hypothesize that *there is a difference* between e.g. the mean of 2 groups, or an association between an exposure and an outcome.

The hypotheses are always stated so that either one or the other (but not both) can be true. On the basis of the hypotheses a statistical decision rule is constructed, e.g.:
- IF the observed value of a statistic takes on a certain range of values;
- THEN reject the null and accept the alternative hypothesis;
- OTHERWISE accept the null and reject the alternative hypothesis.

The range of values for the statistic will be determined by the desired levels of statistical significance. The statistic calculated is known as the *test statistic* and its value is compared to pre-determined *critical values* which are determined by the chosen *significance level*.

Type I errors, type II errors, and the power of tests

There are 4 possible outcomes of a hypothesis test, with probabilities as summarized in Table 9.6.

Table 9.6 Possible outcomes of a hypothesis test

	H_0 is accepted	H_0 is rejected
H_0 is true	$1 - \alpha$	α
H_A is true	β	$1 - \beta$

The significance level of the test is the probability that we (erroneously) reject H_0 when it is true:

$$\text{Prob (reject } H_0 \text{ when } H_0 \text{ is true)} = \alpha$$

This is called a Type I error. A Type II error occurs when we (erroneously) accept H_0 when it is false:

$$\text{Prob (accept } H_0 \text{ when } H_0 \text{ is false)} = \beta$$

The power of the test is the probability that we (correctly) reject H_0 when it is false. The power of a test is defined as $= 1 - \beta$, i.e. the probability that we correctly reject the null hypothesis when it is false and hence H_A is true.

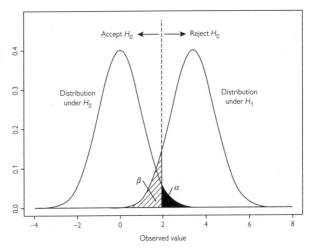

Fig. 9.6 Possible outcomes of a hypotheses test showing Type I (α) and Type II (β) errors.

These errors are shown in Fig. 9.6 which shows the relationship with probabilities from the Normal distribution.

Type I and II errors are inevitable, but their likelihoods α and β are known, either because they were specified in the study design, or by being calculated afterwards.

The quantity $1 - \alpha$ is a similar concept to the sensitivity of a diagnostic test, and $1 - \beta$ is similar to the specificity. They are (almost) never equal to 1, and must often be chosen in a trade off between study size (and expense) and power. A conservative statistical decision rule might want a very small α, e.g. 1% or 0.01, which is analogous to a small chance of a false negative test, but a rather larger β, e.g. 20% or 0.20, which corresponds to a larger chance of a false positive test.

Example

Given the sample of mean PCV from 302 children (see 📖 p.228), if we wanted to test whether the true population mean is equal to 25.5 we would set up the following null and alternative hypotheses.

The null hypothesis, H_0: $\mu = 25.5$, and

The alternative hypothesis, H_A: $\mu \neq 25.5$

We specify the significance level, to be 5%, denoted by $\alpha = 0.05$.

In this case, the alternative hypothesis includes examples where the true population mean, (μ), is <25.5 and those where it is >25.5. This is known as a *two-tailed alternative*.

If we were specifically interested in whether the population mean was >25.5, we would have a one-tailed alternative. The same is true if we were interested only in whether the population mean was <25.5.

We are interested in whether there is any difference between the sample mean and the hypothesized value, and whether any difference is statistically significant. In order to make this assessment, we calculate a test statistic:

Test statistic(z) = (sample mean − hypothesized mean)/standard error

First we divide the difference in means by the standard error to find 'how many standard errors away' the hypothesized true mean (25.5) is from the sample mean (24.9). Then this test statistic is compared to values from a standard probability distribution, in this case the Normal distribution, which 'convert' the test statistic into the probability of obtaining this value or a more extreme value. This probability, or p-value, is a measure of how likely it would be to obtain our sample mean if the true population mean was the hypothesized value of 25.5.

Small values of this probability indicate that this is an unlikely occurrence and so provide evidence that the null hypothesis should be rejected in favour of the alternative hypothesis.

In the PCV example, we have a sample mean of 24.9 and a sample standard deviation of 3.5. With a sample size of 302, the standard error is $3.5/\sqrt{302} = 0.20$. The test statistic (called 'z' when the Normal distribution is used and 't' when the students t distribution is used) is therefore:

$$z = (24.9 − 25.5)/0.20 = −2.98$$

The probability (p-value) of getting this value of the test statistic *or one more extreme* is 0.001 (obtained from standard statistical tables). This is the value we would use in a one-tailed test (where the alternative hypothesis states whether the 'true' value is different from the sample mean in a specified direction). But we are conducting a two-tailed test where the alternative hypothesis is that there is a difference between the sample and hypothesized mean, without specifying which direction the difference is in. We have used a two-tailed alternative hypothesis because there is no reason to suspect that the mean might be higher or lower than 25.5. We therefore need to allow for both the possibility of a value higher than 25.5 and a value lower than 25.5. As the normal distribution is symmetrical, these two probabilities will be equal and so the two-tailed p-value we want is 0.001 × 2 = 0.002.

This p-value is smaller than our pre-specified significance level of $\alpha = 0.05$. We therefore have evidence that the null hypothesis is false and reject it in favour of the alternative hypothesis. Our conclusion is that there is evidence that the true population mean of PCV is not equal to 25.5.

Statistical or clinical significance

In assessing the strength of evidence in medicine we often ask whether a finding was 'significant'. But what does significance mean?

- Statistical significance is a mathematical construction that assesses the probability of the finding having occurred by chance.
- Clinical significance relates to whether a difference is important in practice.

Statistically significant, clinically insignificant

Suppose we are looking at a drug that may have an unwanted side effect of raising BP. A trial comparing the drug with placebo finds that the drug raises BP by an average of 0.1mmHg, with a p-value of 0.023. This means that the difference is deemed statistically significant at a 5% level. This difference may be real, but an increase of 0.1mmHg may not be clinically of interest. Thus it may be statistically significant, but not clinically important.

Statistically insignificant, clinically significant

On the other hand, if a difference is not statistically significant it may still be real, and/or important. A non-significant statistical result does not imply that there is no effect; it just means that we have failed to demonstrate that it could not have occurred by chance. The sample may simply be too small to show that the effect is there. For example, if a new drug appears to increase survival by 20%, but is not statistically significant because there were small numbers in the trial, it is obvious that if the effect is real it would certainly be important. We have no evidence that the difference did not occur by chance, but that doesn't mean we should necessarily stop looking for it. Further research is required to determine whether this difference is real or not.

Hypothesis tests or confidence intervals?

The *British Medical Journal* and some other leading journals now strongly prefer results of statistical testing to be presented in the form of CIs, rather than just p-values as has been common practice in the past.

A CI conveys additional information; it has to do with precision of an estimate, rather than trying to answer the possibly over-simplified question 'is there a significant finding or not?'.

If a hypothesis test is appropriate, rather than just a CI, it is best to report the actual p-value, rather just reporting whether a particular finding is significant or not. For example, is it reasonable that p-values either side of 0.05, i.e. 0.051 and 0.049, should correspond to substantially different inferences?

Multiple comparisons

If we test a single null hypothesis that is in fact true, at the 5% level, then the probability of a non-significant result is 95%. If we test 2 such independent hypotheses, both at the 5% level, the probability of a non-significant result in the first is 95% and the probability of a nonsignificant result in the second is 95%; the probability that neither are significant is $0.95 \times 0.95 = 0.90$. If we were to test 20 such hypotheses the probability that none is significant is $0.95^{20} = 0.36$ and so we are likely to see a significant result that is not true.

In practice, multiple hypothesis tests are not usually independent, so the probabilities given are not quite correct. However, the general rule is that the more you look for, the more likely you are to find something, 'if you torture the data long enough, it will eventually confess!'. Care should be made in attaching too much importance to a single 'significant' result among a sea of non-significant ones.

There are methods that are proposed to correct for multiple testing, the simplest of which is the Bonferroni correction; if you are conducting n significance tests, then for an overall Type I error of α, you should test each hypothesis at a significance level of α/n. This test tends to be conservative, i.e. the true Type I error after Bonferroni correction will be less than α, due to the dependence between hypothesis tests.

P-values and sample size

Given a large enough study even tiny differences can become statistically significant; the larger the study for a given effect size the smaller the p-values will be. For this reason you should be careful when looking at very large datasets, since nearly all differences appear to be significant if you take the standard cut-off point of 0.05. One rule of thumb is to use a lower p-value if the dataset is very large.

Otherwise, be careful of over-interpreting your results and pay close attention to the differences between statistical versus clinical significance.

Sample size and power calculations

One of the most common questions when designing a study is 'how large should my study be?'. To answer this question, we need to know a number of things:

- What is the study aiming to measure?
- What design is suggested?
- What do we know already about the variability in the population(s)?
- What difference do we expect there to be? Or what difference would be clinically relevant to find?

We can then use this information to estimate samples sizes to help design appropriate studies. The sample size will also depend on the analysis to be performed once the data have been collected. For example, if analysis will be performed using a log transformation, then sample size calculations should be based on the log scale.

Estimation and confidence intervals

In a cross-sectional study, when we may be interested in accurate estimation of the mean of a measurement such as body mass index rather than hypothesis tests, we want to choose a sample size which will give an acceptable standard error. A convenient way to do this is to choose the sample size so that the width of CIs is small enough to give sufficient precision to your estimate of the mean.

Hypothesis tests

We are often interested in testing whether, for example, there is a difference between 2 means, as well as estimating the magnitude of such a difference. For significance tests we need to choose a sample size large enough to detect a difference with high confidence if it exists, which will be based on the power of the test. It is also useful to specify the minimum difference, δ, that would be considered clinically important.

Power of a test

Recall that there are 2 types of error we may make in a hypothesis test (see 📖 p.234); rejecting H_0 when it is true (Type I error) and failing to reject H_0 when it is false (Type II error). We control the probability of a Type I error when setting the significance level α of a test. When determining the sample size required to detect a real difference we need to be concerned with the probability of a Type II error.

The power of a test is given by:

$$\text{Power} = 1 - P \text{ (do not reject } H_0 \text{ when } H_A \text{ is true)} = 1 - \beta$$

For a given test, this will depend on the true difference between the 2 groups to be compared, the amount of variability in the outcome measure, the sample size, and the chosen significance level, α.

Other than α, sample size is the factor over which we have most control. It is important to plan a study to have a large enough sample size to detect a clinically meaningful difference, typically power = 0.80 to 0.95 (i.e. 80 to 95%).

Doing a sample size calculation

In a research study it is important to work with a statistician who can perform appropriate and often complex sample size calculations. In smaller projects you may want to work it out on your own. You would need to consult a more comprehensive statistical text for help with this, but may also make use of various online tools or computer packages.

When to consult a statistician

Often statisticians are only consulted at the end of a study when all the data have been collected; however, this can lead to problems if there are aspects of the study design which the statistician is not aware of or require specialist analysis, e.g. if matching has been performed in selecting participants. A good study should involve the statistician from the beginning and they can provide advice on an appropriate design for a study, the most appropriate software to use in addition to helping to analyse the results when they become available.

Further resources

The material presented in this book has aimed to give examples of statistical methods and techniques that may be commonly seen in the epidemiological literature. The scope for detailed descriptions and technical detail is limited here and the reader may wish to supplement the material presented by consulting more specialist texts. There are a wide range of books that cover statistical methods in medicine and epidemiology and we present a very small selection of them here.

Books

- Armitage P et al. *Statistical Methods in Medical Research*. Blackwell; 2001.
- Bland JM. *An Introduction to Medical Statistics*. Oxford: Oxford University Press; 2000.
- Bland JM, Peacock J. *Statistical Questions in Evidence-based Medicine*. Oxford: Oxford University Press; 2000.
- Kirkwood B, Sterne J. *Essential Medical Statistics*. Wiley-Blackwell; 2003.
- Peacock J, Peacock P. *Oxford Handbook of Medical Statistics*. Oxford: OUP; 2010.

Online resources

There are also a number of excellent online resources including the *British Medical Journal's* (BMJ) *Statistics at Square One* (9th edn, 1997), a free online text book on statistics: ℰ http://resources.bmj.com/bmj/readers/statistics-at-square-one

BMJ Statistics Notes series (ℰ http://resources.bmj.com/bmj/topics/other-series).

Software

There are a wide range of tools with which to perform statistical analysis and the choice of which to use will be based on a number of factors, including the complexity of the analysis, the expertise of the user, and the availability of appropriate software. Many, such as Microsoft Excel, will be familiar and can be used for many of the methods described in this book. Others offer a wider range of methods, but are similar in appearance to Excel in terms of the graphical user interface (GUI), such as SPSS. At the other end of the spectrum are command driven languages such as R. The following is a non-exhaustive list of some of the software and packages that can be used to perform statistical analysis together with an indication of their capabilities and ease of use.

Microsoft Excel

Simple descriptive statistics, plots, and regression can be done in the basic installation of Excel. The Analysis Toolpak allows many more methods to be used such as ANOVA and hypothesis tests. Details can be found at: ℘ http://office.microsoft.com/en-us/excel-help/about-statistical-analysis-tools-HP005203873.aspx

This is an add-in program that is available when you install Microsoft Office or Excel, but needs to be specifically loaded as it is not a default option. Details of how to load it can be found at: ℘ http://office.microsoft.com/en-us/excel-help/load-the-analysis-toolpak-HP001127724.aspx

SPSS

A general purpose statistical package that can perform a very wide variety of analyses. It covers everything from initial descriptive analyses to very complex methods. On initial sight it looks very much like Excel and is easy to get started but there are numerous options that are available through sub-menus that mean the user can have very precise control over choices that are made. In addition to the GUI, there is the option to write scripts which can be very useful when analyses have to be repeated, for example on different datasets. Further details can be found at: ℘ http://www.spss.com/software/statistics

SAS

Another general purpose package that provides an extremely wide variety of options. It has particularly good facilities for dealing with very large datasets, including initial manipulation and processing. As with SPSS, there is the option of using a GUI or writing scripts. Further details can be found at: ℘ http://www.sas.com

Stata

A package widely used in education and research. Earlier versions of Stata emphasized a command-line interface, which facilitates replicable analyses, but more recently a GUI which uses menus and dialog boxes to give access to nearly all built-in commands. This generates code which is always displayed, easing the transition to the command line interface and more flexible scripting language. The current dataset can be viewed or edited in spreadsheet format. For further details see: ℘ http://www.stata.com

R

R is a programming and software environment for statistical computing and graphics. The R language has become a de facto standard among statisticians for developing statistical software and is widely used for statistical software development and data analysis. It is freely available for various operating systems. R uses a command line interface; however, several graphical interfaces are available for use with R. It is highly extensible through the use of user-submitted packages, including many specifically dealing with epidemiology, for specific functions or specific areas of study and can produce publication-quality graphs, including mathematical symbols. For further details see: ℘ http://cran.r-project.org

Statistical techniques in clinical medicine

Independent t-test

What is it for?
Comparing the means of 2 groups, i.e. where we have numerical data (e.g. height) in 2 different samples (e.g. girls and boys).

When is it used?
When the 2 groups are independent samples.

What does it do?
It tells you whether the means of the 2 groups are significantly different.

What is the output?
A p-value (which indicates the probability that the data are consistent with the null hypothesis of no difference between the groups).

How do you interpret the output?
If the p-value is small, typically <5% or 0.05, then the null is rejected in favour of the alternative. This will represent a difference in either direction (two-tailed alternative) or in a specific direction (one-tailed).

What restrictions are there on its use?
If the data are severely non-Normal and sample sizes are small, then a non-parametric test such as the Mann–Whitney U-test may be more suitable (see 📖 p.257).

Example
The birth weights of babies (in kg) have been measured for a sample of mothers split into two categories: non-smokers and smokers for which summaries can be seen in Table 10.1.[1]

Table 10.1 Summaries of birth weights (kg) of babies for samples of smoking and non-smoking mothers

	Non-smoker	Smoker
Sample size	115	74
Mean	3.06	2.77
Standard deviation	0.75	0.66

The difference between the sample means is 0.28kg. Could this difference have arisen by chance or is it statistically significant?

We first identify null and alternative hypotheses and specify the required significance level.

- Null hypothesis H_0: birth weight is the same in heavy smokers and non-smokers.
- Alternative hypothesis H_A: birth weight is lower in heavy smokers than non-smokers.
- Significance level $\alpha = 0.05$.

To carry out the test we calculate a t statistic based on the observed difference between the sample means divided by the standard error[*].

$$t = (mean_1 - mean_2) / SE = 0.284 / 0.104 = 2.73$$

The t statistic of 2.73 is then looked up in a table of distributions, in this case giving a p-value of 0.0035 for a one sided α, and 0.007 for a two-sided α.

In this comparison we specified that we were interested in whether birthweight was lower in smokers, so we use the one-sided p-value (we would use the two-sided p-value if we were interested in whether the two weight distributions were different, not specifying a direction).

As this p-value is less than the significance level we specified (0.05) we can conclude that there is evidence to reject the null hypothesis and accept the alternative, namely that birth weights of babies born to mothers who are heavy smokers are lower than those born to non-smoking mothers.

[*]Note a pooled standard error was used, combining the values from both of the groups.

The t-distribution and degrees of freedom

When the variance, and thus standard deviation, is estimated from sample data, we use the t-distribution in preference to the Normal in order to acknowledge the additional uncertainty that is introduced when the true population variance is unknown. If we were to use the Normal distribution, then the interval $\bar{x} \pm 1.96 \times SE$ actually includes the true value slightly less than 95% of the time, i.e. the confidence interval will be too narrow.

Using the t-distribution corrects for this because we use a multiplying factor larger than 1.96, thus making the interval a little wider and restoring the confidence to 95%. The t-distribution has an additional parameter, the degrees of freedom (v), which is based on the sample size, and in the case of a single group is equal to the sample size minus one, $v = N - 1$.

With large enough samples (N >30) the t-distribution becomes approximately Normally distributed, as the estimated standard deviation s will be close to the true value σ and thus the additional error will be small. Therefore the multiplying factors from both distributions will be almost equal.

For hypothesis tests, the t-distribution is used to calculate p-values which correctly reflect the sample size in estimating the variance. When comparing two groups, the required degrees of freedom is a combination of the sample sizes of both groups, $v = ((N_1 - 1) + (N_2 - 1))$.

Reference

1 Hosmer DW, Lemeshow S. *Applied Logistic Regression*. New York: Wiley; 1989.

Paired t-tests

What is it for?

Comparing the means of 2 paired groups, i.e. where we have numerical data in 2 linked samples (e.g. paired observations from before and after an intervention).

When is it used?

When the 2 groups are of equal size and participants in 1 sample are paired with those in the other i.e. they are not independent samples.

What does it do?

It tells you whether the means of the 2 groups are significantly different.

What is the output?

A p-value (which indicates the probability that the data are consistent with the null hypothesis of no difference between the groups).

How do you interpret the output?

If the p-value is small then the null is rejected in favour of the alternative. This will represent a difference in either direction (two-tailed alternative) or in a specific direction (one-tailed).

What restrictions are there on its use?

If the data are severely non-Normal and sample sizes are small, then a non-parametric test such as the Wilcoxon signed rank test may be more suitable (see 📖 p. 258).

Example

A study was performed to assess the effect of different diets on LDL cholesterol in hypercholesterolaemic men.[1] Table 10.2 gives the measurements taken from 12 men after trying each of 2 diets with a 'washout' period in between.

We first identify null and alternative hypotheses and specify the required significance level.

- Null hypothesis H_0: there is no difference in LDL between the 2 diets.
- Alternative hypothesis H_A: there is a difference in LDL between the 2 diets.
- Significance level $\alpha = 0.05$.

In the paired t-test it is the differences between the 2 conditions (diets in this example) that are of interest rather than the distribution of the values in each condition. Therefore the test statistic is based on the mean of the differences between the 2 groups, 0.38. This now reduces to a single sample t-test on the difference, which under the null hypothesis of no difference will be equal to zero.

The test statistics is t = mean difference/SE = $0.38/(0.43/\sqrt{12}) = 3.04$ which with degrees of freedom $v = (12-1)=11$ gives a p-value of 0.022 for a two-sided test. As the p-value is less than our specified significance level of 0.05, we conclude that there is evidence to reject the null hypothesis of no difference between the 2 diets.

When data are paired, performing (incorrectly) an independent t-test will result in a loss of power, i.e. be less likely to indicate a significant difference when there is one. Here, an independent t-test would give a non-significant p-value of 0.289.

Table 10.2 LDL cholesterol levels for a sample of men given 2 different diets

Participant	Diet 1	Diet 2	Difference
1	4.61	3.84	0.77
2	6.42	5.57	0.85
3	5.4	5.85	−0.45
4	5.54	4.8	−0.26
5	3.98	3.68	0.30
6	3.82	2.96	0.86
7	5.01	4.41	0.6
8	4.34	3.72	0.62
9	3.80	3.49	0.31
10	4.56	3.84	0.72
11	5.35	5.26	0.09
12	3.89	3.73	0.16
Mean	4.64	4.26	0.38
SD	0.79	0.91	0.43

Reference

1 Castro IA *et al.* Functional foods for coronary heart disease risk reduction: a meta-analysis using a multivariate approach. *Am J Clin Nutr* 2005 **82**:32–40.

Confidence intervals for a proportion

What is it for?
Quantifying the uncertainty in a proportion that has been measured from a sample of the population (see 📖 p.218).

When is it used?
To test whether a proportion is equal to a particular value or to see if 2 proportions are different.

What does it do?
A CI gives a range of values in which we are confident the true population proportion will lie.

What is the output?
A symmetrical interval centred around the observed sample value. The interval can be for different levels of confidence, but are usually 95% or 99%.

How do you interpret the output?
If the CI is narrow then the proportion has greater precision. If an interval is constructed around the difference in proportions between 2 groups, then if a 95% CI contains zero, we can be 95% confident that there is no difference in the proportions in the underlying populations.

What restrictions are there on its use?
The calculation relies on Normality and crucially symmetry. This may be inappropriate when dealing with proportions that are close to zero or one. In practice, we can use the Normal distribution as an approximation for large N and when p is not too close to zero or 1. Otherwise exact methods based on the true underlying Binomial probability distributions should be used.

How is it done?
An approximate 95% CI for a single proportion can be calculated in a similar fashion to that used for sample means and takes the form of the sample estimate plus/minus 1.96 times the standard error, which in this case is based on properties of the Binomial distribution.

$$p \pm 1.96 \sqrt{\frac{p(1-p)}{N}}$$

Example
Table 10.3 shows data from a study of the effects of smokeless tobacco use and low birth-weight in India.[1]

The frequencies of low birth-weight babies (defined as <2500g) is given by categories of mothers' tobacco usage (non-users, 1–4 times, 5 or more times).

Table 10.3 Frequencies of low birth-weight babies by mothers' tobacco usage

	≥2500g	<2500g	Total
Non-users	646	160	806
1–4 times	85	27	112
5 or more times	35	21	56
Total	766	208	974

The proportion of low birth-weight cases in the non-users group is $160/806 = 0.199$. As this is calculated from a sample, we wish to obtain a CI to indicate a range in which we are confident the true population proportion will lie.

Using the Normal approximation, a 95% CI will be:

$$0.199 \pm 1.96 \times \sqrt{(0.199 \times 0.801 / 806)} = (0.171, 0.226)$$

We are therefore 95% confident that the true population proportion of low birth-weight cases in the non-users group is between 0.171 and 0.226.

This approximate CI is liable to be misleading if sample size is small, or the probability is close to either zero or one. A probability close to zero is often the case for many proportions encountered in epidemiology e.g. disease incidence or death rates, in which case exact methods based on calculating Binomial probabilities should be used.

Reference

1 Gupta, P, Sreevidya S. Smokeless tobacco use, birth weight, and gestational age: population based, prospective cohort study of 1217 women in Mumbai, India. *BMJ* 2004; **328**:1538.

Normal test for difference in proportions

What is it for?

This is a test for comparing the proportions of some outcome between 2 groups.

When is it used?

When there are the same 2 possible outcomes, often deemed success and failure, in both of the groups.

What does it do?

It tells you whether there is a difference in the proportions of successes between the 2 groups.

What is the output?

A p-value which indicates the probability of the data arising from the null hypothesis that there is no difference between the proportions of successes in the 2 groups.

How do you interpret the output?

If the p-value is small then the null is rejected in favour of the alternative. This will represent a difference in either direction (two-tailed alternative) or in a specific direction (one-tailed).

What restrictions are there on its use?

The test relies on a Normal assumption to the Binomial distribution. This is likely to be reasonable, if the proportions are based on a large sample size and are not close to either zero or 1. Otherwise exact methods based on properties of the Binomial distribution should be used.

How is it done?

When performing a hypothesis test to ascertain whether there is a significant difference between the proportions in the 2 groups, the null hypothesis will be that there is no difference between the true proportions in the 2 groups, for example, case/not case or exposed and unexposed categories.

In the example of maternal tobacco usage and low birth weight (see Table 10.3), we are interested in whether the proportion of low birth-weight cases amongst tobacco users is greater than that in non-users. Here we combine the 2 tobacco users groups in order to have a single comparison, as shown in Table 10.4.

Table 10.4 Frequency of low birth-weight babies by mothers' tobacco usage

	≥2500g	<2500g	Total
Non-users	646	160	806
Users	120	48	168
Total	766	208	974

We have a one-tailed alternative with the null and alternative hypotheses being
- H_0: $p_1 = p_2$, i.e. the difference is zero.
- H_A: $p_1 > p_2$, i.e. the difference is greater than zero.

In which case, if the Normal approximation to the Binomial distribution is suitable then a test statistic can be constructed as

$$Z = (\text{proportion}_1 - \text{proportion}_2) / \text{SE}(\text{difference in proportions})$$

Note that the SE is for the difference between the proportions in the two groups, for which the formula can be found on 📖 p.xxvi.

In this case, the difference in proportions is equal to $(160/806) - (48/168) = 0.087$ and the standard error of the difference is 0.019. The test statistic is:

$$z = 0.087 / 0.019 = 4.548$$

That is, the test statistic lies 4.548 standard deviations away from the mean, which corresponds to a p-value of <1% ($p<0.001$). Thus there is strong evidence that there is a difference between the proportions (of low birth-weight) in the 2 groups.

Chi-squared test for association

What is it for?
This is a test for comparing the proportions of outcomes in different groups.

When is it used?
When there are 2 or more possible outcomes in 2 or more groups. In the case of 2 outcomes in 2 groups, it is equivalent to the Normal test between proportions.

What does it do?
It tells you whether there is a difference in the proportions between the groups.

What is the output?
A p-value which indicates the probability of the data arising from the null hypothesis that there is no association between the proportions of each outcome and the group they are in.

How do you interpret the output?
If the p-value is small then the null is rejected in favour of the alternative. This will represent an association between outcome and group.

What restrictions are there on its use?
The test relies on an underlying Normal assumption to the Binomial distribution. This is likely to be reasonable if the proportions are based on a large enough sample. In practice this equates to having the expected number of outcomes >5 in each cell of the table of group-outcome combinations. There are correction factors that can be applied when there are small numbers, such as Yates continuity correction; however, for small numbers it is more accurate to use exact methods based on properties of the true underlying distribution, such as Fisher's exact test.

Example
We refer again to the data from a study of the effects of smokeless tobacco use and low birth weight in India shown in Table 10.3.[1]

Can we detect a difference between birth weight in the different tobacco groups given these data?

Under the null hypothesis there will be no difference in the proportions of each outcome in each of the groups. For example, overall there were 208 cases of low birth weight out of 974, a proportion of 21.4% and we would expect to see this proportion in each of the 3 groups if there is no association. We calculate the χ^2 value for the whole table by summing the individual values in each of the 6 cells, i.e.

$$\chi^2 = \sum (O_i - E_i)^2 / E_i$$

Where E_i denotes the expected number calculated under the null hypothesis of equal proportions.

In this example the χ^2 value is 10.3, which is compared to tables of the χ^2 distribution. In order to use such a table the number of degrees of freedom must be specified. For an r x c table, where r and c are the number of rows and columns, respectively, there are $(r - 1)(c - 1)$ degrees of freedom which is $(3 - 1)(2 - 1) = 2$ for the 3×2 table in the example. This corresponds to a p-value of 0.006 indicating strong evidence that the null hypothesis is false. Larger values of χ^2 indicate larger differences between the observed and expected numbers, and stronger evidence that there is a difference between the groups.

Reference

1 Gupta, P, Sreevidya S. Smokeless tobacco use, birth weight, and gestational age: population based, prospective cohort study of 1217 women in Mumbai, India. *BMJ* 2004; **328**:1538.

Parametric and non-parametric tests

Many statistical tests require that the data can be assumed to follow some underlying distribution, commonly the Normal distribution. However we may have data for which this cannot be assumed, for example,

- The distribution may be clearly non-Normal.
- The distribution might be Normal, but there are not enough data to establish this.
- The data may be categorical and not able to be placed on a numeric scale.

Methods for CIs and hypothesis tests for the comparison of two means, paired or unpaired, are quite robust—it is not critically important that the data analysed should conform very closely to the Normal distribution. These tests are usually fine to use with reasonably-sized samples as long as the data are unimodal and roughly symmetric about the mode.

If, however, the data are severely non-Normal and sample sizes are small, these methods may be unreliable. Non-parametric tests essentially compare medians rather than means, using the rank order of observations, and they make no assumptions about the underlying distributions of values. They may also be suitable for comparing nominal and ordinal data. The test statistic is compared to pre-calculated critical values to give a p-value. These values are calculated using the Binomial distribution.

Mann–Whitney U test

What is it for?
Comparing the distribution of a numeric variable of 2 groups where the conditions for the independent t-test are not met. It is a non-parametric test (see 📖 p.256).

When is it used?
When the 2 groups are independent samples with small sample sizes and evidence of non-Normality.

What does it do?
It tells you whether the distribution of the variable is significantly different between the 2 groups.

What is the output?
A p-value which indicates the probability that the data are consistent with the null hypothesis of no difference between the groups in terms of the ranks of the observations.

How do you interpret the output?
If the p-value is small then the null is rejected in favour of the alternative. This will represent a difference in either direction (two-tailed alternative) or in a specific direction (one-tailed).

What restrictions are there on its use?
Non-parametric tests are usually used where the data are severely non-Normal and sample sizes are small. If this is not the case then an independent t-test is likely to be more powerful.

Using the test
The null hypothesis is that there is no tendency for members of 1 group to have higher values (of the numeric variable) than members of the other. Treating each pair of data, the test statistic is based on the number of pairs in which the first group has higher values than the second (and vice versa). If this is small, then nearly all the first group have greater values than the second, if it is large nearly all the first group have lower scores than the second.

Wilcoxon's signed-rank test

What is it for?
Comparing the distribution of a numeric variable of 2 linked groups where the conditions for the paired t-test are not met. It is a non-parametric test (see 📖 p.256).

When is it used?
When the members of 2 groups are paired, i.e. the samples are not independent, and there is a small sample size and evidence of non-Normality.

What does it do?
It tells you whether the distribution of the variable is significantly different between the 2 groups.

What is the output?
A p-value which indicates the probability that the data are consistent with the null hypothesis of no difference between the groups in terms of the ranks of the observations.

How do you interpret the output?
If the p-value is small then the null is rejected in favour of the alternative. This will represent a difference in either direction (two-tailed alternative) or in a specific direction (one-tailed).

What restrictions are there on its use?
Non-parametric test are usually used where the data are severely non-normal and sample sizes are small. If this is not the case then a paired t-test is likely to be more powerful.

Linear regression

Regression allows us to analyse the relationship between 2 variables. The most simple and widely used form of such an association is a linear, or straight line, relationship. This involves fitting a straight line through our data points. We could do this by hand, but a degree of error would inevitably be introduced.

Straight lines are described by the basic formula:

$$y = mx + c$$

- y refers to values of the response variable.
- x to values of the explanatory variable.
- m is the slope of the line, i.e. it is the increase (or decrease if −ve) of the response variable per unit increase in the explanatory variable.
- c is the intercept, that is the point at which the line cuts the y axis.

The values of m and c are chosen so that the line is a best fit to the data points. This best fit line goes as far as possible through the middle of the scattered points of the observations on the graph. Note that if we mistakenly swap our explanatory and response variables, then the regression coefficients may be very different.

Least squares regression

In mathematical terms the line is found by minimizing the sum of the squares of the vertical distances from the line. For this reason the method is known as least squares regression.

Example

Measurements of percentage body fat and thigh circumference (in cm) were taken from 20 healthy females aged 20–34 years.[1] The body fat measurements were obtained by a procedure requiring the immersion of the person in water. It would therefore be very helpful if a regression model could provide reliable predictions of the amount of body fat from other measurements which are easier to obtain.

Fig. 10.1 shows a scatter plot where the vertical axis (y) represents the response variable (body fat) and the horizontal axis (x) represents the explanatory variable (thigh circumference).

The scatter plot indicates that there is a positive relationship between the two variables, i.e. increased thigh circumferences associated with increased body fat. Analysis shows:
- Number of observations (N) = 20.
- Intercept (c) = −23.6.
- Slope (m) = 0. 0.86.

The equation for this example will therefore be:

$$\text{Body fat} = 0.86 \times \text{thigh circumference} - 23.6$$

This means for every unit increase in thigh circumference we can predict an increase in body fat of 0.86%. We now have an equation with which we can predict body fat from thigh circumference.

For example, the predicted %body fat for a thigh circumference of 50 would be $0.86 \times 50 - 23.6 = 19.4\%$.

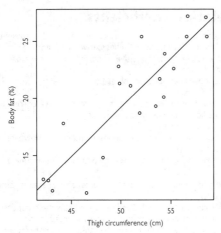

Fig. 10.1 Relationship between thigh circumference (cm) and body fat (%) for a sample of 20 females.

Limitations

There are important limitations which must be considered when drawing conclusions from a regression model such as this.

- We can only use this equation to accurately predict values of body fat within the range 42.3–58.6, i.e. the lowest and highest values of thigh circumference in the range that we are looking at; outside of this range we have no knowledge of what might be happening.
- We have produced this equation from a small sample of the total population. Had we picked a different set of 20 women then we would almost certainly get different values for m and c.
- We can construct a CI for m to see whether it includes zero, which would indicate no relationship between the explanatory and response variables. Again, a larger sample will lead to a smaller confidence interval and thus we will have more confidence in our estimates of the coefficients.

Non-linear regression

It is important to realize that not all relationships will follow such a straightforward pattern. In the example given, within the range of the data given, the relationship appears to be well represented by a linear relationship; however this cannot be the case at very high values (for which the response has an upper limit of 100%) or very low values (where the limit is 0%). For predictions over the entire range of possible values of the explanatory variable we would have to consider possible non-linear relationships. Techniques are available to overcome these problems and it is possible to fit highly complex curves to data.

Reference

1 Neter MH, *et al. Applied linear statistical models* (4th edn). Boston, MA: McGraw-Hill; 1996.

Correlation coefficients

A correlation coefficient is a measure of how well a straight line fits
the data. The coefficient takes values between +1 and −1 depending on
whether the relationship is positive or negative and how close the points
lie to a straight line.

Fig. 10.2 shows examples of correlation coefficients, r, for values close
to +1, −1, and zero.
- +1 indicates that the relationship is a perfect positive correlation, i.e. all
the points lie on the line which slopes up.
- −1 indicates a perfect negative relationship.
- 0 indicates there is no linear relationship; there may however be a non-
linear relationship.
- The further r is from 0, the closer the points will lie around a straight
line.

There are a number of different measures of correlation, examples of
which include:
- Pearson's linear correlation coefficient: probably the most commonly
used as it relates directly to fitting a linear regression model.
- Spearman's rank correlation: uses the ranks of the data rather
than their actual values. This may be advisable where a non-linear
relationship is suspected.
- Kendall's tau: compares the ranks of pairs of observations. This gives a
measure that will be 1 for complete agreement between X and Y and
−1 for complete disagreement.

Values of the correlation coefficients for the body fat and thigh circumfer-
ence data shown in Figure 10.1 are as follows:
- Pearson's correlation coefficient: 0.878.
- Spearman's rank correlation coefficient: 0.850.
- Kendall's tau: 0.653.

In each case, there appears to be strong correlation between the two
variables.

Association and causation

Regression allows us to look at the relationship between two quantitative variables, but it must be remembered that even when we find strong
associations, they are not necessarily causal (see 📖 pp.156–61). It is a
common error to assume that because 2 variables are related, 1 must
cause the other. This is not true; it may be that an apparent relationship
or a strong correlation between the 2 variables is in fact due to a third,
unmeasured variable, or confounder.

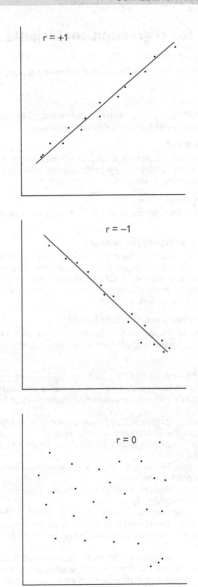

Fig. 10.2 Examples of correlation coefficients.

T-tests for regression coefficients

What is it for?
To assess whether association between 2 variables in a regression model is significant.

When is it used?
When a regression model has been fit to assess the relationship between a response variable and 1 or more explanatory variables.

What does it do?
It tells you whether a regression coefficient (slope) associated with a particular explanatory variable is significantly different from zero and thus a significant relationship exists.

What is the output?
A p-value which indicates the probability that the true value of the coefficient is zero.

How do you interpret the output?
If the p-value is small then the null is rejected in favour of the alternative, that there is a significant association between the response and the explanatory variable in question. One-tailed alternatives refer to an association in a specific direction, either positive or negative, whilst two-tailed alternatives don't make such a distinction.

What restrictions are there on its use?
The test relies on the assumption that the sampling distribution of the estimates of the regression coefficients are Normally distributed.

Example
For the body fat example (see 📖 p.260), the question is whether there is a significant association between thigh circumference and body fat.

We first identify null and alternative hypotheses and significance level we are looking for.

If the response variable is completely unrelated to the explanatory variables, i.e. if the explanatory variable contributes nothing to the prediction of y irrespective of its value, then this would indicate that the slope m is equal to zero.

Null hypothesis, H_0: m = 0, there is no association between thigh circumference and body fat.

Alternative hypothesis, H_A: m ≥0, there is a positive association between thigh circumference and body fat.

To carry out the test we calculate a t-statistic based on the observed difference between the estimate (of the slope, m) from the sample and that under the null hypothesis (zero) divided by the standard error (of the estimate of the slope).

The output from a regression model is often reported in terms of the coefficients (in this case the intercept and the slope associated with thigh circumference) together with their standard errors and possibly t-statistics and associated p-values (Table 10.5).

Table 10.5 Results from a linear regression analysis of body fat (%) against thigh circumference (cm)

	Estimate	SE	t	p-value
Intercept	−23.6345	5.6574	−4.178	0.0006
Thigh	0.8565	0.1100	7.786	<0.001

We are interested in the coefficient (slope) for thigh and not the intercept. The t-statistic is calculated as

$$t = (m \text{ from the sample} - m \text{ from the null hypothesis})/SE = 7.79$$

The degrees of freedom for a test of a regression coefficient is $(N - p)$ where p is the number of parameters that have been fit in the model, in this case 2 (the intercept and slope). Therefore $df = (20 - 2) = 18$, giving a one-sided p-value of <0.001. This means that there is a significant positive association (positive as the sign of the slope is positive) between thigh circumference and body fat in this sample of women.

Multiple regression

Multiple regression is a natural extension of the simple linear regression model which is used to predict values of an outcome from several explanatory variables.

Each explanatory variable has its own coefficient and the outcome variable is predicted from a combination of all the variables multiplied by their respective coefficients.

Example

In the body fat example (see 📖 p.260), in addition to body fat and thigh circumference there were also measurements of mid-arm circumference for the sample of 20 women.

A multiple regression model using the 2 possible explanatory variables will give estimates and standard errors for each variable (plus the intercept). In this example, the coefficient for a particular variable is estimated allowing for the fact that the other variables are also in the model (Table 10.6).

Table 10.6 Results from multiple regression analysis of body fat (%) against thigh circumference (cm) and mid-arm circumference (cm)

	Estimate	SE	t	p-value
Intercept	−25.99695	6.99732	−3.715	0.00172
Thigh	0.85088	0.11245	7.567	7.72E-07
Mid-arm	0.09603	0.16139	0.595	0.55968

We can see that of the 2 variables, thigh has a much stronger relationship with body fat than mid-arm, which is non-significant and thus would not be considered to add any additional explanatory power.

Assessment of the regression model

The output from a regression analysis will often be expressed in terms of an analysis of variance (ANOVA) (see 📖 p.268). The idea is to express the total variability in the response variable into components that can be explained by the regression line and that left as unexplained, or random, variation. We desire as much variability as possible to be explained by the regression line and not left as unexplained. The ratio of the different components of variation can then be assessed by an F-test.

Other summary statistics that are commonly presented for a regression analysis are:
- R^2 = the proportion of the total variation that can be explained by the regression line.
- R^2 (adjusted), which adjusts for the number of explanatory terms in a model.

Unlike R^2, the adjusted R^2 increases only if the new term improves the model more than would be expected by chance.

We are often interested in whether a particular explanatory variable should be included in the regression model, i.e. does it have a significant contribution to the prediction of the response given the other variables in the model? We can assess the contribution of a variable by omitting it from the regression model and seeing whether the explanatory power has decreased, either by comparing the values of R^2 or more formally by performing an ANOVA comparing the residual sum of squares from the 2 models.

Model choice

Dealing with a number of explanatory variables brings into question the important issue of which ones should be included in the model. If adding a particular variable causes a significant improvement in the fit of the model, i.e. a significant reduction in the error, then it should be included in the model.

There are several approaches to this, which include:
- Including all explanatory variables, known as the 'full model'.
- Experimenter decides which variables are included in the model (and in which order they are entered).
- Automatic methods, such as 'stepwise selection' where variables are automatically selected according to pre-defined criteria.

Care is needed because the values of the regression coefficients will depend on which other variables are included in the model and especially when explanatory variables are correlated, the order in which they are entered into the model can have a great effect.

Various stepwise methods are used to determine which variables should be included in the model, but variable selection may depend upon only slight differences between candidates and these slight numerical differences can lead to major differences in the final choice of model. They should therefore only really be used for exploration of the data.

Ideally, variables should be selected on information from past research. In this case, known predictors should be entered into the model first and entered in the order of their importance in predicting the outcome. New predictors are then entered into the model in order of their importance (based on statistical criteria) in predicting the outcome.

Model checking

When assessing the validity of a multiple regression model, it is important to try and check whether the assumptions of the model seem to hold. These include:
- Are the relationships linear?
- Are the deviations (residuals) from the regression line Normally distributed around the line?
- Are the variances constant over all values of the explanatory variables?
- If two explanatory variables are correlated with the outcome but also with each other, which (if any) is having an effect?

Analysis of variance

What is it for?

To assess the relative explanatory power and significance of variables in a regression model.

When is it used?

When a regression model has been fitted to assess the relationship between a response variable and 1 or more explanatory variables.

What does it do?

The idea is to express the total variability in the response variable into components that can be explained by the regression line and that left as unexplained, or random, variation often referred to as residual variation.

What is the output?

The ratio of the different components of variation, which can be assessed by an F-test.

How do you interpret the output?

The F-statistic represents the ratio of the variation explained by an explanatory variable compared with that left unexplained by the regression model. If the ratio is high, it indicates that the explanatory variable in question is an important predictor. The associated p-value indicates whether the ratio is significantly greater than one.

What restrictions are there on its use?

The test relies on the assumption that the sampling distribution of the estimates of the regression coefficients are Normally distributed.

Example

The weight and various physical measurements for 22 male participants aged 16–30 years were recorded. Participants were randomly chosen volunteers, all in reasonably good health from a university in Australia.[1]

Table 10.7 shows the results of running a multiple regression model with mass as response variable against all the variables (known as the full model). Here we can clearly see that the waist circumference is a highly significant predictor and that height is just significant (at the 5% level).

The ANOVA table for this regression line including all of the possible explanatory variables is shown in Table 10.8, with values of R^2 and R^2(adj) being 98% and 96% respectively and the F-statistic giving a p-value of <0.0001. The regression model (as a whole) is clearly a significant predictor of the variability in the response variable.

Often ANOVA is used to assess whether variables need to be included in the model, i.e. do they contribute significant explanatory power. In this example, it does not look as though the width of an individual's shoulders is a powerful predictor of their body mass, at least when the other variables are included in the model.

In addition to the t-test of the coefficient in the model which is non-significant (t = −0.122, p = 0.905), we can compare models with and without shoulder included in the variable list. Table 10.9 gives an ANOVA table for a comparison between two such models.

Table 10.7 Results of a multiple regression analysis of mass against a selection of explanatory variables for a sample of 22 males

	Estimate	SE	t	P-value
Intercept	−69.517	29.037	−2.394	0.036
Foream	1.782	0.855	2.085	0.061
Bicep	0.155	0.485	0.320	0.755
Chest	0.189	0.226	0.838	0.420
Neck	−0.482	0.721	−0.669	0.518
Shoulder	−0.029	0.239	−0.122	0.905
Waist	0.661	0.116	5.679	0.000
Height	0.318	0.130	2.438	0.033
Calf	0.446	0.413	1.081	0.303
Thigh	0.297	0.305	0.974	0.351
Head	−0.920	0.520	−1.768	0.105

Table 10.8 Analysis of variance table for full regression model. Same data as Table 10.7

Source of variation	Sum of squares	Df	Mean squares (SS/df)	F
Regression	2466.63	10	246.663	47.17
Residual	57.52	11	5.229	
Total	2524.15	21		

Table 10.9 Analysis of variance for difference between two models; with and without the inclusion of width of shoulder (cm)

Model	Residual df	Residual sum of squares	Change in sum of squares	F statistic	P-value
Including shoulder	11	57.52	–	–	
Excluding shoulder	12	57.60	−0.08	0.015	0.905

Again, we conclude that the effect of shoulder is non-significant as predictor of body mass when the other variables are included in the model. Note that the p-value for the F-test is the same as that for the t-test of the coefficients. This is because there is a direct relationship between the F and t-statistics, $F = t^2$, i.e. here $0.015 = (-0.122^2)$ and they will always lead to identical conclusions. At the same time, the adjusted-R^2 increased slightly, from 0.957 to 0.960 reflecting the fact that the inclusion of shoulder did not provide enough additional explanatory power to warrant another variable in the model.

In contrast, excluding waist resulted in a significant drop in the variation that could be explained by the model, resulting in more variation being 'left over' or unexplained. Table 10.10 gives the results of excluding waist from the full model.

The same technique can be used to compare the results from omitting groups of variables. For example, omitting the effect of all the variables except for waist and length of forearm can be observed in Table 10.11 which results in a non-significant drop in explanatory power.

Table 10.10 Analysis of variance table for difference between two models; with and without waist (cm)

Model	Residual df	Residual sum of squares	Change in sum of squares	F statistic	P-value
Including waist	11	57.52	–	–	–
Excluding waist	12	226.15	−168.63	32.2	0.000

Table 10.11 Analysis of variance table for difference between two models; full model and model with just waist (cm) and length of forearm (cm)

Model	Residual df	Residual sum of squares	Change in sum of squares	F statistic	P-value
Full model (all variables)	11	57.52	–	–	–
Excluding all but waist and forearm	19	160.536	−103.01	2.46	0.084

Reference
1 Sall, J. *JMP Start Statistics, Third Edition*. Cary, NC: SAS Institute Inc; 2006.

Logistic regression

What is it for?

For predicting probabilities and odds ratios (ORs) from a set of explanatory variables.

When is it used?

Formally, when the logistic function is applied to the response variable in a regression model to ensure that predictions are within the range zero to 1. It is often used to analyse data from case–control studies (see 📖 pp.172–4).

What does it do?

In the simplest case, with a single explanatory variable, the regression line will take the following form:

$$\log(p / 1 - p) = mx + c$$

Where p is the probability of a successful outcome. In case–control stuides $\log(p/1-p)$ represents the log of the OR.

This can be extended to incorporate additional variables as with multiple regression.

What is the output?

Estimates of the parameters in the model, together with associated standard errors (SEs) as with linear regression.

How do you interpret the output?

The coefficient representing the slope represents the increase in $\log(p/1 - p)$, the log of the OR, associated with a unit increase in x. By taking the exponential of this coefficient, exp(m) in the model described, we can estimate the OR associated with a unit increase in x.

What restrictions are there on its use?

The response variable must be between zero and 1 and the error or residual term should follow a Binomial distribution.

Example

High levels of vitamin E are thought to be protective of cancer. This hypothesis was investigated by measuring vitamin E in stored blood samples from 271 men in a large cohort study who subsequently developed cancer. These values were compared with those from 533 control men who at the time had not developed cancer.[1]

The results of running a logistic regression analysis are shown in Table 10.12.

Table 10.12 Results of performing a logistic regression of the relationship between levels of vitamin E (mg/L) and cancer

	Estimate	Standard error
Intercept	0.642	0.161
Vitamin E (mg/L)	−0.028	0.003

It is important to be aware of the precise interpretation of the slope, m, in this case. Here, a decrease of 0.028 is predicted in the log odds of cancer for a unit increase in the explanatory variable, 1mg/L of vitamin E. Taking the exponential of this coefficient gives the odds ratio, exp(−0.028) = 0.972. In order to assess whether this reduction in the odds ratio is significant, we can perform a t-test or construct a confidence interval.

Null hypothesis, H_0: m = 0, there is no association between vitamin E intake and cancer.

Alternative hypothesis, H_A: m ≠ 0, there is an association between vitamin E intake and cancer.

  t = (m from the sample − m from the null hypothesis)/SE
  = −0.028/0.003 = −9.33, which gives a p-value of <0.001.

To calculate a CI for the slope, we assume that the estimate is Normally distributed (as N is large). It is calculated as −0.028 ±(1.96 × 0.003) or −(0.0339, −0.0221). This interval doesn't include zero and so we conclude, as with the t-test, that there is a significant (inverse) association between vitamin E intake and cancer.

This CI is calculated on the log scale. In order to obtain a CI for the odds ratio we need to take the exponential of the limits of this interval, i.e. exp(−0.0339) and exp(−0.0221) or (0.967, 0.978) which notably doesn't include one. As the interval was calculated on the log scale, it is not symmetrical when converted to the ordinal scale.

Reference

1 Wald NJ et al. Serum vitamin E and subsequent risk of cancer. *Br J Cancer*. 1987; **56**(1):69–72.

Measuring survival

We often have data that represent the time from some event, such as diagnosis, or entry into a clinical trial to an outcome of interest, e.g. death, readmission to hospital, recurrence of a tumour. We usually refer to the terminal event as the end-point and people who have not yet experienced the endpoint as 'survivors'.

Censoring

Problems arise in the measurement of survival because often we do not know the exact survival times of all participants; often the end-point has not occurred by the time the data are to be analysed. The exact time of occurrence is therefore censored. Censored observations cannot simply be ignored since they carry important information, e.g. we know that the participant has at least reached the end time point occurrence-free.

An important assumption that is often made is that the censoring is non-informative; that is the actual survival time of a person is independent of any censoring mechanism. So for a group of similar individuals someone who is censored at a given time must be representative of all other people who have survived until that time.

Survivor and hazard functions

The survivor function is the probability that the survival time, T, is at least t, i.e. $\text{Prob}(T \geq t)$. If there is no censoring, then the survivor function can be estimated by:

$$\tilde{S}(t) = \frac{\text{number with survival time} \geq t}{\text{total number of individuals}}$$

The hazard function is the instantaneous death rate for an individual who has survived to time t.

Kaplan–Meier product limit estimator

What is it for?

To estimate the survival of individuals over a period of time based on data comprising times to event, e.g. death or remission.

When is it used?

It is often used when there is right-censored data, which occurs if a patient withdraws from a study, i.e. is lost from the sample before the final outcome is observed.

What does it do?

Estimates the survivor function, i.e. the probability that an individual survives until at least a specified time.

What is the output?

A table or graph showing the probabilities of survival at different points in time, which are defined by the times to event in the data.

How do you interpret the output?

A plot of the Kaplan–Meier estimate is a series of horizontal steps. The rate of decline indicates the rate at which the events occur over time. Often we will want to compare 2 (or more) survival distributions; e.g. does a treatment group have increased survival over a control group? To simply compare 2 survival distributions we can plot Kaplan–Meier estimates of each group on the same plot.

What restrictions are there on its use?

It can be used when actual times to event are known, rather than just (time) intervals in which the event occurred.

Example

Measurements were made on patients with malignant melanoma. Each patient had their tumour removed by surgery. Patients were followed for a period of up to 15 years.[1]

The Kaplan–Meier plots for males and females can be seen in Fig. 10.3 in which the solid (black) line is the estimated survivor function for females and the dashed (blue) line for males. The line for females is clearly higher than that for males, indicating greater survival over time. In order to test whether this apparent difference is statistically significant a *log-rank test* can be performed.

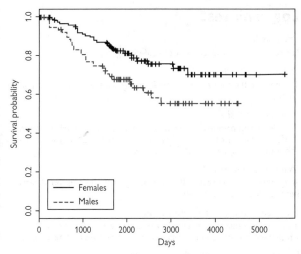

Fig. 10.3 Kaplan–Meier estimates of the survivor functions for patients having surgery for malignant melanoma, by gender.

Reference

1 Andersen PK et al. *Statistical Models Based on Counting Processes*. New York: Springer-Verlag; 1993.

Log-rank test

What is it for?
For comparing survival curves from different groups.

When is it used?
To compare the survival over time from 2 groups, e.g. a treatment and a control group.

What does it do?
Provides a non-parametric test which makes use of the full survival data to detect differences in survival curves. It doesn't make any assumptions about the underlying form of the 2 curves.

What is the output?
A p-value which indicates the probability that there is no difference between the 2 survival curves.

How do you interpret the output?
If the p-value is small then the null is rejected in favour of the alternative under which there is a significant difference between the curves at some time point.

What restrictions are there on its use?
Expected numbers for both groups are calculated for intervals of time and compared to those observed. A chi-squared test is then performed and therefore the expected numbers should be >5.

Example
Using the data on survival after surgery for malignant melanoma (see 📖 p.276):

$$H_0: S_1(t) = S_2(t) \text{ no difference in survival time}$$
$$H_A: S_1(t) \neq S_2(t) \text{ for some t there is a difference}$$

By dividing the time into time intervals in the same way as for the Kaplan–Meier estimator (see 📖 p.276), we calculate the expected number of deaths in each interval under the null hypothesis. A chi-squared test-statistic is then calculated by comparing the observed and expected numbers of deaths.

In this example, the observed and expected numbers are calculated as shown in Table 10.13.

Table 10.13 Log-rank test for differences in survival between genders

	N	Observed	Expected	$(O - E)^2/E$
Females	126	28	37.1	2.25
Males	79	29	19.9	4.21

Therefore the test statistic is $\chi^2 = \Sigma(O_i - E_i)^2/E_i = 6.46$ on 1 df, which gives a p-value of 0.011 and so we conclude that there is a statistically significant difference between the survival of males and females.

Cox proportional hazards model

What is it for?
For comparing survival curves from different groups.

When is it used?
Where it is important to know which explantory variables are associated with survival, and the size of the association, but knowing the actual survival distribution is not as important.

What does it do?
Model the dependence of survival times on explanatory variables without specifying the distribution of survival times.

What is the output?
Estimates of the parameters in the model together with associated standard errors.

How do you interpret the output?
If the p-value associated with a particular explanatory variable is small then it provides evidence that the variable is significantly associated with survival.

What restrictions are there on its use?
It assumes that the hazard at time t for a patient in 1 group is proportional to the hazard at time t for a patient in the second group (known as proportional hazards). It doesn't provide information on the underlying distribution of survival.

Example
Using the data on survival after surgery for malignant melanoma (see 📖 p.276), we fit a Cox proportional hazards model with age and sex as explanatory variables (Table 10.14).

Table 10.14 Results of fitting a Cox proportional hazards model to survival times after surgery for malignant melanoma

	Estimate	Exp(coeff.)	SE(coeff.)	z	p
Sex	0.5983	1.82	0.268	2.24	0.025
Age	0.0165	1.02	0.009	1.91	0.056

Here we see that there is a significant effect of gender but age is just non-significant. The exponentiated coefficients in the third column of Table 10.14 can be interpreted as the multiplicative effects on the hazard. For example, keeping the value of age constant, the increased hazard of being male compared to female is exp(0.598) = 1.82, i.e. an increase of 82%.

Receiver operating characteristic curves

What is it for?

To assess the utility of a test (diagnostic, screening) for distinguishing positive and negative results.

When is it used?

To examine the trade-off between sensitivity and specificity when using different cut-off points to define positive and negative outcomes. Can be used to compare the performance of different tests. This method is also used to assess the validity of different predictive scoring methods.

What does it do?

A curve is plotted of 1 − specificity (x-axis) against the sensitivity (y-axis) for several cut-off points. If this is plotted for different tests for the same condition it can provide a comparison of the test performance.

What is the output?

It produces a graphical demonstration of the trade-off between sensitivity and specificity. It is usually shown with a diagonal line (at 45 degrees) with the receiver operating characteristic (ROC) curve to the left of the line. The area under the curve may be calculated and compared with that from other tests.

How do you interpret the output?

The greater the area under the curve the better the test performs. Good tests therefore have ROC curves which go furthest into the top left corner. When comparing more than one test, additional statistical analyses can be performed including logistic regression (see 📖 p.272).

Example

Clinicians wanted to develop a tool for use in emergency medicine to help distinguish serious from self-limiting infection in febrile children. They used 40 different criteria to develop a clinical decision-making model and compared this with clinical judgement in the prediction of serious bacterial infection.[1]

They used results from 15,000 visits, and used a ROC curve in their analysis. Fig. 10.4 shows results of the predictive model with different cut-off points (solid line) compared with clinician estimation for urinary tract infection (circles (data points) and broken line).

The diagonal line is the reference, in which the test would be ineffective at distinguishing diseased and non-diseased.

The model curve shows how as the sensitivity of the model increases specificity declines, such that as the model reaches 0.9 (or 90%) sensitivity, specificity falls to around 0.4 (i.e. 1 − specificity is 0.6). You can see how the choice of cut-off depends on whether it is more important to pick up most cases, in which case choose a point to the top of the sensitivity distribution, with the recognition that this will lead to overtreatment, or be highly specific and risk missing most cases. The clinicians diagnoses were highly specific at 90–100%, (i.e. 1 − specificity = 0–0.1) but had low sensitivity, thus missing around 50% of the cases at best.

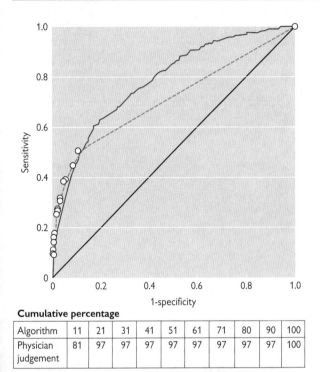

Cumulative percentage

Algorithm	11	21	31	41	51	61	71	80	90	100
Physician judgement	81	97	97	97	97	97	97	97	97	100

Fig. 10.4 ROC curve of the model (solid line) compared with clinician estimation for urinary tract infection (circles (data points) and broken line). Cumulative percentage displays the distribution of the false positive rates. Reproduced from Craig JC et al. *BMJ* 2010; **340**:bmj.c1594, with permission from BMJ Publishing Group Ltd.

Reference

1 Craig J C et al. The accuracy of clinical symptoms and signs for the diagnosis of serious bacterial infection in young febrile children: prospective cohort study of 15 781 febrile illnesses. *BMJ* 2010; **340**:bmj.c1594.

Epidemiology of common diseases

Introduction

This handbook ends with a handy reference section that briefly summarizes what we know about the epidemiology of common diseases.

Chapter 11 provides a brief overview of the distribution of the burden of disease in the world, in Europe, and in the UK, contrasting non-communicable and communicable disease. It uses data from the Global Burden of Disease study and makes use of the concept of disability adjusted life years (DALYs). The definition of DALYs is included here with reference to further reading.

Chapter 12 provides summary epidemiological information on 40 of the most common or important conditions. These are presented in alphabetical order for ease of reference. The choice of conditions to include has been difficult, but they cover the major causes of mortality and morbidity for both chronic and infectious diseases in the UK and other high-income countries, plus a few of the most significant conditions from lower-income countries such as malaria and neglected tropical disease.

For each condition we have provided a structured report, starting with a very brief summary of the condition followed by the descriptive epidemiology that includes estimates of incidence, prevalence, mortality, case fatality, some measure of morbidity, and the broad distribution by time, person, and place. We then report the fixed and modifiable risk factors followed by key approaches to prevention and control. There is no one source of all this information for each disease, so we have collated data from a number of sources which are cited in the text and can be checked for updates over time.

We hope that this section will provide a useful resource for clinicians considering likely diagnoses in their patients, and also for students and doctors in training who are learning about diseases and revising for exams.

Global burden of disease

Terminology

In this final section of the book we describe the epidemiology of diseases in the world. We look at the burden of non-communicable and communicable disease at the global, European, and UK level. These estimates are limited by measurement difficulties, but we present both mortality and a composite measure of morbidity and mortality, the disability-adjusted life year (DALY).

The DALY is a measure combining years of life lost due to premature mortality with years of life lost due to time lived in poor health. It was developed for the World Bank and is now widely used by WHO and other global institutions to compare the health burdens of different diseases across the world:

$$DALY = YLL + YLD$$

(where YLL is years of life lost, YLD is years lived with disability).

1 DALY is a year of perfect health lost. Diseases that cause long-term disability, such as mental health problems, may lead to a large proportion of DALYs without being major causes of mortality.

Further reading

Murray CJL, Lopez AD (eds) *The Global Burden of Disease*. Cambridge, MA: Harvard University Press on behalf of the World Health Organization and the World Bank; 1996.

WHO. *The Global Burden of Disease: 2004 Update*. Geneva: WHO; 2008. ℘ http://www.who.int/healthinfo/global_burden_disease

Global burden of non-communicable disease

Non-communicable disease is the major cause of mortality in high-income countries, and its importance is growing in middle- and low-income countries as the control and treatment of infectious disease improves. This shift from a predominant infectious disease burden to non-infectious conditions is known as the 'epidemiological transition'.

Mortality

Globally non-communicable diseases are responsible for 59.6% of deaths. Cardiovascular disease is the leading cause of death, responsible for 17.1 million deaths a year[1] (Table 11.1); the distribution of chronic disease deaths in Europe is shown in Table 11.2.

Morbidity

The burden of chronic disease morbidity is also high and people are often affected for many years. However, many conditions can be prevented or ameliorated by lifestyle changes including smoking cessation, weight loss, and physical activity (see 📖 pp.60–3).

Although low- and middle-income countries experience most of the global burden of infectious disease, almost half of their burden of disease is caused by non-communicable conditions. The burden of non-communicable disease in middle- and low-income countries is increasing as the prevalence of high BP, high serum cholesterol, smoking, and obesity increases.

Overall burden

When DALYs are used to estimate the overall burden of disease, a number of conditions that are rarely fatal become much more important. For example, mental health problems represent a huge burden of disease while not contributing much to overall mortality.

Inequality

The risk of developing a non-communicable condition often increases with age. Therefore the prevalence of these conditions tends to be higher in the high-income countries due to their older population.

Morbidity and mortality can often be improved with healthcare. Therefore the burden of disease can disproportionately affect lower-income countries where resource scarcity can limit healthcare provision, and they suffer under the dual burden of communicable and non-communicable disease.

As knowledge about the causes of non-communicable conditions continues to grow, richer countries are often able to take action to protect their population. For example, they may introduce stricter controls over occupational chemical exposure, tobacco control interventions, and healthy eating initiatives.

Table 11.1 Global burden of non-communicable diseases, 2004[1]

	Number of deaths (millions)	% of all deaths	% of all DALYs
All causes	58.8	100.0	100
Non-communicable causes			
Cardiovascular disease	17.1	29.1	9.9
Malignant cancer	7.4	12.6	5.1
Injuries	5.8	9.8	12.3
Respiratory diseases	4.0	6.9	3.9
Digestive diseases	2.0	3.5	2.8
Neuropsychiatric disorders	1.3	2.1	13.1
Genitourinary disease	0.9	1.6	1.0
Musculoskeletal disease	0.1	0.2	2.0
Specific conditions			
Coronary heart disease	7.2	12.2	4.1
Cerebrovascular disease	5.7	9.7	3.1
Chronic obstructive pulmonary disease (COPD)	3.0	5.1	2.0
Lung, tracheal, bronchus cancer	1.3	2.3	0.8
Road traffic accidents	1.3	2.2	2.7
Diabetes mellitus	1.1	1.9	1.3
Hypertensive heart disease	1.0	1.7	0.5
Self-inflicted injuries	0.8	1.4	1.3
Stomach cancer	0.8	1.4	0.5
Cirrhosis of the liver	0.8	1.3	0.9
Nephritis and nephrosis	0.7	1.3	0.6
Colon and rectum cancers	0.6	1.1	0.4

Table 11.2 European burden of non-communicable diseases, 2004[1]

	Number of deaths (millions)	% of all deaths	% of all DALYs
All causes	9.5	100.0	100
Non-communicable causes			
Cardiovascular disease	5	50.2	22.9
Malignant cancer	2	19.6	11.3
Injuries	0.8	8.3	13.2
Respiratory diseases	0.4	3.9	3.9
Digestive diseases	0.4	4.4	4.6
Neuropsychiatric disorders	0.3	3.0	19.1
Genitourinary disease	0.1	1.2	0.9
Musculoskeletal disease	0.028	0.3	3.6
Specific conditions			
Coronary heart disease	2.3	24.2	11.1
Cerebrovascular disease	1.4	14.4	6.3
COPD	0.2	2.5	2.0
Lung, tracheal, bronchus cancer	0.4	3.9	2.2
Road traffic accidents	0.1	1.4	2.4
Diabetes mellitus	0	1.6	1.8
Hypertensive heart disease	0.2	1.9	0.8
Self-inflicted injuries	0.2	1.6	2.0
Stomach cancer	0.2	1.6	0.9
Cirrhosis of the liver	0.2	1.9	2.0
Nephritis and nephrosis	0.08	0.8	0.4
Colon and rectum cancers	0.2	2.5	1.3

Reference

1 WHO. *The Global Burden of Disease: 2004 Update*. Geneva: WHO; 2008. ♒ http://www.who.int/healthinfo/global_burden_disease

Burden of non-communicable disease in the UK

Mortality

In 2005 there were 580,000 deaths in the UK.[1] The top categories of causes of death were:
- Circulatory: 36.0%.
- Neoplasm: 27.2%.
- Respiratory: 14.0%.
- Digestive: 5.0%.
- External causes: 3.3%.
- Mental/behavioural: 3.0%.

Infectious and parasitic diseases only accounted for 1.2% of deaths.

Overall burden

In 2004 the UK was assessed as having 7.5 million DALYs overall, of which 87.5% were due to non-communicable diseases.[1] The top 4 global burden of disease categories in the UK account for 68% of total UK DALYs:
- Neuropsychiatric conditions: 1.97 million (26% of total).
- Cardiovascular disease: 1.30 million (17%).
- Malignant neoplasms: 1.17 million (15%).
- Respiratory diseases: 691,000 (9%).

Demands on healthcare

- Chronic diseases are a major burden on the UK NHS.
- This burden will only increase as the population ages.
- Modifiable factors increase the risk of common chronic conditions and the need for healthcare, including obesity, high BP, smoking, and physical inactivity.
- Obesity is common. In England >60% of the adult population and 30% of children are overweight or obese.[2]
- 30% of adults in England have high BP and almost half of these are not being treated for it.[2]
- 22% of adults in England are current cigarette smokers.[2]

Healthcare costs

- Healthcare costs for chronic conditions increase as technologies advance.
- In 2008/09 the UK NHS had a budget of >£100 billion which equates to approximately £1980 per person.[3]
- Over 800 million prescriptions were dispensed in the community by the NHS in 2009, costing >£8.5 billion.[4]
- 18 of the 20 most commonly prescribed drugs treat non-communicable diseases and 4 of the top 5 of these drugs were for cardiovascular disease.[4]

Inequality

- The prevalence of non-communicable conditions increases with age.
- Men are more likely to be a current cigarette smoker than women (24% v 20%).[2]

- Obesity is more common in populations living in the most deprived areas compared to the most affluent areas (27% v 24%).[5]
- Smoking is much more common in the most deprived communities (34%) than the most affluent (14%).[5]

References

1 Green S, Miles R. *The burden of illness and disease in the UK*. London: Department of Health; 2007.
2 The NHS Information Centre. *Health Survey for England 2008 trend tables*. London: The NHS Information Centre for health and social care; 2009. ♒ http://http://www.ic.nhs.uk/pubs/hse08trends
3 NHS website: ♒ http://www.nhs.uk
4 The NHS Information Centre. *Prescriptions dispensed in the community: England, statistics for 1999 to 2009*. The Health and Social Care Information Centre, Prescribing Support Unit. 2010. ♒ http://www.ic.nhs.uk
5 The NHS Information Centre. *A summary of public health indicators using electronic data from primary care*. QRESEARCH and the Health and Social Care Information Centre, 2008. ♒ http://www.ic.nhs.uk

Global burden of communicable disease

Overall, infectious and parasitic diseases cause just under 20% of the global burden of disease (see Table 11.3).

Mortality

The proportion of deaths due to communicable diseases declined in rich countries in the 20th century, but they remain important causes of morbidity and continue to present new challenges such as HIV/AIDS and other emerging infections. Globally infectious and parasitic diseases are responsible for 16.2% of deaths, a large number of which are preventable. HIV/AIDS, for example, is the leading cause of adult deaths in sub-Saharan Africa. More than 90% of deaths from communicable diseases are caused by a handful of diseases: lower respiratory infections, HIV/AIDS, diarrhoeal diseases, TB, malaria, and measles.

Morbidity

The burden of communicable disease morbidity is also high. Infectious diseases in childhood, whilst not always associated with high mortality, can lead to poor development and educational achievement for millions of children in low- and middle-income countries, and to loss of productivity and opportunity for adults. In the UK, communicable diseases place a high level of demand on health services and burden of disease and loss of work for individuals.

Inequality

The burden is unevenly distributed between regions of the world, with a much higher proportion of mortality, ill health, and disability attributable to communicable diseases in poorer regions and countries. Major causes of death and disability in the world, such as diarrhoeal disease, measles, and malaria, are far less important in areas such as Europe, as shown by comparing Tables 11.3 and 11.4. However, inequalities also exist within regions and countries, with the burden of disease falling disproportionately on poorer sections of the population. Within Europe, for example, communicable disease causes 1.5% of deaths in high-income areas compared with 2.9% in low- and middle-income areas. In the poorest regions there is an additional burden from neglected tropical diseases (see pp.356–7) which are estimated to affect >1 billion people.

Table 11.3 Global burden of communicable diseases, 2004[1]

	Number of deaths	% of all deaths	% of all DALYs
All infectious and parasitic diseases	9.5 million	16.2	19.8
Lower respiratory infections	4.2 million	7.1	6.2
Diarrhoeal diseases	2.2 million	3.7	4.8
HIV/AIDS	2.0 million	3.5	3.8
Tuberculosis	1.5 million	2.5	2.2
Malaria	0.9 million	1.5	2.2
Childhood infections* (incl. measles)	0.9 million	1.4	2.0
Measles	0.4 million	0.7	1.0
Hepatitis B & C	0.2 million	0.3	0.2
Neglected tropical diseases**	0.2 million	0.3	1.3
STIs excluding HIV	0.1 million	0.2	0.7

*Childhood infections includes pertussis, polio, diphtheria, measles, tetanus;
**See 🕮 Neglected tropical diseases, p.356 for definitions.

Table 11.4 European burden of communicable diseases, 2004[1]

	Number of deaths (000s)	% of all deaths	% of all DALYs
All infectious and parasitic diseases	219	2.3	4.0
Lower respiratory infections	235	2.5	1.7
Diarrhoeal diseases	39	0.4	0.9
HIV/AIDS	31	0.3	0.8
Tuberculosis	77	0.8	1.1
Meningitis	11	0.1	0.2
Hepatitis B & C	12	0.1	0.1
STIs excluding HIV	1	0.01	0.2
Childhood infections** (incl. measles)	1	0.01	0.04

Reference

1 WHO. *The Global Burden of Disease: 2004 Update.* Geneva: WHO; 2008. 🔗 http://www.who.int/healthinfo/global_burden_disease

Burden of communicable disease in the UK

Mortality from infectious disease declined over the last century from 20% of deaths in 1911 to around 6.6% today. This includes 1% from infections and parasitic diseases such as TB, HIV, and meningitis, and 5.5% from influenza and pneumonia.[1] However, infections are still responsible for a significant amount of illness placing a strain on individuals, health services, and the economy.

Demands on healthcare

- 20% of the population suffer from an infectious intestinal disease each year (although only 3% consult a GP).
- Almost 1% of calls to NHS Direct are related to colds or flu-like illness.
- 35% of all GP consultations in England are infectious disease related, and approximately half of those made by children.
- 40% of people in the UK consult their GP at least once a year because of some infectious disease.
- 4% of admissions and 5% of bed-days are attributable to infectious diseases.

Healthcare costs

- The HPA estimates the annual cost of treating communicable disease in England at £6 billion:[2]
  - Primary care bears the highest burden of costs at £3.5 billion.
  - Hospital admissions costs are around £900 million.
  - Infectious intestinal disease (IID) such as food poisoning, with 20% of the population annually suffering from an IID (only 3% of these consult.
- Respiratory infections such as cold and influenza account for 5.5 million GP visits each year costing £170 million.
- HIV/AIDS costs an estimated £400 million pa.

Mortality

1.2% of all deaths in England and Wales are due to infectious and parasitic diseases (ICD-10 A00-B99, 2005 data);[1] including 3% of deaths in children under 16.

Inequality

Gastrointestinal infection leading to hospital admission was 2.4x higher in the poorest fifth of the population than in the most affluent quintile.

References

1 Office for National Statistics, *Review of the Registrar General on deaths by cause, sex and age, in England and Wales, 2005.* London: ONS; 2006. ℘ http://www.statistics.gov.uk
2 HPA. *Health Protection in the 21st Century.* London: HPA; 2005. ℘ http://www.hpa.org.uk

Epidemiology of diseases

Arthritis

Summary

Arthritis is the term used to describe a group of conditions characterized by inflammation of the joints. The two commonest types are osteoarthritis (OA) and rheumatoid arthritis (RA). OA is caused by local inflammation at the synovial joints often caused by overactivity of the body's normal repair processes. RA is a systemic disease caused by chronic inflammation that most commonly affects synovial joints but can affect almost any part of the body. The specific symptoms depend on the type of arthritis, but in general they include pain, stiffness, inflammation or swelling of the joint, and a progressive deformity or loss of function.

Descriptive epidemiology

- *Incidence* It is difficult to estimate incidence as people present at all stages of disease.
- *Prevalence* Worldwide there are estimated to be 151.4 million people with OA and 23.7 million people with RA.[1] In the UK 9 million people are estimated to have arthritis including 8.5 million who are estimated to have joint pain caused by OA.[2] In England, there were 290 000 admissions to hospital with arthritis in 2008/09.[3]
- *Case fatality* Very low, but depends on the severity of disease and the presence of other related conditions and extra-articular manifestations.
- *Mortality* Globally there were 7000 deaths from OA and 26 000 deaths from RA in 2004; most deaths occurred in women.[1] There were 1257 deaths from arthritis and arthrosis in 2008 in England and Wales.[4]
- *Disability* Worldwide arthritis was responsible for 20.6 million DALYs in 2004 when there were an estimated 55.3 million people with moderate or severe disability as a result of arthritis.[1]
- *Time* The prevalence of OA is likely to increase as the population ages.
- *Person* OA is predominantly a disease of middle to late age and is more commonly seen in women. RA can present at any age, but is most common between 30–50 years. Pre-menopausal women are 3x more likely to be affected by RA than men, but this difference disappears post-menopause.
- *Place* Occurs worldwide, but most cases are found in Europe and the Western Pacific region (including Australia, China, and Japan).[1]

Risk factors

- *Fixed risk factors* Sex (women are more commonly affected); age (OA is rare before 40 years and RA most commonly presents between 30–50 years); genetic (HLA genotypes associated with RA); family history.[2]
- *Modifiable risk factors* OA: obesity; previous trauma or preexisting joint damage.

Prevention

- *Primary prevention* OA: weight loss.
- *Secondary prevention* RA: disease-modifying antirheumatic drugs; corticosteroids; surgery.
- *Treatment/tertiary prevention* OA: joint replacement; physiotherapy. RA: physiotherapy; surgery.

Common types of arthritis

- Osteoarthritis.
- Rheumatoid arthritis.
- Seronegative spondyloarthritis:
  - Ankylosing spondylitis.
  - Psoriasis.
  - Inflammatory bowel disease.
  - Reactive arthritis (post-infection).
- Septic arthritis.
- Crystal arthritis, e.g. gout and pseudogout.
- Trauma, e.g. haemarthritis.

References

1 WHO *The global burden of disease: 2004 update.* Geneva: WHO; 2004. http://www.who.int/healthinfo/global_burden_disease/GBD_report_2004update_full.pdf
2 NHS CKS http://www.cks.nhs.uk
3 NHS HES Online 2008/9 http://www.hesonline.nhs.uk
4 ONS Mortality statistics 2008 http://www.statistics.gov.uk

Asthma

Summary

Asthma is a chronic respiratory disease characterized by reversible narrowing of the airways in response to an allergen or other stimulus (e.g. cold air, atmospheric pollution, or exercise). Symptoms are often worse at night and include wheeze, cough, chest tightness, and episodes of shortness of breath.

Descriptive epidemiology

- *Incidence* Most new cases occur in children.
- *Prevalence* Worldwide there are estimated to be 234.9 million people with asthma of whom 28.8 million are in Europe.[1] In the UK there are estimated to be 5.4 million people with asthma.[2] In England, there were 64 000 admissions to hospital for asthma in 2008/09.[3]
- *Case fatality* Overall very low, but depends on the severity of disease. Deaths mainly occur during an acute episode of airway narrowing. Acute attacks can be prevented with adequate medical care and the outcome of an attack is often dependent on urgent access to medical treatment.
- *Mortality* Globally 287 000 deaths were caused by asthma in 2004.[1] Most deaths occurred in middle- and low-income countries.[1] There were 1036 deaths from asthma in 2008 in England and Wales.[4]
- *Disability* Worldwide asthma was responsible for 16.3 million DALYs in 2004 when there were an estimated 19.4 million people with moderate or severe disability as a result of asthma.[1]
- *Time* The number of new cases of asthma has increased dramatically over the last 40 years; however this trend is now levelling off.[5] Prevalence is likely to remain high as it is a chronic condition that often presents in childhood.
- *Person* Asthma is predominantly a disease of childhood and symptoms often decrease with age. However a proportion of people will develop asthma later in life.
- *Place* Worldwide, but most morbidity and mortality is seen in middle- and low-income countries.[1]

Risk factors

- *Fixed risk factors* Age (young); family history of atopy.
- *Modifiable risk factors* Maternal smoking; environmental tobacco smoke;[6] occupational exposure to allergens (cause 9–15% of adult-onset asthma).[7]

Prevention

- *Primary prevention* Maternal smoking cessation.
- *Secondary prevention* Avoid exposure to allergen (e.g. house dust mite, environmental tobacco smoke, occupational agent); smoking cessation.[2]
- *Treatment/tertiary prevention* Bronchodilators; corticosteroids; anti-inflammatory agents and antibiotics in some cases.

References

1 WHO The global burden of disease: 2004 update. Geneva: WHO; 2004. ℘ http://www.who.int/healthinfo/global_burden_disease/GBD_report_2004update_full.pdf

2 Asthma UK ℘ http://www.asthma.org.uk

3 NHS HES Online 2008/9 ℘ http://www.hesonline.nhs.uk

4 ONS Mortality statistics 2008 ℘ http://www.statistics.gov.uk

5 Anderson H. Prevalence of asthma. *BMJ* 2005; **330**:1037–8.

6 Gilliland FD. Effects of maternal smoking during pregnancy and environmental tobacco smoke on asthma and wheezing in children. *Am J Respir Crit Care Med* 2001; **163**(2):429–36.

7 SIGN and BTS (2009) ℘ http://www.sign.ac.uk

Bladder cancer

Summary

Bladder cancer typically presents with painless haematuria, abnormal micturition (painful, sudden, frequent) or recurrent urinary tract infections. It is more common in men than women. Worldwide, its distribution reflects the prevalence of smoking, occupational exposure to chemicals, and schistosomiasis.

Descriptive epidemiology

- *Incidence* Worldwide, it is the 6th commonest cancer with 323 000 new cases in 2008.[1] In the UK it is the 7th commonest cancer with 10 100 new cases in 2007.[3]
- *Prevalence* Worldwide, an estimated 1.1 million people were alive in 2002 having been diagnosed with bladder cancer within the previous 5 years.[2] In England, there were 86 000 admissions to hospital with bladder cancer in 2008/09.[4]
- *Survival* Depends on grade and stage at presentation. In the UK 5-year survival is 66% for men and 57% for women.[3]
- *Mortality* Worldwide it is the 10th commonest cause of cancer death with 150 000 deaths in 2008.[5] In the UK it is the 8th commonest cause of cancer death.[3] There were 4475 deaths in England and Wales in 2009.[6]
- *Time* Age-specific incidence rates have fallen over the last 10 years in the UK and mortality rates have declined over the last 30 years, partly due to the reduction in smoking prevalence.[3]
- *Person* In developed countries it tends to affect men over the age of 40 who smoke or have had occupational exposure to chemicals. In the Middle East and Africa it tends to affect people with schistosomiasis.[3]
- *Place* In developed countries distribution reflects smoking and occupational chemical exposure while in developing countries distribution reflects prevalence of schistosomiasis. It is the 2nd commonest cause of cancer deaths in men in the Eastern Mediterranean region[5] and the highest death rate is seen in Egypt.[7]

Risk factors

- *Fixed risk factors* Age (85% aged >65 years); ethnicity (highest risk in white); family history.[3]
- *Modifiable risk factors* Smoking; environmental tobacco smoke; occupational chemical exposure (polycyclic hydrocarbons,[8] e.g. oil refining; arylamines, e.g. manufacture of plastics or rubber); schistosomiasis; recurrent bladder infection.

Prevention

- *Primary prevention* Smoking cessation; control occupational exposure to chemicals (e.g. see the UK Health and Safety Executive website: ℘ http://www.hse.gov.uk); early recognition and treatment of schistosomiasis and other bladder infections.
- *Secondary prevention* Screening is not currently recommended.
- *Treatment/tertiary prevention* Surgery; chemotherapy; radiotherapy; regular cystoscopy to identify recurrence.

References

1 WHO GLOBOCAN 2008 ℅ http://globocan.iarc.fr
2 WHO GLOBOCAN 2002 ℅ http://www-dep.iarc.fr
3 Cancer Research UK ℅ http://www.cancerresearchuk.org
4 NHS HES Online2008/9 ℅ http://www.hesonline.nhs.uk
5 WHO *The global burden of disease: 2004 update.* Geneva: WHO; 2004. ℅ http://www.who.int/
   healthinfo/global_burden_disease/GBD_report_2004update_full.pdf
6 Death registrations in England and Wales 2009 ℅ http://www.statistics.gov.uk
7 Parkin DM. The global burden of urinary bladder cancer. *Scand J Urol Nephrol* 2008; **42**(S218):12–20.
8 HPA Hydrocarbons ℅ http://www.hpa.org.uk

Brain and CNS cancer

Summary

Cancer of the brain, central nervous system (CNS), or meninges is rare. It typically presents with headache or seizure but symptoms can be more specific depending on the site of the tumour. Better imaging has led to an increase in diagnosis but mortality has remained fairly constant.

Descriptive epidemiology (meninges, brain, and CNS)

- *Incidence* Worldwide there were 238 000 new cases of brain and CNS cancer in 2008.[1] In the UK it is the 16th most common cancer with 4676 cases in 2007.[2]
- *Prevalence* Worldwide, an estimated 277 000 people were alive in 2002 having been diagnosed with cancer of the brain and CNS within the previous 5 years.[5] In England and Wales, there were 17 079 admissions to hospital with cancer of the brain, meninges, and CNS in 2008/09.[3]
- *Survival* Depends on age, type of tumour, grade, and stage at presentation. In the UK 5-year survival is 11% in men and 16% in women.[2] Survival is much higher in people <40 years (~50% 5-year survival).[2]
- *Mortality* Worldwide, there were 175 000 deaths from cancer of the brain and CNS in 2008.[1] In the UK it is the 13th most common cause of cancer death.[2] There were 3313 deaths in England and Wales in 2009.[4]
- *Time* In the UK there was a slight increase in age standardized incidence from 1970–1990 but since then, rates have been relatively constant.[2] This increase is in part due to better imaging techniques (CT and MRI) leading to more and earlier diagnoses.
- *Person* It is the commonest site of solid tumours in children but most cases occur in adults.[2]
- *Place* Highest age-standardized incidence rates are seen in North America, Europe, Australasia, and Brazil.[1]

Risk factors

- *Fixed risk factors* Age; genetic (e.g. neurofibramatosis).
- *Modifiable risk factors* Radiation; immunosuppression (cerebral lymphoma).

Prevention

- *Primary prevention* No prevention.
- *Secondary prevention* Screening is not recommended.
- *Treatment/tertiary prevention* Surgery; radiotherapy; chemotherapy; physiotherapy; occupational therapy.

References

1 WHO GLOBOCAN 2008 ℗ http://globocan.iarc.fr
2 Cancer Research UK ℗ http://www.cancerresearchuk.org
3 NHS HES Online2008/9 ℗ http://www.hesonline.nhs.uk
4 Death registrations in England and Wales 2009 ℗ http://www.statistics.gov.uk
5 WHO GLOBOCAN 2002 ℗ http://www-dep.iarc.fr

Breast cancer

Summary
Almost 1 in 3 cancers diagnosed in women in the UK is a breast cancer. The introduction of screening has led to cancer being detected at an earlier stage and a related fall in mortality. The global trend is towards an increase in incidence as women have fewer children, later in life.

Descriptive epidemiology

- *Incidence* Worldwide, it is the 2nd commonest cancer in women with 1.1 million new cases in 2004.[1] In the UK it is the commonest cancer in women with 47 700 new cases in 2009.[2]
- *Prevalence* Worldwide, an estimated 4.4 million women were alive in 2002 having been diagnosed with breast cancer within the previous 5 years.[3] In England, there were 167 000 admissions to hospital with breast cancer in 2008/09.[4]
- *Survival* Depends on grade and stage at presentation. In the UK 5-year survival is 82%.[2]
- *Mortality* Worldwide it is the commonest cause of cancer death in women with 519 000 deaths overall in 2004 (<0.4% of deaths occurred in men).[1] In the UK it is the 3rd commonest cause of cancer death.[2] There were 10 440 deaths in England and Wales in 2009.[5]
- *Time* Since the introduction of screening in the UK, 20 years ago, there has been an increase in age-standardized incidence and a decline in mortality.
- *Person* <1% of all cases occur in men.
- *Place* Most cases occur in Europe and the Americas and it is the 9th commonest cause of death in high-income countries.[1] Rates are traditionally lower in low-income countries and Eastern Asia, which partly reflects the different trends in family size and breastfeeding. However incidence is anticipated to increase in all countries as women change their reproductive and lifestyle patterns.

Risk factors

- *Fixed risk factors* Age (80% of cases in women >50 years)[2]; sex (>99% in women); family history; genetic (e.g. BRAC1 and 2); exposure to oestrogen (increased risk with early menarche and late menopause); certain benign breast conditions.
- *Modifiable risk factors* Hormone replacement therapy (HRT); oral contraceptive pill (OCP); reduced risk in parous women and those who breastfeed; alcohol; post-menopausal obesity.

Prevention

- *Primary prevention* Breastfeeding; weight control; sensible alcohol consumption; prophylactic mastectomy in women with genetic high risk.
- *Secondary prevention* Most high-income countries have a population-based screening programme for breast cancer. In the UK, the NHS Breast Screening programme was established in 1988. It offers screening to all women over the age of 50 and uses a call and recall system to invite women aged 50–70 registered with a GP for screening every 3 years.[6]

- ***Treatment/tertiary prevention*** Surgery; chemotherapy; hormonal therapy; radiotherapy; post-mastectomy surgical reconstruction or prosthesis.

References

1 WHO *The global burden of disease: 2004 update.* Geneva: WHO; 2004. ℘ http://www.who.int/healthinfo/global_burden_disease/GBD_report_2004update_full.pdf
2 Cancer Research UK ℘ http://www.cancerresearchuk.org
3 WHO GLOBOCAN 2002 ℘ http://www-dep.iarc.fr
4 NHS HES Online2008/9 ℘ http://www.hesonline.nhs.uk
5 Death registrations in England and Wales 2009 ℘ http://www.statistics.gov.uk
6 NHS Breast Cancer Screening ℘ http://www.cancerscreening.nhs.uk

Cardiovascular disease

Summary

Cardiovascular disease (CVD) is used to describe all disorders of the heart and blood vessels (including cerebrovascular disease, coronary heart disease, and peripheral vascular disease). Worldwide it was the leading cause of death in 2004, responsible for 31.5% of deaths in females and 26.8% of deaths in males.[1] CVD is also the commonest cause of death in the UK and is responsible for approximately 200 000 deaths per year, 35% of all deaths.[2] This section covers the major types of CVD associated with atherosclerosis. Raised BP and hypertension are important risk factors for the development of atherosclerosis, which is in turn the commonest underlying disease process in cerebrovascular disease and coronary heart disease.

Atherosclerosis

A build-up of fatty deposits (atheroma) in the arteries is called atherosclerosis. Raised BP and hypertension can increase the risk of atheroma forming in arteries by damaging the lining of the vessels and disrupting blood flow. When formed, atheroma narrow or stiffen vessels further disrupting blood flow. Atherosclerosis is ubiquitous; it begins to appear in teenagers and continues to increase with age.[3] It is often clinically silent but it presents when an artery has been narrowed to the point that the blood flow is insufficient to meet the metabolic demands of the tissue. The clinical presentation depends on which artery is most affected but the commonest presentations are cerebrovascular disease (stroke), coronary heart disease and peripheral arterial disease.

Prevention

- *Primary prevention* Low-fat diet; smoking cessation; NHS Health Check;[4] US Medicare provides screening for total and HDL cholesterol and triglycerides every 5 years in people without CVD;[5] physical activity; sensible alcohol intake.
- *Secondary prevention* Smoking cessation; low-fat diet; physical activity; control of hypertension; cholesterol control.
- *Treatment/tertiary prevention* Smoking cessation; hypertension and cholesterol control; interventional procedures to widen narrowed arteries.

Risk factors

- *Fixed risk factors* Age; sex (more common in men); family history.
- *Modifiable risk factors* Smoking; high BP; high cholesterol; high saturated fat intake; diabetes; physical inactivity; obesity.

NHS Health Check[4]

NHS health checks were introduced in England in 2009. All adults aged 40–74 years without a history of heart disease, kidney disease, diabetes, or stroke are invited, every 5 years, to attend a health check to assess their risk of developing these conditions. By offering appropriate early intervention, this scheme is expected to save 650 lives and prevent 1600 heart attacks and strokes each year.

References

1 WHO *The global burden of disease: 2004 update.* Geneva: WHO; 2004. ℘ http://www.who.int/
   healthinfo/global_burden_disease/GBD_report_2004update_full.pdf
2 BHF ℘ http://www.heartstats.org
3 Rose G. Epidemiology of atherosclerosis. *BMJ* 1991; **303**:1537–9.
4 NHS ℘ http://www.nhs.uk
5 Medicare ℘ http://www.cms.gov

Cerebrovascular disease

Summary

The term cerebrovascular disease describes a range of conditions characterized by abnormal, damaged, or blocked blood vessels that lead to disrupted blood flow to the brain. Stroke is the commonest clinical presentation of cerebrovascular disease and is an important cause of morbidity and mortality worldwide. Raised BP is the commonest modifiable risk factor for stroke.[1] The main categories of cerebrovascular disease are:

- Cerebral infarct.
- Intracerebral haemorrhage.
- Subarachnoid haemorrhage.
- Other non-traumatic intracranial haemorrhage.

Descriptive epidemiology

- *Incidence* In 2004 there were estimated to be 9 million first instances of stroke worldwide.[2]
- *Prevalence* Worldwide it is estimated that there were 30.7 million people alive in 2004 who had survived a stroke.[2] In England, there were 98 200 admissions to hospital with cerebrovascular disease in 2008/09.[3]
- *Case fatality* A systematic review found that early case fatality from stroke (21–30 days) was between 17–30% in high-income countries and between 18–35% in low- and middle-income countries depending on the cause.[4]
- *Mortality* Worldwide it was responsible for 5.7 million deaths in 2004, almost 10% of all deaths, making it the 2nd commonest cause of death.[2] Although the mortality is high, it is only responsible for 4.2% of all years of life lost (this measure takes into account the age at death).[2] There were 46 446 deaths in England and Wales in 2008.[5]
- *Disability* Worldwide cerebrovascular disease was the 6th most common cause of disability, responsible for 46.6 million DALYs in 2004. At this time there were an estimated 12.4 million people worldwide with moderate or severe disability as a result of cerebrovascular disease.[2]
- *Time* By 2030, cerebrovascular disease is predicted to grow in importance and become the 4th leading cause of DALY's worldwide.[2] In high-income countries age-adjusted stroke incidence has fallen by >40% in the last 40 years but has more than doubled in low- and middle-income countries.[4]
- *Person* More common with age; more common in people with raised BP.
- *Place* Cerebrovascular disease occurs worldwide. Although it is a commoner cause of mortality and morbidity in high-income countries, the majority of deaths and DALYs are found in middle- and low-income countries.[2] It is expected to grow in importance in low- and middle-income countries, partly related to the prevalence of smoking in these regions and the general shift from infectious to chronic conditions.[2]

Risk factors

- *Fixed risk factors* Age; family history.
- *Modifiable risk factors* High BP; smoking; obesity; physical inactivity; diet (high salt, high saturated fat); excess alcohol consumption; diabetes; psychosocial stress; relevant cardiac disease (e.g. atrial fibrillation); apolipoprotein ratio.[1] Evidence for the role of cholesterol in the aetiology of stroke is equivocal.[6]

Prevention

- *Primary prevention* BP control; smoking cessation; maintain healthy weight; healthy diet (reduced salt (<6g/day), high fruit and vegetables (5-a-day), low saturated fat); diabetes control; sensible alcohol consumption.
- *Secondary prevention* Prompt treatment of transient ischaemic attack (TIA) or minor stroke can reduce the risk of an early recurrent stroke by 80%;[7] BP control; smoking cessation; statin therapy; diabetes control.
- *Treatment/tertiary prevention* Thrombolytic treatment (where appropriate); physiotherapy; occupational therapy; regular exercise; smoking cessation.

References

1 O'Donnell MJ et al. Risk factors for ischaemic and intracerebral haemorrhagic stroke in 22 countries (the INTERSTROKE study): a case-control study. *Lancet* 2010; **376**:112–23.

2 WHO *The global burden of disease: 2004 update.* Geneva: WHO; 2004. ♒ http://www.who.int/healthinfo/global_burden_disease/GBD_report_2004update_full.pdf

3 NHS HES Online2008/9 ♒ http://www.hesonline.nhs.uk

4 Feigin VL. Worldwide stroke incidence and early case fatality reported in 56 population-based studies: a systematic review. *Lancet Neurol* 2009; **8(4)**:355–69.

5 ONS Mortality statistics 2008 ♒ http://www.statistics.gov.uk

6 Amarenco P, Labreuche J. Lipid management in the prevention of stroke: review and updated meta-analysis of statins for stroke prevention. *Lancet Neurol* 2009; **8**:453–63.

7 Rothwell, PM et al. Effect of urgent treatment of transient ischaemic attack and minor stroke on early recurrent stroke (EXPRESS study): a prospective population-based sequential comparison. *Lancet* 2007; **370**:1432–42.

Cervix cancer

Summary

Cancer of the cervix is the commonest cancer in Africa and South East Asia, despite it only occurring in women. And in these regions it is the commonest cause of cancer death in women. Many high-income countries have introduced screening programmes which have led to a considerable fall in the number of cases. The main cause of cervix cancer is infection with a high risk type of human papillomavirus (HPV) and vaccination against this infection is now available in some countries.

Descriptive epidemiology

- *Incidence* Worldwide, there were 489 000 new cases in 2004.[1] It is the only cancer with a higher incidence in Africa and South East Asia than in developed countries.[1] In the UK it is the 11th most common cancer in women with 2830 cases in 2007.[2]
- *Prevalence* Worldwide, an estimated 1.4 million women were alive in 2002 having been diagnosed with cancer of the cervix within the previous 5 years.[3] In England, there were 8891 admissions to hospital with cancer of the cervix in 2008/09.[4]
- *Survival* Depends on grade and stage at presentation. In the UK 5-year survival is around 2/3 overall, but it is >85% in women <40 years.[2]
- *Mortality* Globally it is the 5th commonest cause of cancer death in women with 268 000 deaths overall in 2004 but it was the commonest cause of cancer death in women in Africa and South East Asia.[1] There were 830 deaths in England and Wales in 2009.[5]
- *Time* Since the introduction of screening in the UK, incidence rates have almost halved (in last 20 years).[2]
- *Person* A disease of women, over half the cases in the UK are diagnosed in women <50 years.[2]
- *Place* Occurs predominantly in lower-income countries. Despite this being a disease only seen in women, it was the commonest cancer in Africa and South East Asia in 2004.[1]

Risk factors

- *Fixed risk factors* Sex.
- *Modifiable risk factors* HPV including types 16 and 18; condom use/delayed sexual debut/fewer partners; tobacco smoking; immunosuppression; long-term use of oral contraception; early pregnancy; number of pregnancies; vaccination.

Prevention

- *Primary prevention* Most high-income countries have a population-based screening programme. In the UK, the NHS Cervical Screening programme was established in 1988. It offers screening to all sexually active women aged 25–64 years and uses a call and recall system to invite women registered with a GP, for screening every 3–5 years.[6] Unlike other screening programmes, it is not designed to detect cancer, but instead looks for early abnormalities that can develop into cancer without intervention.[6] HPV vaccination has recently been developed to help prevent cancer of the cervix and is approved for use by many countries.[7] In 2008 the UK began to offer the HPV vaccine routinely to girls aged 12–13 years.[8]

- *Secondary prevention* Cervical screening.
- *Treatment/tertiary prevention* Surgery; chemotherapy; radiotherapy.

References

1 WHO *The global burden of disease: 2004 update*. Geneva: WHO; 2004. http://www.who.int/healthinfo/global_burden_disease/GBD_report_2004update_full.pdf
2 Cancer Research UK http://www.cancerresearchuk.org
3 WHO GLOBOCAN 2002 http://www-dep.iarc.fr
4 NHS HES Online2008/9 http://www.hesonline.nhs.uk
5 Death registrations in England and Wales 2009 http://www.statistics.gov.uk
6 NHS Cervical Cancer Screening http://www.cancerscreening.nhs.uk
7 National Cancer Institute http://www.cancer.gov/search/results.aspx
8 NHS Immunisations http://www.immunisation.nhs.uk/Vaccines/HPV

Chronic obstructive pulmonary disease

Summary

Chronic obstructive pulmonary disease (COPD) includes emphysema and chronic bronchitis. It is characterized by airflow obstruction, defined as a FEV_1* <80% predicted or FEV_1/FVC** <0.7. As it is predominantly caused by smoking, global and temporal distributions mainly reflect patterns in smoking prevalence. Smoking cessation is the most important intervention. At any stage it can slow down disease progression and postpone disability.

*FEV_1, forced expiratory volume in 1 second. ** FVC, forced vital capacity.

Descriptive epidemiology

- *Incidence* It is difficult to estimate incidence as many cases are undiagnosed and people present at all stages of disease. It is estimated that 20% of all smokers will develop COPD.[1]
- *Prevalence* Worldwide it is estimated that there were 63.6 million people with symptomatic COPD in 2004.[2] Based on information from primary care, the prevalence of COPD in adults in England was 1.5% (834 000 people) in 2008.[3] However it is thought that there are an additional 450 000 undiagnosed people in the UK.[4] In England, there were 119 000 admissions to hospital with COPD in 2008/09.[5]
- *Case fatality* Depends on severity of underlying disease and the occurrence of acute exacerbations.
- *Mortality* Worldwide it was responsible for 3 million deaths in 2004 making it the 4th commonest cause of death.[2] There were 24 816 deaths in England and Wales in 2008, approximately 1 in every 20 deaths.[6]
- *Disability* Worldwide COPD was the 13th most common cause of disability, responsible for 30.2 million DALYs in 2004 when there were an estimated 26.6 million people worldwide with moderate or severe disability as a result of COPD.[2]
- *Time* The burden of disease caused by COPD is expected to dramatically rise. It is predicted that in 2030 it will be the 5th leading cause of global DALYs.[2]
- *Person* Rare in people <40 years, but it is the amount of tobacco and duration of smoking that is the most important factor.
- *Place* Most deaths occur in middle-income countries and most cases are found in the Western Pacific region.[2] The disease is relatively uncommon in Africa.[2] It is a leading cause of disability in middle- and high-income countries, specifically the Americas and the Western Pacific Region.[2] The distribution of COPD is likely to shift from high- and middle to middle- and low-income countries as smoking patterns change.

Global smoking prevalence[7,8] (Fig. 12.1)

- *Men* 35% of men in developed countries and 50% of men in developing countries smoke. In China alone there are >300 million male smokers.
- *Women* The pattern is reversed in women. 22% of women in developed countries and 9% of women in developing countries smoke.
- It is anticipated that by 2030 there will be >3 billion smokers worldwide.
- 1 in 2 smokers will die from smoking related disease.

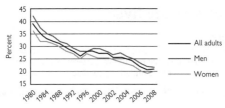

Fig. 12.1 Prevalence of cigarette smoking in adults in England (1980–2008). Source: NNS (2010) ℘ http://www.ic.nhs.uk/webfiles/publications/Health%20 and%20Lifestyles/Statistics_on_Smoking_2010.pdf, data unweighted 1980–1996.

Risk factors

- *Fixed risk factors* Genetic (alpha-1 antitrypsin deficiency).
- *Modifiable risk factors* Smoking (80% of cases in UK); environmental tobacco smoke; occupational chemical exposure (e.g. coal dust, cadmium—estimated to cause or make worse 15% of cases);[9,10] indoor air pollution (in low-income countries indoor air pollution from biomass fuels used in heating and cooking causes large burden of COPD);[11] outdoor air pollution triggers acute exacerbations.

Prevention

- *Primary prevention* Smoking cessation (℘ http://www.smokefree.nhs. uk); control of tobacco (see 🕮 Lung cancer, p.346).
- *Secondary prevention* Smoking cessation; control outdoor air pollution.
- *Treatment/tertiary prevention* Smoking cessation; drug treatment (can include beta-2 agonists, mucolytics, theophylline, corticosteroids depending on severity[12]); home oxygen; pulmonary rehabilitation; non invasive ventilation.

References

1 Waterer GW, Temple SE. Do we really want to know why only some smokers get COPD? *Chest* 2004; **125**(5):1599–600.
2 WHO *The global burden of disease: 2004 update*. Geneva: WHO; 2004. ℘ http://www.who. int/healthinfo/global_burden_disease/GBD_report_2004update_full.pdf
3 QOF 2008/09 ℘ http://www.ic.nhs.uk
4 NHS Choices ℘ http://www.nhs.uk/conditions
5 NHS HES Online2008/9 ℘ http://www.hesonline.nhs.uk
6 ONS Mortality statistics 2008 ℘ http://www.statistics.gov.uk
7 WHO *The Tobacco Atlas*. Geneva: WHO; 2002 ℘ http://www.who.int/tobacco/statistics/ tobacco_atlas/en
8 ONS *Cigarette Smoking*.London: ONS; 2006 ℘ http://www.statistics.gov.uk/cci/nugget. asp?id=866
9 HSE COPD ℘ www.hse.gov.uk
10 Blanc PD, Torén K. Occupation in chronic obstructive pulmonary disease and chronic bronchitis: an update. *Int J Tuberc Lung Dis* 2007; **11**(3):251–7.
11 WHO ℘ http://www.who.int
12 NHS ℘ http://www.cks.nhs.uk

Cirrhosis of the liver

Summary

Cirrhosis is the result of chronic liver damage from any cause. This diverse aetiology can make it difficult to interpret patterns in this diagnosis and often more detailed analysis of the underlying conditions is more informative.

Examples of conditions that cause cirrhosis of the liver:

- Alcohol (60–80%).[*]
- Chronic viral hepatitis (10–20%).[*]
- Autoimmune hepatitis.
- Drugs e.g. methotrexate.
- Primary/secondary biliary cirrhosis (5–10%).[*]
- Inherited conditions including haemochromatosis (5%)[*], Wilson disease, alpha-1 antitrypsin deficiency.
- Non-alcoholic fatty liver disease.
- Cryptogenic.

[*]Source of prevalence data[1]

Descriptive epidemiology

- **Incidence and prevalence** Difficult to determine as the condition can remain clinically silent for many years.
- **Mortality** Worldwide it was responsible for 772 000 deaths in 2004, making it the 18th commonest cause of death.[2] There were 2660 deaths from cirrhosis of the liver in England and Wales in 2008.[3]
- **Disability** Worldwide, cirrhosis of the liver was outside the top 20 leading causes of DALYs in 2004, but it was a significant cause of disability, responsible for 13.6 million DALYs.[2]
- **Time** In the USA, the liver cirrhosis age-adjusted death rate gradually increased from 1950, peaked in 1973 and has been in decline since.[4]
- **Person** Worldwide, it causes more deaths in men than women (510 000 compared to 262 000 in 2004).[2]
- **Place** The highest burden is seen in the European region where cirrhosis of the liver was the 9th leading cause of DALYs in 2004.[2]

Risk factors

- Related to the underlying cause of liver damage.

Prevention

- **Primary prevention** Prevent conditions that progress to cirrhosis (e.g. hepatitis B and C infection; excessive alcohol consumption; obesity) and prompt recognition of liver disease with appropriate treatment to reduce progression to cirrhosis (e.g. haemochromatosis).
- **Secondary prevention** Avoid alcohol; vaccination for hepatitis B; specific management of the underlying condition.
- **Treatment/tertiary prevention** Liver transplant (the British Liver Trust report that 700 people a year, in the UK, undergo a transplant to survive).[5]

References

1 ℘ http://www.gpnotebook.co.uk
2 WHO *The global burden of disease: 2004 update.* Geneva: WHO; 2004. ℘ http://www.who.int/healthinfo/global_burden_disease/GBD_report_2004update_full.pdf
3 ONS Mortality statistics 2008 ℘ http://www.statistics.gov.uk
4 ℘ http://www.cdc.gov
5 ℘ http://www.britishlivertrust.org.uk

Colorectal cancer

Summary

Colorectal cancer presents with either general symptoms such as weight loss or anaemia or specific symptoms including altered bowel habit, abdominal mass, abdominal pain, or blood in the stool. Incidence is anticipated to rise in low- and middle-income countries as rates of obesity and physical inactivity increase.

Descriptive epidemiology

- *Incidence* Worldwide, it is the 3rd commonest cancer with 1.1 million new cases in 2004.[1] In the UK it is the 3rd commonest cancer with 38 610 new cases in 2007.[2]
- *Prevalence* Worldwide, an estimated 2.8 million people were alive in 2002 having been diagnosed with colorectal cancer within the previous 5 years.[3] In England, there were 137 600 admissions to hospital with colorectal cancer in 2008/09.[4]
- *Survival* Depends on grade and stage at presentation. In England and Wales 5-year survival is ~50%.[2]
- *Mortality* Worldwide it is the 4th commonest cause of cancer death in men and women and the 20th cause of death overall with 639 000 deaths in 2004.[1] In the UK it is the 2nd commonest cause of cancer death.[2] There were 13 934 deaths in England and Wales in 2009.[5]
- *Time* Rates are likely to increase in low- and middle-income countries as obesity levels rise. Incidence and mortality have fallen in the USA over the last 10 years.[6]
- *Person* In the UK, 84% of cases occur in people aged >60 years.[2] Men and women are equally affected.
- *Place* Occurs worldwide, higher rates in high-income countries.[1]

Risk factors

- *Fixed risk factors* Age (>80% cases aged >60 years); family history (lifetime risk of death from colorectal cancer is 1 in 6 for people with 2 1st-degree relatives with the condition and 1 in 10 for people with one 1st-degree relative aged <45 with the condition)[7]; genetic (FAP (familial adenomatous polyposis) and HNPCC (hereditary non-polyposis colorectal cancer) cause 1 in 20 cases[2] and the lifetime risk of death from colorectal cancer is 1 in 2.5 for people with FAP and 1 in 2 for people with HNPCC[7]); inflammatory bowel disease (1 in 100 cases).[2]
- *Modifiable risk factors* Diet (low in fibre, fruit and vegetables and high in processed and red meat all increase risk); obesity; smoking; physical inactivity.

Prevention

- *Primary prevention* Diet; exercise; smoking cessation.
- *Secondary prevention* The NHS Bowel Cancer Screening programme was introduced in England in 2006.[8] All adults aged 60–69 years are invited to participate using a call and recall system based on GP registers. Participants provide a sample for faecal occult blood (FOB) testing every 2 years. Participants with a positive FOB, estimated to be 2%, proceed to colonoscopy where a polyp is found in 40% and

a cancer in 10%. (NB in Scotland, adults aged 50–74). The UK British Society of Gastroenterology recommends screening for people at high risk of colorectal cancer, including people with colonic adenomas, inflammatory bowel disease, acromegaly, a uretero-sigmoidostomy, a family history of colorectal cancer or a genetic predisposition.[7]

- *Treatment/tertiary prevention* Surgery; chemotherapy; radiotherapy; regular colonoscopies (5-yearly until aged 75[7]).

References

1 WHO *The global burden of disease: 2004 update*. Geneva: WHO; 2004. ℰ http://www.who.int/healthinfo/global_burden_disease/GBD_report_2004update_full.pdf
2 Cancer Research UK ℰ http://www.cancerresearchuk.org
3 WHO GLOBOCAN 2002 ℰ http://www-dep.iarc.fr
4 NHS HES Online2008/9 ℰ http://.hesonline.nhs.uk
5 Death registrations in England and Wales 2009 ℰ http://www.statistics.gov.uk
6 CDC Colorectal Cancer Trends ℰ http://www.cdc.gov
7 Cairns S, Scholefield JH (eds). Guidelines for colorectal cancer screening in high risk groups. [Special Issue] *Gut* 2002; **51**(Suppl V):v28.
8 NHS Bowel Cancer Screening ℰ http://www.cancerscreening.nhs.uk

Coronary heart disease

Summary

Coronary heart disease (CHD) occurs when blood flow to the heart through the coronary arteries is impaired. The main clinical syndromes are angina and acute myocardial infarction (MI). Smoking is a major modifiable risk factor for CHD. Mortality is high following an acute MI but this can be improved with prompt medical treatment.

Descriptive epidemiology

- *Incidence* There were estimated to be 100 883 MIs in England in 2007[1] and 1.1 million MIs per year in the USA.[2]
- *Prevalence* Worldwide it is estimated that there were 54 million people with angina in 2004.[3] There were 303 500 admissions to hospital in England with CHD in 2008.[4]
- *Case fatality* In the USA almost half of all people who have an acute MI will die.[2]
- *Mortality* Worldwide it was the commonest cause of death in 2004, responsible for 7.2 million deaths, over 12% of all deaths[3]. It is responsible for 5.8% of all years of life lost.[3] There were 76 985 deaths in England and Wales in 2008 from CHD.[5]
- *Disability* Worldwide it was the 4th most common cause of disability, responsible for 62.6 million DALYs in 2004. At this time there were an estimated 23.2 million people worldwide with moderate or severe disability as a result of CHD.[3]
- *Time* The burden of disease caused by CHD is expected to rise by 2030, making it the 2nd commonest cause of global DALYs.[3] In the UK the incidence of MI is estimated to be reducing by 2% per year in people <70 years.[1]
- *Person* Incidence increases with age.[1] Men have a higher incidence than women, but this difference reduces after the menopause.[1] More common in South Asian men and women in UK.[1]
- *Place* CHD is the commonest cause of death in high-income countries and the 2nd commonest cause of death in middle- and low-income countries.[3] It contributes a higher proportion of DALYs in high- and middle income countries compared to low-income countries.[3] In the UK, studies have shown that MI incidence and mortality is higher in Northern England, Scotland, Northern Ireland, and Wales.[1]

Risk factors

- *Fixed risk factors* Age; family history; sex (men >women).
- *Modifiable risk factors* Smoking; cholesterol; physical inactivity; diet (high fat, low fruit and vegetables); high BP; diabetes.

Prevention

- *Primary prevention* Smoking cessation; BP control; maintain healthy weight; healthy diet (high fruit and vegetables (5-a-day), low saturated fat, reduce salt); diabetes control; physical activity.
- *Secondary prevention* Smoking cessation; BP control; cholesterol control; diabetes control; coronary artery intervention.
- *Treatment/tertiary prevention* Smoking cessation; drug treatment; surgery.

References

1 BHF ✍ http://www.heartstats.org
2 NIH ✍ http://www.nhibi.nih.gov
3 WHO *The global burden of disease: 2004 update*. Geneva: WHO; 2004. ✍ http://www.who.int/healthinfo/global_burden_disease/GBD_report_2004update_full.pdf
4 NHS HES Online 2008/9 ✍ http://www.hesonline.nhs.uk
5 ONS Mortality statistics 2008 ✍ http://www.statistics.gov.uk

Dementia

Summary

Dementia is a group of conditions that cause progressive decline in higher cortical function without affecting consciousness. There are multiple aetiologies but age is the main risk factor and epidemiological trends reflect the age distribution of populations.

Descriptive epidemiology

- *Incidence* It is difficult to estimate incidence as many cases are undiagnosed and people present at different stages of disease.
- *Prevalence* Worldwide, there were an estimated 24.2 million people with dementia in 2004.[1] The NHS estimates that there are 570 000 people in England with dementia (Fig. 12.2).[2] In England, there were 14 000 admissions to hospital with dementia in 2008/09.[3]
- *Mortality* Worldwide there were 492 000 deaths from dementia in 2004.[1] Dementia is the 6th commonest cause of death in high-income countries.[1] There were 16 610 deaths in England and Wales in 2008.[4]
- *Disability* Worldwide dementia was responsible for 11.2 million DALYs in 2004 when there were an estimated 14.9 million people with moderate or severe disability as a result of dementia.[1] It is the 4th leading cause of DALYs in high-income countries.[1]
- *Time* The prevalence and burden of disease will increase as the population ages.
- *Person* As age is the major risk factor, most cases are women.
- *Place* Most cases are seen in countries with aging populations: the Americas, Europe and the Western Pacific.[1]

Risk factors

- *Fixed risk factors* Age; genetic (e.g. Huntingdon's disease, tau protein in frontotemporal dementia).
- *Modifiable risk factors* Vascular dementia—smoking; obesity; physical inactivity; excess alcohol; thyroid abnormalities; B vitamin deficiency.

Prevention

- *Primary prevention* Vascular dementia—smoking cessation, weight loss, sensible alcohol intake, physical activity; some evidence for remaining physically and mentally active.[2]
- *Secondary prevention* No screening available.
- *Treatment/tertiary prevention* Behavioural therapy; cognitive stimulation; drug treatment; occupational therapy; physical therapy.

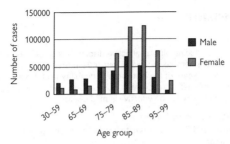

Fig. 12.2 Numbers of diagnosed and undiagnosed cases of dementia in the UK (2006). Alzheimer's Research Trust ⅊ http://www.dementia2010.org

References

1 WHO *The global burden of disease: 2004 update*. Geneva: WHO; 2004. ⅊ http://www.who.int/healthinfo/global_burden_disease/GBD_report_2004update_full.pdf
2 NHS Choices ⅊ http://www.nhs.uk/conditions
3 NHS HES Online2008/9 ⅊ http://www.hesonline.nhs.uk
4 ONS Mortality statistics 2008 ⅊ http://www.statistics.gov.uk

Depression

Summary

Depression (excluding bipolar affective disorder) is a common condition that causes considerable morbidity, but little mortality. It is the world's leading cause of years of life lost through disability (YLD) but simple life-style changes can help to prevent it. Many people do not seek healthcare, but talking therapies can be effective in mild disease.

Descriptive epidemiology

- *Incidence* It is difficult to estimate incidence as many people do not seek healthcare.
- *Prevalence* Worldwide there were an estimated 151.2 million people with depression in 2004.[1] In the UK, it is estimated that 1 in 4 women and 1 in 10 men will have an episode of depression that requires treatment and up to 15% will have severe depression.[3] In England, there were 21 300 admissions to hospital with depression in 2008/09.[4]
- *Case fatality* Depends on severity of disease but is generally very low. Depression is a risk factor for suicide; >90% of all suicides occur in people with mental illness.[3]
- *Mortality* Worldwide there were 15 000 deaths from depression in 2004.[1] There were 124 deaths in England and Wales in 2008.[5]
- *Disability* Worldwide depression was the 3rd most common cause of disability, responsible for 65.5 million DALYs in 2004 when there were an estimated 98.7 million people with moderate or severe disability as a result of depression.[1] Depression is the leading cause of YLD in men and women in high-, middle-, and low-income countries.[1]
- *Time* Depression is predicted to become the leading cause of disability worldwide in 2030.[1]
- *Person* Although depression is widespread, young adult women are disproportionately affected. It is more common in people with physical disease.
  - *Childhood and adolescence*[6] Prevalence: in prepubescent children 1% and in adolescence 3%, 2F:1M. Outcome: spontaneous recovery 10% at 3 months but 50% remain depressed at 1 year.
  - *Adult*[6] Lifetime prevalence: 67% for a depressive episode and 15% for severe depression. 2F:1M but suicide is more common among men. Outcome: on average an episode will last 6–8 months, chronic or persistent symptoms occur in 10%.
  - *Post-partum*[6] Prevalence: there is uncertainty around the prevalence of depression during pregnancy and child rearing. One study found that during pregnancy almost 1 in 5 women will have symptoms of depression, 10% will be affected during the first 2 postpartum months, increasing to over half of all women within the 1st postpartum year.
  - *Elderly* Common in elderly adults, partly due to life events, e.g. retirement with loss of routine, bereavement, or chronic illness. Many conditions can lead to depression, e.g. vitamin B12 or folate deficiency, malignancy, stroke. Depression should be excluded before dementia is diagnosed.

- *Place* A major cause of disability across the globe, but the leading cause of DALYs in high- and middle-income countries.[1]

Risk factors
- *Fixed risk factors* Sex (F > M); family history; genetic (e.g. 5-HTT gene); pregnancy; stressful event.
- *Modifiable risk factors* Alcohol; substance abuse; drug treatment (e.g. Beta-blockers)

Prevention
- *Primary prevention* Physical activity; sensible alcohol consumption; smoking cessation; refrain from illicit drugs.
- *Secondary prevention* Low index of suspicion in at risk groups can lead to early diagnosis.
- *Treatment/tertiary prevention* Cognitive behavioural therapy (CBT); drug treatment (antidepressant e.g. selective serotonin reuptake inhibitor[6]); suicide prevention.

References
1 WHO *The global burden of disease: 2004 update.* Geneva: WHO; 2004. ℘ http://www.who.int/healthinfo/global_burden_disease/GBD_report_2004update_full.pdf
2 Patient UK ℘ http://www.patientuk.co.uk
3 NHS Choices ℘ http://www.nhs.uk/conditions
4 NHS HES Online2008/9 ℘ http://www.hesonline.nhs.uk
5 ONS Mortality statistics 2008 ℘ http://www.statistics.gov.uk
6 NHS CKS: ℘ http://www.cks.nhs.uk

Diabetes

Summary

Diabetes mellitus is a chronic disease characterized by hyperglycaemia caused by insufficient production of, or an inadequate response to, insulin. There are 2 main types of diabetes: Type 1, an autoimmune condition that presents mainly in childhood and Type 2, an acquired condition that presents mainly in adults. Obesity is a significant risk factor for Type 2 diabetes and as the prevalence of obesity rises, diabetes is becoming a major international public health concern.

Descriptive epidemiology

- *Incidence* It is difficult to estimate incidence of type 2 diabetes as many cases are undiagnosed.
- *Prevalence* Worldwide, there were an estimated 220.5 million people with diabetes in 2004.[1] Over 90% of all diabetes is Type 2.[2] Gestational diabetes can occur in up to 14% of women during pregnancy.[3] In the UK there are estimated to be 2.8 million people with diabetes, but 35% of these are undiagnosed.[3] In the US in 2007 there were estimated to be 23.6 million people with diabetes of whom over 1 in 4 were undiagnosed.[4] In England, there were 60 000 admissions to hospital with diabetes in 2008/09.[5]
- *Case fatality* Diabetes is underreported as a cause of death. Diabetes increases the risk of CVD. A person with diabetes is twice as likely to die as a person of the same age without the disease.[4]
- *Mortality* Worldwide it was the 12th commonest cause of death in 2004 when there were 1.1 million deaths.[1] There were 5541 deaths in England and Wales in 2008.[6]
- *Disability* Worldwide, diabetes was responsible for 19.7 million DALYs in 2004.[1]
- *Time* Diabetes is predicted to become the 10th highest cause of disability worldwide in 2030[1] and it is predicted that diabetes deaths will double from 2005 to 2030.[2]
- *Person* Type 1 usually presents in childhood or adolescence. Type 2 usually presents in adults.
- *Place* The majority of disability and deaths occur in middle- and low-income countries.[1] But it was the 6th leading cause of disability in the Americas in 2004.[1]

Risk factors

- *Fixed risk factors* Type 1: genetic; family history; environmental. Type 2: age; family history; genetic; ethnicity.
- *Modifiable risk factors* Type 2: healthy diet; physical activity; weight management.

Prevention
- *Primary prevention for Type 2* Healthy diet; physical activity; weight management. No prevention for Type 1.
- *Secondary prevention*
  - *General population* Population-based screening for diabetes is not recommended.[7]
  - *Patients with diagnosed diabetes* Screening for retinopathy, foot problems, renal disease, hypertension, hyperlipidaemia.
- *Treatment/tertiary prevention* Weight loss; smoking cessation (to reduce risk of CVD); glucose control; BP control; lipid control; sensible alcohol consumption; patient education programmes.

References
1 WHO *The global burden of disease: 2004 update.* Geneva: WHO; 2004. ℘ http://www.who.int/healthinfo/global_burden_disease/GBD_report_2004update_full.pdf
2 WHO Diabetes ℘ http://www.who.int
3 NHS Choices ℘ http://www.nhs.uk/conditions
4 NIH Diabetes ℘ http://www.diabetes.niddk.nih.gov
5 NHS HES Online 2008/9 ℘ http://www.hesonline.nhs.uk
6 ONS Mortality statistics 2008 ℘ http://www.statistics.gov.uk
7 UK NSC (2006) ℘ http://www.screening.nhs.uk/diabetes

Emerging infectious disease

The influenza pandemic of 2009 was a timely reminder of the potential risk from novel infectious agents. Emerging infectious diseases (EIDs) pose challenges in terms of surveillance, control, and treatment. They can overwhelm public health systems and undermine previous health improvements. The increase in EIDs is thought to be related to a number of environmental, social, and scientific changes including:

- Changes in causative organisms, e.g. allowing the organism to cross the species barriers from animals to humans.
- Introduction into new populations due to changes in the environment (e.g. climate change) or population mixing (e.g. as a result of globalization with increased travel and interconnectedness of populations).
- Recognition of previously unknown infectious agents.
- Discoveries of infectious agents causing known diseases.
- Re-emergence of previously controlled infectious (e.g. due to development of antibiotic resistance, new environmental conditions, or failures of established control mechanisms).

Examples

Severe acute respiratory syndrome (SARS) Caused by the SARS coronavirus, emerged in China in late 2002 and led to a series of outbreaks before being controlled in mid-2003. It caused respiratory disease and had a high case fatality. During the course of the epidemic there were 8098 reported cases with a high case fatality (almost 10%) leading to 774 deaths.

SARS was a test for the international public health community as it spread rapidly across different states in a short space of time. It demonstrated the potentially explosive mix of a new infection with rapid travel in a globalized world.

Unlike many respiratory infections, SARS is most infectious after the onset of symptoms. Therefore the strict quarantine imposed was effective in controlling the spread of the infection.

West Nile virus Caused by a flavivirus and transmitted from mosquitoes. Until the 1990s it was mainly seen in Africa and Asia, but then started to occur as outbreaks in Europe and north America in humans, horses and birds. It can lead to fatal encephalitis. It is now an important health problem in the USA, with 3630 cases and 124 deaths in 2007.

Over the past four decades a number of new infectious diseases have been recognized (Table 12.1).

Table 12.1 Emerging infectious agents[1,2]

Date	Infectious agents
1970s	Ebola virus (Ebola haemorrhagic fever), *Campylobacter jejuni, Cryptosporidium parvum*, Hantaan virus, *Legionella pneumophila* (Legionnaires' disease), *Monkeypox virus*, Parvovirus B19 (Erythema infectiousum)
1980	Human T-lymphotropic virus (HTLV1)
1981	Toxin producing *Staphylococcus aureus* (Toxic shock syndrome)
1982	*Escherichia coli* O157:H7, *Borrelia burgdorferi* (Lyme disease), HTLV2
1983	HIV, *Helicobacter pylori*
1985	*Enterocytozoon bieneusi*
1986	*Cyclospora cayatenensis*, Bovine Spongiform Encephalopathy (BSE) (prion disease)
1988	Hepatitis E virus, Human Herpesvirus 6
1989	Hepatitis C virus, *Ehrlichia chafeensis, Photorhabdus asymbiotica*
1991	Guanarito virus (Venezuelan haemorrhagic fever)
1992	*Vibrio cholerae* O139, *Bartonella henselae* (Cat scratch disease)
1993	Sin Nombre virus (Hantavirus pulmonary syndrome)
1994	Sabia virus (Sabia associated haemorrhagic fever), Hendra virus (Hendra virus disease)
1995	Human Herpesvirus 8 (Kaposi's sarcoma)
1996	New variant Creutzfeldt–Jakob disease (nvCJD), bat lyssaviruses
1997	Avian Influenza virus in humans (H5N1)
1999	West Nile virus (Nipah virus) found in USA
2003	SARS coronavirus
2004	Simian foamy retrovirus (zoonotic retrovirus found in humans)
2005	HTLV4, HTLV5, human bocavirus
2008	*Plasmodium knowlesi* (Malaria), Lujo virus (Viral haemorrhagic fever)
2009	H1N1 influenza virus (Pandemic influenza)

References

1 *Emerging Infectious Disease* [journal] ℘ http://www.cdc.gov/ncidod/eid/index.htm
2 HPA webpage on emerging infections ℘ http://www.hpa.org.uk/Topics/InfectiousDiseases/InfectionsAZ/EmergingInfections

Gastroenteritis

Summary

Acute gastroenteritis is a term used to describe diarrhoea and/or vomiting of short duration. Causes of acute gastroenteritis include a range of viruses, bacteria, and parasites, plus less commonly toxins or chemicals (Box 12.1).

Descriptive epidemiology

- *Incidence* Commonest cause of illness worldwide with an estimated 4620 million cases in 2004.[1] In the UK gastroenteritis is one of the most common reasons for consulting in primary care, with about 1 in 30 people attending for this reason each year. Many more people will be affected and not present to their GP. In the USA each year there are an estimated 76 million cases of food-borne diseases, and 325 000 hospital admissions.[2]
- *Prevalence* As a short-lived condition the point prevalence is generally low, but period prevalence is high, affecting between 1/3 and 1/5 of the population each year.[3]
- *Case fatality* Low, but dependent on the causative agent, the vulnerability of the person, and the availability of re-hydration therapy.
- *Mortality* Globally 2.2 million deaths attributable to diarrhoeal disease in 2004.[1] It causes 17% of deaths in children <5 years, 45% of these are in Africa, 35% in South East Asia, and 20% in the rest of the world.[1] 90% of deaths are in children <5 years mostly in developing countries. In the USA there are around 5000 deaths per year from food-borne diseases.[2]
- *Morbidity* Diarrhoeal disease was the 2nd leading cause of morbidity in 2004 with 72.8 million DALYs worldwide.[1]
- *Time* Many causative agents are seasonal. Diarrhoeal disease is predicted to fall to the 23rd leading cause of death worldwide by 2030.[1]
- *Person* Anyone can be affected, but infants, the elderly and others who are unable to maintain hydration are most vulnerable to severe disease.
- *Place* Occurs everywhere, but the brunt of the morbidity and mortality is in developing countries, particularly those with poor sanitation.

Risk factors

- *Fixed risk factors* Age (young and old); seasonal (dependent on organism).
- *Modifiable risk factors* Unsafe water (affects more than one billion people in the world); sanitation; hygiene; food preparation, storage, distribution and handling.

Prevention

- *Primary prevention* Improved water supply, sanitation and hygiene. WHO estimate that improved sanitation reduces diarrhoea morbidity by 32%, and hygiene education can reduce cases by up to 45%. Food safety in production, distribution and preparation are effective. Vaccines are available against some causative organisms.
- *Secondary prevention* Identification of outbreaks; follow-up cases; investigate potential sources.
- *Treatment/tertiary prevention* Oral re-hydration therapy reduces mortality; antibiotic treatment for some.

Box 12.1 Causes of enteric infections (UK)

- Adenovirus.
- Astrovirus.
- Botulism.
- Calicivirus.
- *Campylobacter spp.*
- Cryptosporidium.
- *Escherichia coli* O157.
- *Entamoeba histolytica.*
- *Giardia lamblia.*
- *Listeria monocytogenes.*
- Norovirus.
- Rotavirus.
- *Salmonella.*
  - *Salmonella enteritidis.*
  - *Salmonella typhimurium.*
  - *Salmonella typhi, paratyphi* A, and *paratyphi.*
- *Shigella* spp.
- *Yersinia* spp.

References

1 WHO *The global burden of disease: 2004 update.* Geneva: WHO; 2004. ℘ http://www.who.int/healthinfo/global_burden_disease/GBD_report_2004update_full.pdf
2 WHO Food safety and foodborne illness (2007) ℘ http://www.who.int/mediacentre/factsheets/fs237/en
3 HPA Gastrointestinal disease. ℘ http://www.hpa.org.uk/infections/topics_az/gastro/menu.htm

Healthcare associated infections

Healthcare associated infections (HCAIs) are infections acquired by patients (or staff) as a result of some healthcare contact (e.g. hospital admission) or other intervention (e.g. outpatient procedure).

Major HCAIs

The following can cause bacteraemia, chest infections, urinary tract infections, peripheral or central line infection etc.
- *Escherichia coli*.
- *Staphylococcus aureus*, including meticillin-resistant *Staphylococcus aureus* (MRSA).
- *Acinetobacter baumannii*.
- Glycopeptide-resistant enterococci (GRE).
- Norovirus and *Clostridium difficile* cause gastrointestinal infection.

Burden

HCAIs cause considerable morbidity and mortality. Estimates of the burden:
- European Union: 3 000 000 HCAIs and up to 50 000 deaths each year.
- UK: estimate 300 000 HCAIs per year, causing 5000 deaths and contributing to over 15 000 deaths per year.
- England: prevalence of HCAIs 8.2% in 2006.
- USA: 1.7 million infections and 99 000 associated deaths each year.

Risk factors for HCAIs

- Underlying illnesses in the patient that increase their susceptibility to infection (e.g. heart disease, critical illness, cancer, AIDS).
- Some treatments may increase susceptibility to infection (e.g. immunosuppressive therapy).
- Invasive procedures provide a portal of entry for organisms (e.g. surgery, intravenous therapy, catheterization).
- Use of antibiotics to treat infection may facilitate the growth of others (e.g. *Candida*, *Clostridium difficile*).
- Widespread use of antibiotics for infection or prophylaxis promotes antibiotic resistance.
- Proximity of patients and high-throughput facilities provide opportunities for transmission between patients.
- Needlestick injury.

Minimizing the risk of HCAI

- Handwashing/ decontamination between patients to prevent the transfer of micro-organisms.
- Use of protective clothing including gloves, aprons, and dress codes to reduce transmission on clothing.
- Appropriate systems to reduce the risk of transmitting infection during invasive procedures (e.g. sterilization, decontamination of equipment).
- Universal and specific precautions for patients with an infection (e.g. enteric or respiratory precautions).
- Correct use of antibiotics to minimise the risk of antibiotic resistant micro-organisms emerging and to reduce the risk of *Clostridium difficile*.

Further reading

Health Protection Agency. *Surveillance of Healthcare Associated Infections Report: 2008*. London: HPA; 2008.

High blood pressure and hypertension

Summary

In >95% of cases (primary) the cause of high BP and hypertension is not known although lifestyle factors are closely related to risk.[1] Hypertension is defined by NICE as a persistent raised BP above 140/90mmHg (systolic/diastolic pressure).[2] Hypertension can directly cause morbidity and mortality but its major contribution to ill health is as a risk factor for cardiovascular disease, stroke in particular. Hypertension is often clinically silent but prompt recognition and treatment can prevent serious consequences. This topic considers disease directly attributable to hypertension; primary and secondary hypertension and hypertensive renal and heart disease.

Descriptive epidemiology

- *Incidence* Difficult to measure as the condition is often clinically silent. Incidence rates of 3–18% have been reported depending on population studied.[3] Worldwide, 8.4 million pregnancies were affected by hypertension in 2004.[4]
- *Prevalence* Worldwide it is estimated that there were almost 1 billion people with hypertension in 2000.[5] In the UK in 2006, 31% of men and 28% of women had hypertension.[6] There were 35 000 admissions to hospital in England in 2008 with hypertensive disease.[7]
- *Mortality* Worldwide there were 1 million deaths from hypertensive heart disease in 2004, which was the 13th most common cause of death[4] and there were a further 62 000 maternal deaths caused by hypertensive disease. There were 4473 deaths in England and Wales in 2008 from hypertensive disease.[8]
- *Disability* Worldwide hypertensive heart disease was responsible for 8 million DALYs in 2004.[4]
- *Time* The prevalence of hypertension is predicted to rise to >1.5 billion adults by 2025.[5]
- *Person* Increases with age (30% of people aged 45–54 and 70% of people aged >70); More common in Black African and Black Caribbean ethnic groups.[1]
- *Place* Hypertensive heart disease is a leading cause of death in middle-income countries where the majority of the burden of disability from this condition is also found.[4]

Risk factors

- *Fixed risk factors* Age; family history; genetic; ethnicity.
- *Modifiable risk factors* Obesity; high salt intake; low potassium intake; excessive alcohol intake; physical inactivity; diabetes.
- *Specific risk factors for secondary hypertension* Dependent on cause.

Prevention for primary hypertension

- *Primary prevention* Maintain healthy weight; reduce salt intake; sensible alcohol intake; physical activity.
- *Secondary prevention* Maintain healthy weight; reduce salt intake; sensible alcohol intake; physical activity; drug treatment.
- *Treatment/tertiary prevention* Dependent on clinical syndrome that results.

References

1 NHS ✍ http://www.cks.nhs.uk
2 National Institute for Health and Clinical Excellence. *Hypertension* (Clinical Guideline 127). London: NICE; 2011. ✍ http://www.nice.org.uk/CG127
3 Hajjar I *et al.* Hypertension: trends in prevalence, incidence, and control. *Annu Rev Public Health* 2006; **27**:465–90.
4 WHO *The global burden of disease: 2004 update.* Geneva: WHO; 2004. ✍ http://www.who.int/healthinfo/global_burden_disease/GBD_report_2004update_full.pdf
5 Kearney PM *et al.* Global burden of hypertension: analysis of worldwide data. *Lancet* 2005; **65**(9455):217–23.
6 BHF ✍ http://www.heartstats.org
7 NHS HES Online2008/9 ✍ http://www.hesonline.nhs.uk
8 ONS Mortality statistics 2008 ✍ http://www.statistics.gov.uk

HIV/AIDS

Summary

HIV is a human retrovirus that causes AIDS, a syndrome that was first recognized clinically in 1981. Two decades later it became the 4th leading cause of death in the world.

Descriptive epidemiology

- *Incidence* In 2009, there were an estimated 2.6 million new cases of HIV globally[1] and 6630 new cases in the UK.[2] Incidence rate of 3.0 per 1000 in men who have sex with men (MSM) in the UK.[2]
- *Prevalence* Globally 33.3 million people are living with HIV,[1] with population prevalence of up to 40% in some parts of sub-Saharan Africa. In the UK it is estimated that 86 500 people were living with HIV in 2009.[2] The population prevalence is estimated at 0.45% in London, 0.08% in the rest of the UK.
- *Case fatality* Without treatment, the majority of people with HIV develop AIDS. Survival from AIDS diagnosis to death <1 year in resource-poor settings. In richer countries 80–90% of patients die within 3–5 years. With treatment the long-term prognosis is much better.
- *Mortality* Globally an estimated 1.8 million deaths in 2009, down from over 2 million in 2004.[1] Declining in the UK: 1743 deaths in 1995 to 527 in 2009 (see Fig. 12.3).
- *Time* Worldwide, incidence has fallen by 19% since the peak in 1999.[1] But HIV is increasing rapidly in many countries (e.g. India, China) while it has reached a plateau in some parts of Africa (e.g. Uganda). It is predicted to fall to the 10th leading cause of worldwide deaths by 2030 with 1.2 million deaths per year.[3] In the UK incidence is increasing due to in-migration of infected people and increased acquisition in MSM.
- *Person* HIV affects sexually active people, recipients of unscreened blood products, injection drug users, and children (vertical transmission).
- *Place* A global disease but unevenly distributed. In 2004 it was the leading cause of adult mortality in Africa and >90% of child deaths caused by HIV/AIDS occurred in Africa.[3]

Risk factors

- *Fixed risk factors* Age (women aged 15–24, men aged 25–34); geographical area.
- *Modifiable risk factors* Unprotected vaginal or anal sex; multiple sex partners; untreated sexually transmitted infections (STIs) (ulcerative, inflammatory); lack of circumcision (men); shared equipment for injecting drugs; occupational exposure (needlestick injuries); blood products (unscreened); breast feeding (infected mother).

Prevention

- *Primary prevention* School sex education; condom distribution and promotion of consistent use; effective STI diagnosis and treatment; targeted harm minimization for groups at increased risk; screening of pregnant women to prevent mother-to-child transmission through use

of anti-retrovirals (ARV) and avoidance of breast feeding; safe blood/
blood product supply through restrictions on donors and screening
of blood; distribution of clean injecting equipment; drug treatment
programmes; pre- and post-exposure prophylaxis for occupational and/
or sexual exposure; poverty reduction programmes, education and
employment, particularly for women.

- *Secondary prevention* Early detection of disease can prevent or delay
  progression to AIDS and can prevent onward transmission. Promotion
  of voluntary testing and counselling (VCT) for early detection of
  disease plus effective partner notification.
- *Treatment/tertiary prevention* ARV therapy substantially reduces morbidity
  and mortality. Treatment of infected individuals with ARVs also
  reduces transmission.[1]

There were over 7000 new HIV infections every day in 2009

- 97% were in low- and middle-income countries.
- 1000 were in children <15 years of age.
- 6000 were in adults aged 15 years and older of whom:
  - 51% were women.
  - 41% were young people aged 15–24 years.

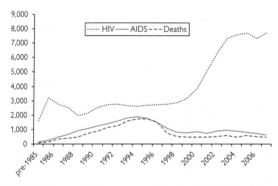

Fig. 12.3 HIV diagnoses, AIDS case reports and deaths in HIV infected individuals,
UK reports to mid-2008 (Data: HPA ℘ http://www.hpa.org.uk).

References

1 UNAIDS ℘ http://www.unaids.org
2 HPA ℘ http://www.hpa.org.uk
3 WHO *The global burden of disease: 2004 update.* Geneva: WHO; 2004. ℘ http://www.who.int/
  healthinfo/global_burden_disease/GBD_report_2004update_full.pdf

Influenza

Summary
Influenza is caused by a virus which attacks mainly the upper-respiratory tract. The virus circulates worldwide and, due to ongoing mutation, varies from season to season. Infection with seasonal influenza confers some degree of immunity to infection by similar viruses which circulate during the following season, limiting the number of new infections. Influenza pandemics occur when new viruses emerge to which there is no pre-existing immunity in the global population. There were 3 pandemics in the 20th century, which resulted in millions of deaths and the most recent was in 2009.

Descriptive epidemiology
- **Incidence** Globally 3–5 million serious cases annually. Up to 30–200 per 100 000 persons per week in the UK, reported through visits to GPs for influenza-like-illness (ILI).
- **Prevalence** In England, there were 135 376 admissions to hospital with influenza in the year 2008/09.[1]
- **Subtype** Most human influenza cases are caused by subtypes A and B, with subtype A causing serious cases more often. Of those influenza cases characterized in the UK in 2007, 60% were subtype A and 36% were subtype B. A small minority of cases are caused by subtype C.
- **Mortality** Globally 250 000–500 000 deaths per year. There were 78 deaths from influenza in England and Wales in 2009 with a further 26 741 deaths from pneumonia.[2] Millions of deaths were attributed to the 1918–19 pandemic, where the case fatality rate was much higher than for seasonal influenza.
- **Transmission** Person-to-person spread via droplets and particles excreted when infected individuals cough or sneeze.
- **Time** Influenza occurs throughout the year, but cases are concentrated over winter months in temperate areas.
- **Person** Incidence of disease is highest amongst infants, the elderly and the immunosuppressed.

Risk factors
- **Fixed risk factors** Immunodeficiency, lung disease, diabetes, cancer, kidney or heart problems; age (infants and elderly); climate (season).

Prevention
- **Primary prevention** Respiratory hygiene: covering mouth and nose with a tissue when coughing and sneezing, proper disposal of used tissues and thorough hand washing. Vaccination: each year a vaccine is produced against the strain which is assessed by WHO to be the most likely major circulating virus in the following season. The efficacy of the vaccine depends on how closely matched the vaccine strain is to the seasonal strain that year. It is unlikely that a strain-specific vaccine will be available quickly enough in the event of pandemic. The seasonal vaccine is currently offered to at-risk groups in the UK. In 2007/08 there was 73.5% coverage of those aged 65 and over, and 45.3% coverage of younger at risk groups.

- *Secondary prevention* Prophylactic treatment of contacts of cases with antiviral drugs; exclusion from school/workplace while infectious.
- *Treatment/tertiary prevention* Antiviral drugs for the treatment of symptomatic influenza are particularly effective if they are taken early in an infection (within two days of the onset of symptoms). Antibiotic treatment of secondary bacterial infections may be necessary for severe cases.

References

1 NHS HES Online 2008/9 ℘ http://www.hesonline.nhs.uk
2 ONS Mortality statistics 2008 ℘ http://www.statistics.gov.uk

Further reading

HPA National Influenza Reports ℘ http://hpa.org.uk
WHO Influenza ℘ http://www.who.int/topics/influenza/en

Kidney cancer

Summary

Kidney cancer includes all cancers of the renal parenchyma, renal pelvis, and ureter. In the UK 90% of kidney cancers are renal cell cancers. Symptomatic patients typically present with haematuria, flank pain, abdominal mass, or systemic effects, e.g. weight loss, lethargy, or anaemia. Advances in diagnostic imaging have meant that it is increasingly diagnosed incidentally in patients undergoing scans (CT/MRI) for other indications.

Descriptive epidemiology (kidney and renal pelvis)

- *Incidence* Worldwide, there were 274 000 new cases in 2008.[9] In the UK it is the 8th commonest cancer with 8228 new cases in 2007.[3]
- *Prevalence* Worldwide, an estimated 586 000 people were alive in 2002 having been diagnosed with kidney cancer within the previous 5 years.[1] In England, there were 13 000 admissions to hospital with kidney cancer in 2008/09.[4]
- *Survival* Depends on grade and stage at presentation. In England and Wales, overall 5-year survival is approximately 50%, but this falls to 10% in people with metastatic disease at diagnosis (approximately 1 in 4 new cases).[2,3]
- *Mortality* Worldwide there were 116 000 deaths from kidney cancer in 2008.[9] In the UK it is the 12th commonest cause of cancer death.[3] There were 3059 deaths in England and Wales in 2009.[5]
- *Time* Incidence is increasing worldwide, in part due to better diagnostic techniques (e.g. CT and MRI).[3]
- *Person* Predominantly occurs in adults, more common in men (possibly due to higher smoking prevalence).[2]
- *Place* Occurs worldwide, but highest age-standardized incidence rates seen in high-income countries.[1]

Risk factors

- *Fixed risk factors* Age; genetic (e.g. tuberous sclerosis, von Hippen–Lindau disease).
- *Modifiable risk factors* Smoking; acquired cystic renal disease;[3] obesity; occupational chemical exposure (e.g. cadmium in manufacture of dyes, plastics, fertilizer, soldering/welding,[7] and printing, rubber, and chemical industries[8]); analgesic (phenacetin, now withdrawn).

Prevention

- *Primary prevention* Smoking cessation; weight loss; control occupational exposure to chemicals.
- *Secondary prevention* Screening using regular imaging (ultrasound, CT, or MRI) is offered to people with certain genetic conditions.
- *Treatment/tertiary prevention* Surgery; chemotherapy; radiotherapy; biological therapy; arterial embolization; regular follow-up with ultrasound, CT or MRI for 5 years.

References

1 WHO GLOBOCAN 2002 ℬ http://www-dep.iarc.fr
2 NICE Guidance TA169 (2009) ℬ http://www.nice.org.uk
3 Cancer Research UK ℬ http://www.cancerresearchuk.org
4 NHS HES Online 2008/9 ℬ http://www.hesonline.nhs.uk
5 Death registrations in England and Wales 2009 ℬ http://www.statistics.gov.uk
6 HPA Cadmium ℬ http://www.hpa.org.uk
8 Pesch B et al. Occupational risk factors for renal cell carcinoma. Int J of Epidemiol 2000; **29**:1014–24.
9 WHO GLOBOCAN 2008 ℬ http://globocan.iarc.fr

Leukaemia

Summary

Leukaemia describes a range of conditions characterized by a malignant proliferation of white blood cells (Table 12.2). Leukaemias are classified as acute or chronic depending on how well-differentiated the malignant clone is and as lymphocytic or myeleogenous depending on which cell type is affected.

Descriptive epidemiology

- *Incidence* Worldwide, there were 375 000 new cases of leukaemia in 2004.[1] In the UK it is the 13th commonest cancer with 7000 new cases in 2007.[2]
- *Prevalence* Worldwide, an estimated 512 000 people were alive in 2002 having been diagnosed with leukaemia within the last 5 years.[3] In England, there were 92 100 admissions to hospital with leukaemia in 2008/09.[4]
- *Survival* Depends on type of leukaemia, age of patient (decreases with age) and stage at presentation. In England and Wales, 5-year survival has increased steadily since the 1970s and is now around 40% overall.[2]
- *Mortality* Worldwide it is the 9th commonest cause of cancer death in men and the 11th commonest cause in women with 277 000 deaths in 2004.[1] There were 3990 deaths from leukaemia in England and Wales in 2009.[5]
- *Time* Age-specific incidence rates have been stable in UK over the last 15 years and mortality has declined since the 1970s as treatment has improved.[2]
- *Person* Slight male preponderance. In the UK, childhood incidence highest aged 0–4 years and adult rates increase from mid-40s to peak in people >85 years.[2] In high-income countries most deaths occur in people >60 while in middle and low-income countries most deaths occur in people aged 15–59 years.[1]
- *Place* Occurs worldwide, lowest incidence seen in Africa and Eastern Mediterranean.[1]

Risk factors

- *Fixed risk factors* Age (mainly ALL in children, CML 40–60 years, AML and CLL >60 years); family history; genetic.
- *Modifiable risk factors* Radiation; radon (see 📖 Lung cancer, p.346)[7]; smoking (see 📖 COPD, p.314); benzene (used to manufacture chemicals[6]).

Prevention

- *Primary prevention* Smoking cessation; control exposure to radiation and radon; control occupational exposure to benzene.
- *Secondary prevention* Screening is not used. Chronic leukaemia is often identified during routine blood tests.
- *Treatment/tertiary prevention* Chemotherapy; biological therapy; radiotherapy; bone marrow and stem cell transplants.

Table 12.2 Overview of leukaemias (UK)

	Acute myeloid leukaemia (AML)	Acute lymphoblastic leukaemia (ALL)	Chronic myeloid leukaemia (CML)	Chronic lymphocytic leukaemia (CLL)
Cases/year	2200	700	600	2600
Age	Increases with age, most cases >65 years	Commonest leukaemia in children	40–60 years	Rare <40 years, increases with age
Risk factors	Radiation Benzene Smoking Genetic (e.g. Fanconi anaemia) Autoimmune Chemotherapy	As AML, plus: Male >female HTLV-1	Male >female Radiation Benzene Smoking Overweight	Family history
5-year survival	Children >66% Adults 8–9% overall (up to 40% in <40 years)	Children >80% Adults 40%	90% if imatinib responsive	Male 44% Female 52%

Source: Data from Cancer Research UK

References

1 WHO *The global burden of disease: 2004 update*. Geneva: WHO; 2004. ℘ http://www.who.int/healthinfo/global_burden_disease/GBD_report_2004update_full.pdf
2 Cancer Research UK ℘ www.cancerresearchuk.org
3 WHO GLOBOCAN 2002 ℘ http://www-dep.iarc.fr
4 NHS HES Online 2008/9 ℘ www.hesonline.nhs.uk
5 Death registrations in England and Wales 2009 ℘ http://www.statistics.gov.uk
6 HPA Benzene ℘ www.hpa.org.uk
7 HPA Radon ℘ http://www.hpa.org.uk

Liver cancer

Summary

The liver is a common site for metastatic cancer deposits. In the UK primary liver cancers are 30x rarer than secondary tumours.[1] Hepatocellular carcinoma is the commonest primary liver cancer. Most cases occur in Asia but their incidence is likely to increase worldwide.

Descriptive epidemiology

- **Incidence** Worldwide, it is the 5th commonest cancer with 632 000 new cases in 2004.[2] In the UK it is the 18th most common cancer with approximately 3400 new cases in 2007.[3]
- **Prevalence** Worldwide, an estimated 386 000 people were alive in 2002 having been diagnosed with liver cancer within the previous 5 years.[4] In England, there were 7600 admissions to hospital with cancer of the liver or intrahepatic bile duct in 2008/09.[5]
- **Survival** Depends on grade and stage at presentation. In the UK 5-year survival is 5%.[3]
- **Mortality** Worldwide, it is the 3rd commonest cause of cancer death in men and the 6th commonest cause in women with 610 000 deaths in 2004.[2] In the UK it is the 14th commonest cause of cancer death. There were 3202 deaths in England and Wales in 2009.[6]
- **Time** Cases are likely to increase as prevalence of alcoholism, obesity related fatty liver disease and hepatitis B and C increase.[7] In the USA the incidence has increased by 80% in the last 20 years.[7]
- **Person** It is rare before 50 years in the USA and Western Europe.[7]
- **Place** Occurs worldwide; most cases occur in the Western Pacific region and it is the 2nd commonest cause of cancer death in the African region.[2]

Risk factors

- **Fixed risk factors** Family history;[3] genetic disorders that cause liver disease including alpha-1 antitrypsin deficiency and haemachromatosis;[3] diabetes (2–3x increased risk).[7]
- **Modifiable risk factors** Underlying liver disease (cirrhosis) from any cause e.g. viral infections (e.g. hepatitis B and C); toxins (alcohol and aflatoxins, produced by *Aspergillius flavus* contamination of nuts, cereals and dried fruit);[8] smoking and alcohol increase the risk of cancer in people with hepatitis B or C;[3] arsenic found in drinking water.

Prevention

- **Primary prevention** Reduce risk of infection with hepatitis B and C (hepatitis B vaccination; protected sexual intercourse; no needle sharing); sensible alcohol consumption; smoking cessation; reduce risk of aflatoxin in food chain.[8]
- **Secondary prevention** AFP (alpha fetoprotein) is produced by some hepatocellular cancers. The British Society for Gastroenterology recommends that people who are at high risk of hepatocellular carcinoma are screened every 6 months with an abdominal ultrasound scan and serum AFP measurement.[9]
- **Treatment/tertiary prevention** Surgery; transplant; chemotherapy; radiotherapy.[3]

References

1 British Society of Gastroenterology ♫ http://www.bsg.org.uk
2 WHO *The global burden of disease: 2004 update.* Geneva: WHO; 2004. ♫ http://www.who.int/healthinfo/global_burden_disease/GBD_report_2004update_full.pdf
3 Cancer Research UK ♫ http://www.cancreresearch.org
4 WHO GLOBOCAN 2002 database ♫ http://www-dep.iarc.fr
5 HES 2008/9 ♫ http://www.hesonline.nhs.uk
6 Death registrations in England and Wales 2009 ♫ http://www.statistics.gov.uk
7 Gomaa AI *et al.* Hepatocellular carcinoma: Epidemiology, risk factors and pathogenesis. *World J Gastroenterol* 2008; **14**(27):4300–8.
8 Food Standards Agency ♫ http://www.food.gov.uk
9 Ryder SD. UK Guidelines for the diagnosis and treatment of hepatocellular carcinoma (HCC) in adults. *Gut* 2003; **52**:iii1–iii8.

Lung cancer

Summary

Over 90% of all lung cancer is caused by tobacco smoking. It is the commonest type of cancer in the world and is responsible for 1.3 million deaths a year. Lung cancer carries a poor prognosis as it often presents at an advanced stage with shortness of breath, cough, and weight loss.

Descriptive epidemiology (trachea, bronchus and lung)

- *Incidence* Worldwide it is the commonest cancer with 1.6 million new cases in 2008.[1] In the UK it is the 2nd commonest cancer with 39 470 new cases in 2007.[2]
- *Prevalence* Worldwide, an estimated 1.4 million people were alive in 2002 having been diagnosed with lung cancer within the previous 5 years.[3] In the UK there are an estimated 65 000 people alive who have ever been diagnosed with lung cancer.[2] In England, there were 83 600 admissions to hospital with lung cancer in 2008/09.[4]
- *Survival* Depends on grade and stage at presentation. In England and Wales 5-year survival is 7%.[2]
- *Mortality* Worldwide it is the commonest cause of cancer death in men and the 2nd commonest cause in women.[5] It caused 1.3 million deaths worldwide in 2004 making it the 8th commonest cause of death overall.[5] In the UK, it is the commonest cause of cancer death.[2] There were 30 018 deaths in England and Wales in 2009.[6]
- *Time* Incidence reflects historical smoking patterns. In the UK new diagnoses have fallen dramatically in men since the 1970s and in women they stopped increasing in the 1990s.[2] Rates are still expected to rise in low- and middle-income countries.
- *Person* Rare before 40 years and more common in men (3M:2F).[2]
- *Place* Current distribution reflects historical patterns of smoking. Occurs worldwide, but predominantly seen in middle and high-income countries with most cases occurring in Europe and the Western Pacific region.[5] Within the UK rates are higher in Northern England and Scotland and lower in the Midlands, South England, and Wales.[2]

Risk factors

- *Fixed risk factors* Age (>80% of cases in over 60s);[2] family history.
- *Modifiable risk factors* Smoking causes 90% of cases;[2] environmental tobacco smoke; radon;[7] occupational chemical exposure (e.g. asbestos, polycyclic hydrocarbons, silica);[2] outdoor air pollution.[8]

Prevention

- *Primary prevention* Tobacco control including: (a) reduce exposure to environmental tobacco smoke—smoking in enclosed public places and workplaces in England became illegal in 2007; (b) reduce number of smokers—in England the legal age for purchasing tobacco increased from 16 to 18 in 2007; (c) reduce tobacco advertising—in 2003 virtually all forms of tobacco advertising were banned in the UK; smoking cessation; maintain safe levels of indoor radon; control occupational chemical exposure.

- *Secondary prevention* Screening is not recommended. A Cochrane review has found that population based screening using sputum, chest X-ray or CT has little impact on treatment or mortality and repeated chest X-rays may actually cause harm.[9]
- *Treatment/tertiary prevention* Small cell cancers: chemotherapy or radiotherapy. Non-small cell cancers: surgery, radiotherapy, chemotherapy.

Radon exposure[7]

Radon is a natural radioactive gas that is released from the uranium found naturally in rocks and soil. Found throughout UK but highest background levels from granite in Cornwall. Radon disperses in the open air but it can accumulate in enclosed spaces (including uranium mines and houses). The UK Government has set targets for indoor radon levels and it is possible to fit a radon sump to reduce indoor levels.

References

1 WHO GLOBOCAN 2008 ⟡ http://globocan.iarc.fr
2 Cancer research UK ⟡ http://www.cancerresearch.org
3 WHO GLOBOCAN 2002 ⟡ http://www-dep.iarc.fr
4 NHS HES Online2008/9 ⟡ http://www.hesonline.nhs.uk
5 WHO *The global burden of disease: 2004 update.* Geneva: WHO; 2004. ⟡ http://www.who.int/healthinfo/global_burden_disease/GBD_report_2004update_full.pdf
6 Death registrations in England and Wales 2009 ⟡ http://www.statistics.gov.uk
7 HPA Radon ⟡ http://www.hpa.org.uk
8 Vineis P *et al.* Lung cancers attributable to environmental tobacco smoke and air pollution in non-smokers in different European countries: a prospective study. *Environ Health* 2007, **6**:7.
9 Manser R *et al.* Screening for lung cancer. *Cochrane Database of Syst Rev*, 2004; **1**: CD001991.

Malaria

Summary

Malaria is an infectious disease caused by 5 species of protozoan parasites of the genus *Plasmodium* spread by the female *Anopheles* mosquito. The species of malaria differ in their geographic distribution and clinical severity.[1] *P. falciparum* is most common in sub-Saharan Africa, Papua New Guinea, and the Solomon Islands and causes most malaria deaths; *P. vivax* found mainly in Central and South America, North Africa, the Middle East, and the Indian subcontinent, causes less severe disease but can relapse; *P. ovale* is found almost exclusively in West Africa and can be asymptomatic; *P. malariae* occurs worldwide, although mainly in Africa and *P. knowlesi* has been recently documented in Borneo and Southeast Asia.[2] The emergence of drug resistance to chloroquine has thwarted control and treatment programmes, but the advent of the use of insecticide treated bednets (ITBNs) and artemisinin-combined therapies (ACTs) appear to be showing some promise.

Descriptive epidemiology

- **Incidence** There were an estimated 2471.3 million new cases of malaria worldwide in 2004.[3] Most cases were caused by falciparum malaria (estimated at 88.4% in 2004[3]). In the UK there were 1370 cases of malaria in 2008.[1]
- **Prevalence** Difficult to measure, but half of the world's population are reported to be at risk.[4]
- **Case fatality** Despite effective therapy, about 1% of all cases of falciparum malaria die. In cases with WHO case definition severe malaria, between 30–50% die.
- **Mortality** It caused 889 000 deaths worldwide in 2004 making it the 14th commonest cause of death overall.[3] It was responsible for 7% of deaths in children <5 years worldwide, increasing to 16% in the African region where 90% of all malaria deaths in children <5 years occured.[3] There were 6 deaths from malaria in the UK in 2008.[1]
- **Morbidity** Worldwide malaria was the 12th commonest cause of disability, responsible for 34 million DALYs in 2004.[3] But it was the 4th commonest cause of disability in low-income countries.
- **Time** In the UK the number of cases and deaths have increased since the early 1970s reflecting trends in travel.
- **Person** People who live in or travel to malarial areas.
- **Place** Malaria predominantly occurs in Africa. 85% of all malaria cases were in the African region in 2004.[3]
- **Transmission** Malaria is spread by the female *Anopheles* mosquito in areas where the temperature exceeds the 16 ^{0}C isotherm. Rare cases occur in temperate climates, for example 'airport malaria' where infected mosquitoes are brought to the country aboard aircraft or where local summer temperatures increase allowing transmission in susceptible local mosquito vectors. Malaria cannot be transmitted directly from person to person, except in rare cases via blood and blood products.

Risk factors

- *Fixed risk factors* Age (young children); ethnicity (white and Asian have increased risk of severe malaria compared to black ethnicity);[5] HIV infection poses relative, but not pronounced risk.
- *Modifiable risk factors* International travel to high prevalence areas; mosquito-avoidance behaviour; adherence to appropriate antimalarial chemoprophylaxis.

Prevention

- *Primary prevention* Improvement of living conditions; vector control (reduction of mosquito breeding sites); sleeping under ITBNs; education of the public on the modes of transmission; appropriate prophylaxis for travellers; vaccination: still in development.
- *Secondary prevention* Screening of blood donors.
- *Tertiary prevention* Prompt seeking of medical treatment; treatment of cases with appropriate antimalarials especially with ACTs which appear to reduce transmission in the mosquito.

References

1 NHS ℘ http://www.nhs.uk
2 Cox-Singh J, Singh B. Knowlesi malaria: newly emergent and of public health importance? *Trends Parasitol* 2008; **24**(9):406–10.
3 WHO *The global burden of disease: 2004 update.* Geneva: WHO; 2004. ℘ http://www.who.int/healthinfo/global_burden_disease/GBD_report_2004update_full.pdf
4 WHO ℘ http://www.who.int
5 Phillips A et al. Risk factors for severe disease in adults with falciparum malaria. *Clin Infect Dis* 2009; **48**(7):871–8.

Further reading

CDC Guidelines: ℘ http://www.cdc.gov/malaria/control_prevention/index.htm
UK data and advice: ℘ http://www.hpa.org.uk/webw/HPAweb&HPAwebStandard/HPAweb_C/12 03496943315?p=1153846674367
World Health Organization Malaria site ℘ http://www.who.int/malaria/malariaandtravellers.html

Malignant melanoma

Summary

Malignant melanoma is the most aggressive type of skin cancer. A leading cause is exposure to UV radiation and it is most commonly seen in fair-skinned people who live or holiday in sunny climates. In the UK incidence is rising faster than any other cancer and it is now the commonest cancer in young adults. It is a major public health problem and as population awareness increases, earlier diagnosis is leading to a fall in mortality.

Descriptive epidemiology

- *Incidence* Worldwide there were 200 000 new cases of malignant melanoma in 2008.[6] In the UK it is the 2nd commonest cancer in people 15–34 years and the 6th commonest cancer overall with 10 670 new cases in 2007.[2]
- *Prevalence* Worldwide, an estimated 643 000 people were alive in 2002 having been diagnosed with malignant melanoma within the previous 5 years.[1] In England, there were 12 300 admissions to hospital with malignant melanoma in 2008/09.[3]
- *Survival* Depends on site, thickness, and stage at presentation. In the UK 5-year survival has increased dramatically since the 1970s and is now 81% in men and 90% in women.[2]
- *Mortality* Worldwide, there were 46 000 deaths from melanoma in 2008.[6] In the UK it is the 17th commonest cause of cancer death.[2] There were 1858 deaths in England and Wales in 2009.[4]
- *Time* In fair-skinned Caucasian populations the incidence of melanoma is increasing rapidly (3–7% per year).[5] There has been a 4-fold increase in cases in the UK since the 1970s.[2]
- *Person* Fair-skinned people who have high exposure to UV either through sunbathing, use of sun-beds, or living in hot climates. More common in young women than young men, but mortality is higher in men.[2]
- *Place* Occurs worldwide, but highest rates are found in fair-skinned Caucasian populations in temperate or tropical climates, e.g. Australia and New Zealand.

Risk factors

- *Fixed risk factors* Fair skin/hair; naevi; family history.
- *Modifiable risk factors* UV exposure (e.g. sunbathing, sun-beds); sunburn; previous non-melanoma skin cancer.

Prevention

- *Primary prevention* Sensible UV exposure (e.g. 'Slip-Slap-Slop' campaign in Australia, regulation of tanning salons).
- *Secondary prevention* Regular checking of skin for moles/change in moles (*A*–asymmetry, *B*–border, *C*–colour, *D*–diameter).
- *Treatment/tertiary prevention* Surgery; chemotherapy; radiotherapy; biological therapy.

References

1 WHO GLOBOCAN 2002 ℘ http://www-dep.iarc.fr
2 Cancer research UK ℘ http://www.cancerresearch.org
3 NHS HES Online2008/9 ℘ http://www.hesonline.nhs.uk
4 Death registrations in England and Wales 2009 ℘ http://www.statistics.gov.uk
5 Lens MB, Dawes, M. Global perspectives of contemporary epidemiological trends of cutaneous malignant melanoma. *Br J Dermatol* 2004; **150**:179–85.
6 WHO GLOBOCAN 2008 ℘ http://globocan.iarc.fr

Measles

Summary

Measles is a viral illness that was common in childhood in high-income countries before the introduction of vaccination. Common symptoms are fever, cough and rash.[1] The incidence of measles in the UK increased when vaccination rates fell in response to discredited research linking the vaccine to autism and inflammatory bowel disease.

Descriptive epidemiology

- *Incidence* Worldwide there were 27.1 million cases of measles in 2004, almost 2/3 of which were in South East Asia.[2]
- *Prevalence* The prevalence of infection is closely linked to vaccination rates.
- *Case fatality* In the UK, 1 in 5000 children with measles die.[3]
- *Mortality* Mortality has fallen in recent years. Estimated to caused 424 000 deaths worldwide in 2004 >99% of which were in children under the age of 15. Measles was responsible for 4% of all deaths in children under 5, of which 45% occurred in Africa, 45% in South East Asia and 5% in the rest of the world.[2]
- *Morbidity* Measles was responsible for 14.9 million DALYs in 2004, almost 90% of which were in Africa and South East Asia.[2]
- *Time* As vaccination becomes more available, the incidence of infection will fall. The WHO Western Pacific Region has a goal for measles elimination by 2012.[4]

Risk factors

- *Fixed risk factors* None.
- *Modifiable risk factors* Unvaccinated; travel to an endemic area or to an area affected by an outbreak.

Prevention

- *Primary prevention* Vaccination in the UK, the MMR (measles, mumps, rubella) vaccine is recommended at 13 months with a booster before the start of school.[1]
- *Secondary prevention* Exclusion during the infectious period; vaccination of contacts of cases; human normal immunoglobulin in contacts of cases where vaccine is contraindicated.
- *Tertiary prevention/treatment* No specific treatment.

References

1 NHS ⅏ http://www.nhs.uk
2 WHO *The global burden of disease: 2004 update*. Geneva: WHO; 2004. ⅏ http://www.who.int/healthinfo/global_burden_disease/GBD_report_2004update_full.pdf
3 NHS CKS ⅏ http://www.cks.nhs.uk
4 WHO ⅏ http://www.wpro.who.int

Meningococcal disease

Summary

Meningococcal disease* is caused by the bacteria *Neisseria meningitidis*. The bacteria is frequently carried in the throat without causing disease but occasionally causes a systemic disease with septicaemia and meningitis. The organism is categorized into serogroups (B, C, A, Y, and W135) based on the polysaccharide outer capsule.

Descriptive epidemiology

- *Incidence* Worldwide there were estimated to be 700 000 cases of meningitis (all causes) in 2004.[1] Globally the incidence of meningococcal disease varies, but during outbreaks in Africa the incidence is around 100–800 per 100 000.[2] Systemic disease incidence is 2–6 per 100 000 person years in the UK.[3]
- *Prevalence* 10% of the population will carry the organism in their throats,[4] higher in 15–19-year-olds (up to 25%).[3]
- *Subtype* Most disease in the UK was caused by serogroups B (60–65%) and C (35–40%) before the introduction of a vaccine against C. Currently >90% of cases are group B and ≤2% are group C.[3]
- *Case fatality* 50% of untreated cases.[2] 10% even with healthcare available,[3] increasing to 40% in patients who present in shock. Most deaths in meningococcal infection are due to meningococcal septicaemia rather than meningitis.
- *Mortality* Globally 340 000 deaths were attributed to meningitis (all causes) in 2004.[1]
- *Morbidity* Up to 20% of meningitis survivors may have neurological sequelae including mental retardation and hearing loss.[2]
- *Transmission* Person-to-person spread via droplet, aided by prolonged (e.g. household) contact.
- *Time* Meningococcal disease occurs mostly as sporadic cases with <5% occurring in clusters and occasional outbreaks. Seasonal variation with a peak in winter in temperate areas. Large outbreaks can occur with W135 serogroup, mostly in Africa.
- *Person* Highest incidence in children <5, with a 2nd peak in young adults 15–19 years old. Rates are slightly higher in males.
- *Place* Industrially developed countries have low endemicity. In parts of Africa meningococcal disease is hyperendemic.

Risk factors

- *Fixed risk factors* Age (children); sex (male); immunodeficiency; asplenia; respiratory tract infections; anaemia; climate (seasons).
- *Modifiable risk factors* Overcrowding; close contact with infected individuals; travel to hyperendemic areas; military recruits; passive smoking; influenza A.

---

*Meningitis refers to inflammation of the brain or spinal cord from any cause.

Prevention

- *Primary prevention* Polysaccharide vaccines exist against serogroups A, C, Y, W135 in various combinations. A monovalent conjugate vaccine against serogroup C was introduced in 1999 in the UK;[5] immunization uptake levels of 85% in target age groups (12 months to 17 years) led to an 80% reduction in the incidence of meningococcal meningitis group C in these groups within 18 months.[3]
- *Secondary prevention* Vaccination/prophylactic antibiotics for close contacts of cases. Parents of young children and university students should be aware of and recognize the symptoms of meningitis. This requires more education and public awareness as if left untreated, meningitis is fatal.
- *Treatment/tertiary prevention* A range of antibiotics may be used for treatment of bacterial meningitis. Hospitalization and intensive support for established disease.

References

1 WHO *The global burden of disease: 2004 update*. Geneva: WHO; 2004. ℘ http://www.who.int/healthinfo/global_burden_disease/GBD_report_2004update_full.pdf
2 WHO ℘ http://www.who.int
3 HPA ℘ http://www.hpa.org.uk
4 Van Deuren, M et al. Update on meningococcal disease with emphasis on pathogenesis and clinical management. *Clin Microbiol Rev* 2000; **13**:144–66.
5 Department of Health. *The Green Book*. London: DH; 2006. ℘ http://www.dh.gov.uk/en/Publicationsandstatistics/Publications/PublicationsPolicyAndGuidance/DH_079917

Further reading

HPA Meningococcus and Haemophilus Forum. *Guidance for public health management of meningococcal disease in the UK, Updated January 2011*. ℘ http://www.hpa.org.uk/web/HPAwebFile/HPAweb_C/1194947389261

Neglected tropical diseases

Summary
The introduction to this chapter described how the burden of infectious disease disproportionately falls on low- and middle-income countries. Within these regions there are a group of infectious diseases, collectively known as neglected tropical diseases (NTDs). It is estimated that >1 billion people have 1 or more of these infections[1]. 7* of the NTDs can be controlled by annual doses of safe and effective drugs which cost <25 pence per person per year.

The major neglected tropical diseases
- *Protozoan* Leishmaniasis; trypanosomiasis (sleeping sickness); Chagas disease.
- *Helminthic* Ascariasis*; trichuriasis*; hookworm*; lymphatic filariasis* (elephantiasis); onchocerciasis* (River blindness); schistosomiasis*; dracunculiasis (Guinea worm); cysticercosis.
- *Bacterial* Leprosy; trachoma*; Buruli ulcer.

Morbidity and mortality (Table 12.3)

Table 12.3 DALYs and deaths arising from NTDs in 2004[2]

	DALYs	Deaths
Leishmaniasis	1 974 000	47 000
Trypanosomiasis	1 673 000	52 000
Chagas disease	430 000	11 000
Ascariasis	1 851 000	2000
Trichuriasis	1 012 000	2000
Hookworm	1 092 000	0
Lymphatic filariasis	5 941 000	0
Onchocerciasis	389 000	0
Schistosomiasis	1 707 000	41 000
Leprosy	194 000	5000
Trachoma	1 334 000	0

Prevention
- *Primary prevention* Specific to condition, but includes vector control (black flies; mosquitos etc.); clean water; sanitation; hygiene practice.
- *Secondary prevention* Specific to condition, but can include mass drug administration (MDA).
- *Treatment/tertiary prevention* Specific to condition, but can include MDA; antimicrobials/antihelminthics; iron supplementation.

References
1 CDC 2011 ℰ http://www.cdc.gov/parasites/ntd.html
2 WHO *The global burden of disease: 2004 update.* Geneva: WHO; 2004. ℰ http://www.who.int/ healthinfo/global_burden_disease/GBD_report_2004update_full.pdf

Further reading
Fenwick A. Waterborne infectious diseases – could they be consigned to history? *Science* 2006; **313**:1077–81.
Hotez P et al. Recent progress in integrated neglected tropical disease control. *Trends in Parasitology* 2007; **23**:511–14.

Non-Hodgkin lymphoma

Summary

Non-Hodgkin lymphoma (NHL) includes all malignant proliferations of lymphocytes, excluding Hodgkin lymphoma. NHL can affect B cells or T cells. They divide abnormally and accumulate in the lymph nodes, most commonly in the neck. People typically present with a persistent palpable lymph node, systemic symptoms (fever, weight loss, itch) or the effects of the cancer (pressure symptoms from mass, anaemia or infection from loss of normal bone marrow function).

Descriptive epidemiology

- *Incidence* Worldwide, there were 356 000 new cases of NHL in 2009.[5] In the UK, it is the 5th commonest cancer with 10 920 new cases in 2007.[2]
- *Prevalence* Worldwide, an estimated 751 000 people were alive in 2002 having been diagnosed with NHL within the previous 5 years.[1] In England, there were 77 300 admissions to hospital with NHL in 2008/09.[3]
- *Survival* Depends on age of patient, type of NHL, and stage at presentation. In the UK 5-year survival is ~55% overall.[2]
- *Mortality* Worldwide, there were 192 000 deaths from NHL in 2008.[5] In the UK it is the 9th commonest cause of cancer death.[2] There were 3993 deaths in England and Wales in 2009.[4]
- *Time* Dramatic increase in age-standardized incidence rates over last 30 years in UK (>40%) and other high-income countries, partly due to change in diagnosis and classification.[2]
- *Person* Affects slightly more males than females and tends to occur in older adults (>60 years).[2]
- *Place* Worldwide, but most cases are in high-income countries.[2] HIV is associated with Burkitt's lymphoma (an aggressive form of NHL).

Risk factors

- *Fixed risk factors* Sex ($\male$>$\female$); age (70% of cases in over 60s);[2] family history; coeliac disease (T cell lymphoma of gut).
- *Modifiable risk factors* Immunosuppression e.g. HIV, autoimmune disease, post-transplant, previous chemotherapy; infection (e.g. EBV in Burkitt's lymphoma).

Prevention

- *Primary prevention* No known prevention.
- *Secondary prevention* Screening is not used.
- *Treatment/tertiary prevention* Radiotherapy; chemotherapy; biological therapy.

References

1 WHO GLOBOCAN 2002 ♒ http://www-dep.iarc.fr
2 Cancer research UK ♒ www.cancerresearch.org
3 NHS HES Online2008/9 ♒ www.hesonline.nhs.uk
4 Death registrations in England and Wales 2009 ♒ http://www.statistics.gov.uk
5 WHO GLOBOCAN 2008 ♒ http://www.globocan.iarc.fr

Oesophageal cancer

Summary

Oesophageal cancer commonly presents with difficulty swallowing. Many patients present with advanced disease which carries a very poor prognosis. Oesophageal cancer is strongly associated with smoking and alcohol consumption. It is particularly common in Eastern Asia.

Descriptive epidemiology

- *Incidence* Worldwide, there were 482 000 new cases of oesophageal cancer in 2008.[8] In the UK it is the 9th commonest cancer with 7970 new cases in 2007.[2]
- *Prevalence* Worldwide, an estimated 424 000 people were alive in 2002 having been diagnosed with oesophageal cancer within the previous 5 years.[1] In England, there were 33 100 admissions to hospital with oesophageal cancer in the year 2008/09.[3]
- *Survival* Depends on grade and stage at presentation. In the UK 5-year survival is 8%.[2]
- *Mortality* Worldwide it is the 5th commonest cause of cancer death in men and the 7th commonest cause in women with 508 000 deaths overall in 2004.[4] In the UK it is the 6th commonest cause of cancer death.[2] There were 6645 deaths in England and Wales in 2009.[5]
- *Time* Age-standardized incidence has steadily increased over the last 30 years in the UK.[2] This could be due to the increase in the prevalence of smoking, gastro-oesophageal reflux disease, obesity, and the decline in fruit and vegetable intake.[6]
- *Person* More common in men[1] and tends to present in people >40 years.[2]
- *Place* An area of Iran has the highest age-standardized incidence rate.[2] Most deaths occur in middle income countries and it is the 3rd commonest cause of cancer death in men in Africa and South East Asia and the 2nd commonest cause of cancer deaths in women in the Eastern Mediterranean.[4]

Risk factors

- *Fixed risk factors* Age (80% of cases in over 60s)[2]; genetic (e.g. Plummer–Vinson syndrome, tylosis); Barrett's oesophagus.
- *Modifiable risk factors*[6] Adenocarcinoma—obesity; diet (low in fruit and vegetables); gastro-oesophageal reflux. Squamous cell carcinoma—smoking and alcohol (increase risk independently and have a multiplicative effect); diet (low fruit and vegetable).

Prevention

- *Primary prevention* Smoking cessation; sensible alcohol consumption.
- *Secondary prevention* Screening is not currently recommended. No evidence to suggest endoscopic screening in people with Barrett's oesophagus is clinically effective.[7]
- *Treatment/tertiary prevention* Surgery; chemotherapy; radiotherapy; dietary advice.

References

1 WHO GLOBOCAN 2002 ✍ http://www-dep.iarc.fr
2 Cancer research UK ✍ http://www.cancerresearch.org
3 NHS HES Online2008/9 ✍ http://www.hesonline.nhs.uk
4 WHO *The global burden of disease: 2004 update.* Geneva: WHO; 2004. ✍ http://www.who.int/healthinfo/global_burden_disease/GBD_report_2004update_full.pdf
5 Death registrations in England and Wales 2009 ✍ http://www.statistics.gov.uk
6 Engel LS. Population attributable risks of esophageal and gastric cancers. *J Natl Cancer Inst* 2003; **95**(18):1404–13.
7 Sommerville M. Surveillance of Barrett's oesophagus: is it worthwhile? *Eur J Cancer* 2008; **44**(4):588–99.
8 WHO GLOBOCAN 2008 ✍ http://globocan.iarc.fr

Pancreatic cancer

Summary

Pancreatic cancer has a very high mortality as the majority of people present with advanced disease. The symptoms are mostly non-specific including weight loss, lethargy, and back pain. Obstructive jaundice can occur when the tumour compresses the bile duct, therefore cancer in the head of the pancreas often presents earlier than more distal tumours.

Descriptive epidemiology

- *Incidence* Worldwide there were 279 000 new cases of pancreatic cancer in 2008.[6] In the UK, it is the 11th commonest cancer with 7680 new cases in 2007.[2]
- *Prevalence* Worldwide, an estimated 143 000 people were alive in 2002 having been diagnosed with pancreatic cancer within the previous 5 years.[1] In England, there were 22 600 admissions to hospital with pancreatic cancer in 2008/09.[3]
- *Survival* Depends on grade and stage at presentation, but generally survival is very low. In the UK 5-year survival is 3%.[2]
- *Mortality* Worldwide it is the 11th commonest cause of cancer death in men and the 10th commonest cause in women with 265 000 deaths overall in 2004.[4] In the UK it is the 5th commonest cause of cancer death.[2] There were 7416 deaths in England and Wales in 2009.[5]
- *Time* In the UK, the age standardized incidence rate in women has not changed, but there has been a steady decline in incidence in men over the last 30 years which may reflect changes in smoking prevalence.[2]
- *Person* Usually affects adults over the age of 60.
- *Place* Worldwide, most cases are in high/middle income countries.[4]

Risk factors

- *Fixed risk factors* Age (80% of cases in over 60s)[2]; type 1 diabetes; chronic pancreatitis (depending on cause); genetic (10% of cases e.g. BRAC2, MEN-1); family history.
- *Modifiable risk factors* Smoking; obesity; type 2 diabetes.

Prevention

- *Primary prevention* Smoking cessation; weight loss; sensible alcohol consumption (prevent chronic pancreatitis).
- *Secondary prevention* Screening is not recommended at present on a population scale, but screening in people at risk of familial/genetic cancer may be developed.
- *Treatment/tertiary prevention* Surgery; chemotherapy; radiotherapy.

References

1 WHO GLOBOCAN 2002 ॐ http://www-dep.iarc.fr
2 Cancer research UK ॐ http://www.cancerresearch.org
3 NHS HES Online 2008/9 ॐ http://www.hesonline.nhs.uk
4 WHO *The global burden of disease: 2004 update*. Geneva: WHO; 2004. ॐ http://www.who.int/healthinfo/global_burden_disease/GBD_report_2004update_full.pdf
5 Death registrations in England and Wales 2009 ॐ http://www.statistics.gov.uk
6 WHO GLOBOCAN 2008 ॐ http://www-dep.iarc.fr

Peptic ulcer disease

Summary

Peptic ulcer disease (ulcers in the stomach and duodenum) (PUD) is often asymptomatic but can present with epigastric burning and/or blood loss. Perforated ulcers were a major cause of morbidity and mortality before Helicobactor pylori (H. pylori) (a risk factor) and proton-pump inhibitors (a treatment) were discovered. In places where diagnosis and treatment is readily available, PUD is rapidly coming under control.

Descriptive epidemiology

- *Incidence* It is difficult to estimate incidence as many cases are asymptomatic and therefore go undiagnosed.[1]
- *Prevalence* It is difficult to estimate prevalence. In England, there were 25 500 admissions to hospital with PUD in the year 2008/09.[2]
- *Case fatality* 15–20% of people with PUD develop internal bleeding and 2–10% of people will have a perforated ulcer.[1]
- *Mortality* Worldwide there were 270 000 deaths from PUD in 2004.[3] There were 2192 deaths directly attributed to gastric and duodenal ulcers in England and Wales in 2008.[4]
- *Disability* Worldwide, PUD was responsible for 5 million DALYs in 2004.[3]
- *Time* In the UK admissions with advanced disease (perforation and haemorrhage) have increased in older adults despite the advent of medication.[5]
- *Person* Men are disproportionately affected by morbidity and mortality.[3] Mainly a disease of adults, but children experience an increasing burden of disease from high- to low-income countries.[3]
- *Place* Low-income countries contribute most of the worldwide DALYs and most deaths occur in middle- and low-income countries.[3]

Risk factors

- *Fixed risk factors* None
- *Modifiable risk factors* H. pylori (80% of gastric ulcers and 95% of duodenal ulcers)[7]; non-steroidal anti-inflammatory drugs (NSAIDs) (20% of gastric ulcers and 5% of duodenal ulcers)[7]; other medications (e.g. bisphosphonates).

Prevention

- *Primary prevention* Cautious use of NSAIDs; treatment of H. pylori.
- *Secondary prevention* Avoid NSAIDs if possible.
- *Treatment/tertiary prevention* H. pylori eradication; proton pump inhibitors; surgery.

Helicobacter pylori[6]

- Gram-negative rod that infects the gastric mucosa (of humans).
- Discovered in 1982.
- Causes chronic inflammation of the gastric mucosa.
- Rates of infection are falling as hygiene standards improve.
- Seroprevalence studies in adults suggest that prevalence in developing countries is up to 70% while prevalence in developed countries is lower, <40%.
- Risk factors: age (infection usually occurs in childhood); ABO blood group; high density housing or overcrowding; socio-economic deprivation.
- The mode of transmission has not been elucidated therefore public health interventions are not yet possible.

References

1 NHS Choices ₰ http://www.nhs.uk/conditions
2 NHS HES Online 2008/9 ₰ http://www.hesonline.nhs.uk
3 WHO *The global burden of disease: 2004 update.* Geneva: WHO; 2004. ₰ http://www.who.int/healthinfo/global_burden_disease/GBD_report_2004update_full.pdf
4 ONS Mortality statistics 2008 ₰ http://www.statistics.gov.uk
5 Higham J et al. Recent trends in admissions and mortality due to peptic ulcer in England: increasing frequency of haemorrhage among older subjects. *Gut* 2002; **50**:460–4.
6 Brown LM. Helicobacter pylori: epidemiology and routes of transmission. *Epidemiol Rev* 2000; **22**(2):283–97.
7 NHS CKS ₰ http://www.cks.nhs.uk

Prostate cancer

Summary

1 in 4 cancers diagnosed in men in the UK is a prostate cancer. Worldwide differences in the use of prostate specific antigen (PSA) as a screening test and TURP (transurethral resection of the prostate) make it difficult to compare trends across countries. Screening can identify cancers before they present symptomatically, although the evidence suggests that many prostate cancers detected through screening would not have developed into clinical disease if left undetected.[10] Countries with widespread use of PSA screening have higher incidence rates and longer survival. The impact of screening on mortality is less clear.

Descriptive epidemiology

- *Incidence* Worldwide, there were 899 000 new cases in 2008.[9] In the UK it is the commonest cancer in men and the 4th commonest cancer overall with 36 100 cases in 2007.[1]
- *Prevalence* Worldwide, an estimated 2.4 million people were alive in 2002 having been diagnosed with prostate cancer within the previous 5 years.[3] In England, there were 47 900 admissions to hospital with prostate cancer in 2008/09.[4]
- *Survival* Depends on grade and stage at presentation. In the UK 5-year survival is 77%.[1]
- *Mortality* Worldwide, it is the 6th commonest cause of cancer death in men with 308 000 deaths in 2004.[2] It is the 4th commonest cause of cancer death in the UK.[2] There were 9402 deaths in England and Wales in 2009.[5] However, in many cases, men live with their prostate cancer and die from an unrelated condition.
- *Time* In the UK, age-standardized incidence rates have increased dramatically over the last 30 years while over the last 10 years, mortality has declined and survival has increased.[1] It is difficult to determine the relative contribution of better diagnostic tests and improvements in treatment.
- *Person* Rarely occurs in men under the age of 50 and it is more common in black ethnic groups compared to white or Asian.
- *Place* Occurs worldwide, but most cases are seen in Europe and the Americas.[2] It is the commonest cause of cancer death in men in Africa and men in low- and middle-income countries in the Americas, including the Caribbean.[2]

Risk factors

- *Fixed risk factors* Sex; age (60% of cases in those >70 years)[1]; ethnicity (black >white and Asian); genetic (BRAC1 and 2).
- *Modifiable risk factors* None identified.

Prevention
- *Primary prevention* No known prevention.
- *Secondary prevention* Screening is possible using PSA but it is controversial. In the US, Medicare provides annual PSA screening for all men aged >50,[6] while in the UK population-wide screening is not recommended.[7] PSA is not specific to cancer and can be elevated in benign conditions of the prostate. A Cochrane review in 2006 concluded that there was insufficient evidence to determine the impact of prostate screening on mortality.[8] Further research is needed.
- *Treatment/tertiary prevention* TURP; surgery; radiotherapy; chemotherapy; hormone treatment.

References
1 Cancer research UK ✍ http://www.cancerresearch.org
2 WHO *The global burden of disease: 2004 update.* Geneva: WHO; 2004. ✍ http://www.who.int/healthinfo/global_burden_disease/GBD_report_2004update_full.pdf
3 WHO GLOBOCAN 2002 ✍ http://www-dep.iarc.fr
4 NHS HES Online 2008/9 ✍ http://www.hesonline.nhs.uk
5 Death registrations in England and Wales 2009 ✍ http://www.statistics.gov.uk
6 Center for Medicare and Medicaid services ✍ http://www.cms.gov/ProstateCancerScreening
7 NHS Prostate Cancer Screening ✍ http://www.cancerscreening.nhs.uk
8 Ilic D et al. Screening for prostate cancer. *Cochrane Database Syst Rev* 2006; **3**:CD004720.
9 WHO GLOBOCAN 2008 ✍ http://globocan.iarc.fr
10 National Cancer Institute ✍ http://www.cancer.gov

Road traffic accidents

Summary

Road traffic accidents are a major public health problem. They are predicted to increase in importance, as motor vehicle ownership increases in middle and low-income countries, to become the 5th leading cause of death worldwide by 2030.[1]

Descriptive epidemiology

- *Incidence* Worldwide, in 2004 there were estimated to be 24.3 million injuries caused by road traffic accidents.[1] In the UK the Department for Transport reported that 230 905 people were injured on Britain's roads in 2008.[2]
- *Mortality* Worldwide, road traffic accidents were the 9th leading cause of death with 1.3 million deaths in 2004.[1] In 2008, there were 2538 deaths from road accidents in Britain.[2]
- *Disability* Worldwide road traffic accidents were the 9th most common cause of disability, responsible for 41.2 million DALYs in 2004.[1]
- *Time* By 2030, road traffic accidents are predicted to become the 5th leading cause of death worldwide, when they will result in 2.4 million deaths a year and be the 3rd leading cause of DALYs. This increase is predicted to result from increased motor-vehicle ownership in middle- and low-income countries.[1] Over the same period, road traffic accident deaths are predicted to fall by 27% in high-income countries.[3]
- *Person* Children, the elderly, pedestrians, and cyclists are the most affected type of road user.[3] Over half of road traffic accident deaths occur in people aged 15–44. In this age group they are also the 3rd leading cause of disease burden.[1,3]
- *Place* 90% of road traffic deaths occur in low- and middle-income countries.[3] Middle-income countries are most affected; in these countries road traffic accidents were the 4th leading cause of DALYs in 2004.[1]

Risk factors

- *Fixed risk factors* Age (children and elderly).
- *Modifiable risk factors* Pedestrians and cyclists; speeding (in 2008 in the UK 14% of accidents involved people driving above the speed limit or too fast for the conditions on the road);[2] alcohol (in 2008 in the UK 6% of all casualties occurred during an accident where one driver was over the legal limit).[2]

Prevention

- *Primary prevention* Road safety campaigns to promote helmet and seat-belt wearing; speed restrictions; visibility and drink driving awareness; transport policy to encourage safer modes/routes of transport; vehicle safety development.[3]
- *Secondary prevention* (i.e. preventing further damage after the accident has occurred) Seat belt use; helmet wearing; vehicle safety features (e.g. airbags).
- *Treatment/tertiary prevention* Prompt access to effective healthcare.

Examples of Road Safety Campaigns

- UK 2010: THINK![4]
- Australia 2007: 'Speeding, no one thinks big of you'.[5]
- UK 1972: Clunk Click Every Trip.[6]

References

1 WHO *The global burden of disease: 2004 update.* Geneva: WHO; 2004. ℘ http://www.who.int/healthinfo/global_burden_disease/GBD_report_2004update_full.pdf
2 UK Department for Transport ℘ http://www.dft.gov.uk
3 WHO ℘ http://www.who.int
4 UK Department for Transport ℘ http://www.dft.gov.uk/think
5 New South Wales Government ℘ http://www.rta.nsw.gov.au
6 The National Archives ℘ http://www.nationalarchives.gov.uk

Self-inflicted injuries

Summary

Self-inflicted injuries include harm resulting from intentional self-poisoning or overdosing including the use of drugs, alcohol, or other chemicals; hanging; strangulation; drowning; firearm use; jumping; use of a motor vehicle or other object; electrocution. They are usually broadly classified into 2 groups; self-harm and suicide*.

*Suicide defined as death from self-inflicted injury.

Descriptive epidemiology

- **Incidence** Worldwide there were 844 000 suicides in 2004, making it the 16th commonest cause of death.[1] There were 3438 suicides in England and Wales in 2008[2] and 34 598 suicides in the US in 2007.[3]
- **Disability** In 2004 they were also the 20th commonest cause of disability worldwide with 19.6 million DALYs.[1] The highest burden of disease was seen in people aged 15–44 years, where it was the 8th leading cause of DALYs worldwide in 2004.[1]
- **Time** From 1950–95 the death rate from suicide increased almost 50% in men and 33% in women.[4] By 2020, the number of deaths from suicide worldwide is predicted to increase to 1.53 million.[4]
- **Person** Men have a 3x higher death rate from suicide than women globally. China is reported to be the only country where women have the higher death rate.[4] The death rate from suicide increases with age, but 15–44-year-olds have more deaths from suicide than people >45.[4]
- **Place** The highest rates of suicide are seen in Europe, particularly Eastern Europe.[4] In Europe they were the 10th leading cause of DALYS in 2004.[1]

Risk factors

- **Fixed risk factors** Age (increases with age); male
- **Modifiable risk factors** Mental illness (depression, schizophrenia, alcohol use disorders); chronic physical illness; social isolation; abuse, violence or loss of cultural and social background.

Prevention

- **Primary prevention** Reduce availability of means (e.g. paracetamol packaging; firearm regulations; improved safety at suicide 'hot spots'); identification and treatment of mental illness; responsible reporting by the media.

References

1 WHO *The global burden of disease: 2004 update*. Geneva: WHO; 2004. ⅏ http://www.who.int/healthinfo/global_burden_disease/GBD_report_2004update_full.pdf
2 ONS Mortality statistics 2008 ⅏ http://www.statistics.gov.uk
3 FASTSTATS ⅏ http://www.cdc.gov
4 Bertolote J, Fleischmann A. A global perspective in the epidemiology of suicide. *Suicidologi* 2002 7(2):6–8.

Sexually transmitted infections

Summary

Sexually transmitted infections (STI) are common and cause considerable morbidity and mortality in the world. The major conditions are shown in Table 12.4. In developing countries, STIs and their complications rank in the top five disease categories for which adults seek health care.

Descriptive epidemiology

- *Incidence* WHO estimates that there were 340 million new cases of curable STI globally in 1999 and an estimated 23.6 million new HSV-2 infections.[1] In the UK in 2009 there were >217 000 cases of chlamydia, 91 000 cases of genital warts, 30 000 cases of genital herpes, 17 000 cases of gonorrhoea, and 3200 cases of syphilis diagnosed in genitourinary medicine clinics (and community-based settings for chlamydia screening).[2]
- *Prevalence* The prevalence of STI is higher than the reported incidence as many are asymptomatic, may remain undiagnosed and become chronic. For curable, bacterial STIs, the estimated prevalence ranges from 2% (for 15–49-year-olds) in Western Europe to 12% in Sub-Saharan Africa.[2] In England, the prevalence of genital chlamydia is 5–7% in 15–24-year-olds (chlamydia screening programme).[2] The number of adults living with HSV-2 infection worldwide is estimated to be 536 million in 2003.[1]
- *Case fatality* STI (excluding HIV) has a low case fatality rate, although untreated syphilis may in the long term lead to fatal cardiovascular or neurological disease.
- *Mortality* An estimated 0.1 million deaths globally each year from STI (other than HIV).[1]
- *Morbidity* STI (excluding HIV) morbidity is primarily measured in terms of reproductive morbidity. Global estimates of YLDs for STI in 2002 were 5.1 million for women and 1.9 million for men. [1]
- *Time* Incidence of STI varies over time. In the UK gonorrhoea reached an all time low in the mid 1990s, thought to be due to behaviour change in response to AIDS but rates have since increased.

Risk factors

- *Fixed risk factors* Age (women aged 15–24, men aged 25–34); geographical area.
- *Modifiable risk factors* Unprotected vaginal or anal sex; multiple sex partners.

Prevention

- *Primary prevention* Similar to HIV/AIDS (see 📖 HIV/AIDS, pp.336–7). School sex education programmes; condom distribution programmes and promotion of consistent use; peer education programmes with vulnerable groups; vaccination for HPV and hepatitis B.

- *Secondary prevention* Avoidance of sexual intercourse during infectious period; screening for asymptomatic disease may facilitate early treatment before serious sequelae. Antenatal screening for syphilis has proved effective in reducing congenital syphilis. Population screening for chlamydia is widely recommended and was introduced in England in 2007 but impact on incidence of disease and on sequelae is unclear. Screening can also lead to case finding through partner notification, and focused behavioural intervention to reduce reinfection rates. Type-specific screening for HSV followed by suppressive therapy may reduce transmission to uninfected partners.
- *Treatment/tertiary infection* Appropriate antimicrobial therapy.

Table 12.4 Major STIs: organisms and diseases

	Organism	Disease
Bacterial	*Neisseria gonorrhoeae*	Cervicitis, urethritis, pelvic inflammatory disease, proctitis, epididymitis, pharyngitis, conjunctivitis
	Chlamydia trachomatis	Serovars D-K: cervicitis, urethritis, pelvic inflammatory disease, proctitis, epididymitis, conjunctivitis
		Serovars L1,2,3: lymphogranulcoma venereum (inguinal or anorectal syndrome)
	Mycoplasma genitalium	Cervicitis, urethritis, pelvic inflammatory disease (possibly)
	Treponema pallidum	Syphilis
	Haemophilus ducreyi	Chancroid
	Klebsiella granulomatis	Granuloma inguinale (Donovanosis)
Viral	Herpes simplex virus	Genital or labial herpes
	Human papillomavirus	Genital warts, genital tract cancers
	Human immunodeficiency virus	AIDS
	Hepatitis A,B,C	Hepatitis
Protozoal	Trichomonas vaginalis	Vaginitis

References
1 WHO ℞ http://www.who.int
2 HPA ℞ http://www.hpa.org.uk

Stomach cancer

Summary

Stomach cancer is the commonest type of infection-related cancer world-wide.[1] It is the commonest cause of cancer death in Japan where there is a nationwide screening programme. Generally, incidence is decreasing as *Helicobacter pylori* (*H. pylori*, see also 📖 p.365) prevalence falls.

Descriptive epidemiology

- *Incidence* Worldwide, there were 989 000 new cases in 2008.[8] In the UK it is the 10th commonest cancer with 7780 new cases in 2007.[3]
- *Prevalence* Worldwide, an estimated 1.5 million people were alive in 2002 having been diagnosed with stomach cancer within the previous 5 years.[4] In England, there were 22 200 admissions to hospital with stomach cancer in 2008/09.[5]
- *Survival* Depends on grade and stage at presentation. In the UK 5-year survival is now 15–18%.[3]
- *Mortality* Worldwide it is 2nd commonest cause of cancer death and the 17th commonest cause of death overall with 803 000 deaths in 2004.[2] In the UK it is the 7th commonest cause of cancer death.[3] There were 4366 deaths in England and Wales in 2009.[6]
- *Time* In the UK, over the last 30 years, age-standardized incidence has fallen by 50%, mortality has fallen by 70% and survival has increased 3-fold.[3] This steady fall in incidence is attributed to the decline in *H. pylori* prevalence due to better living conditions and less overcrowding.[3]
- *Person* Usually occurs in people over the age of 50.[3]
- *Place* Occurs worldwide, but most cases occur in the Western Pacific region where it is the commonest cause of cancer death in women.[2] It is an important cause of death in high- and middle-income countries.

Risk factors

- *Fixed risk factors* Age (95% of cases in over 50s);[3] family history; pernicious anaemia.
- *Modifiable risk factors* *H. pylori* and smoking (act independently and multiplicatively); alcohol only when combined with smoking; Barrett's oesophagus and gastro-oesophageal reflux disease (GORD).

Prevention

- *Primary prevention* Identification and eradication of *H. pylori* infection; smoking cessation; diet high in fruit and vegetables.
- *Secondary prevention* Stomach cancer is the commonest cause of cancer death in Japan. Population based screening using photofluorography was introduced in 1983, annually for people >40 years.[7]
- *Treatment/tertiary prevention* Surgery; chemotherapy; radiotherapy.

References

1 American Cancer Society Global Cancer Facts and Figures 2007 🔗 http://www.cancer.org
2 WHO *The global burden of disease: 2004 update.* Geneva: WHO; 2004. 🔗 http://www.who.int/healthinfo/global_burden_disease/GBD_report_2004update_full.pdf
3 Cancer research UK 🔗 http://www.cancerresearch.org
4 WHO GLOBOCAN 2002 🔗 http://www-dep.iarc.fr
5 NHS HES Online 2008/9 🔗 http://www.hesonline.nhs.uk
6 Death registrations in England and Wales 2009 🔗 http://www.statistics.gov.uk
7 Hamashima C *et al.* The Japanese guidelines for gastric cancer screening. *Jpn J Clin Oncol* 2008; **38**(4):259–67.
8 WHO GLOBOCAN 2008 🔗 http://www.globocan.iarc.fr

Tuberculosis

Summary

Tuberculosis (TB) is an infectious disease caused by *Mycobacterium tuberculosis*. Although treatment and control programmes have been in place for many decades, it remains the leading global cause of death for curable infectious diseases. In recent years the emergence of multidrug-resistant (MDR)-TB and extensively drug-resistant (XDR)-TB is undermining control and treatment programmes.

Descriptive epidemiology

- *Incidence* Worldwide in 2007, there were an estimated 7.8 million new cases of TB[1], a rate of 4.1 per 100 000 per year.[2] In the UK, in 2009, the rate of TB was 14.6 per 100 000.[2] (See Fig. 12.4.)
- *Prevalence* There were estimated to be 13.9 million people with TB in 2004.[1] 1/3 of the world's population is infected with TB, between 5–10% of whom will become ill with the disease.[3]
- *Case fatality* 65% of patients with smear-positive pulmonary TB will die within 5 years unless treated.
- *Mortality* TB is the leading cause of death for curable infectious disease and the 7th commonest cause of death worldwide with 1.5 million deaths in 2004.[1] For treated patients, mortality is highest in drug resistant TB and where people are co-infected with HIV. TB is the commonest cause of death in people with HIV.[3]
- *Morbidity* TB was the 11th leading cause of disability in 2004 with 34.2 million DALYs.[1]
- *Time* In the UK the number of cases and deaths declined dramatically in the 20th century, but started to rise again in the 1980s. Globally, incidence is reportedly stable in most areas, but absolute numbers of cases are rising with population growth. Areas with high HIV prevalence have seen an increase in morbidity and mortality from TB.
- *Person* Anyone may be affected, but in the UK the disease is most common in young adults (15–44 years) and in non-UK born people (63% of cases).
- *Place* More cases in urban than rural areas. In the UK, London accounts for 39% of cases, with a rate of 44.3 cases per 100 000 in 2008.[2] Global distribution is shown in Table 12.5.
- *Transmission* TB is transmitted person to person through droplets. Bovine TB (now rare) is contracted through ingestion of unpasteurized milk from an infected cow.

Risk factors

- *Fixed risk factors* Age (young adults); sex (men >women); geographic area. Children <3 years, older people and those with immune suppression more likely to develop clinical disease.
- *Modifiable risk factors* Overcrowding; residential accommodation (including prisons and refugee camps); alcohol and drug misuse; health care work; international travel to high prevalence areas; poor nutrition; poor control of HIV epidemics; personal hygiene; non-pasteurization of milk.

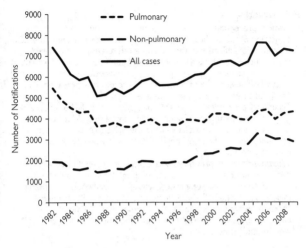

Fig. 12.4 Tuberculosis notifications by site of disease (pulmonary/non-pulmonary), England and Wales, 1982–2009. Data from http://www.hpa.org.uk/Topics/ InfectiousDiseases/InfectionsAZ/Tuberculosis/TBUKSurveillanceData/ TBUKSurveillanceViaNOIDs/TBNOIDs021982.

Table 12.5 Global estimated TB incidence, prevalence and mortality, 2005[5]

| WHO region | Incidence | | | | TB mortality | |
| | All forms | | Smear-positive[*] | | | |
	number (000s)	per 100 000	number (000s)	per 100 000	number (000s)	per 100 000
Africa	2 529	343	1 088	147	544	74
The Americas	352	39	157	18	49	5.5
Eastern Med	565	104	253	47	112	21
Europe	445	50	199	23	66	7.4
South-East Asia	2 993	181	1 339	81	512	31
Western Pacific	1 927	110	866	49	295	17
Global	**8 811**	**136**	**3 902**	**60**	**1 577**	**24**

[*] Smear-positive cases are confirmed by smear microscopy.

Prevention

- *Primary prevention* Improve living conditions; reduce overcrowding; education of the public in modes of transmission; vaccination: the BCG is around 75% effective in the UK and is offered using a risk-based system including targeted vaccination of babies born to mothers linked to high prevalence areas, and people in high risk occupations.[4] Hospital control of infection procedures including respiratory precautions for admitted cases who are smear positive.
- *Secondary prevention* Target screening and case finding to ensure early diagnosis and treatment of people at increased risk. Contact tracing: detailed guidelines are available from the British Thoracic Society. Screening and/or chemoprophylaxis of people who have been in contact with TB.
- *Treatment/tertiary prevention* Most cases of susceptible TB will require 6 months of a combination of drugs. Patients should be monitored to ensure compliance, including directly observed therapy. MDR-TB and XDR-TB and patients who also have HIV will need complex and extended therapy, sometimes up to 24 months. In the UK, 6.8% of cases were resistant to at least 1 first-line drug and 1.1% were multidrug resistant in 2008.[2]

References

1 WHO *The global burden of disease: 2004 update*. Geneva: WHO; 2004. ℳ http://www.who.int/healthinfo/global_burden_disease/GBD_report_2004update_full.pdf
2 HPA ℳ http://www.hpa.org.uk
3 WHO ℳ http://www.who.int
4 Department of Health. *The Green Book*. London: DH; 2006. ℳ http://www.dh.gov.uk/en/PublicationsandstatisticsPublications/PublicationsPolicyAndGuidance/DH_079917
5 WHO ℳ http://www.who.int/mediacentre/factsheets/fs104/en

Further reading

British Thoracic Society Guidelines available through ℳ http://www.hpa.org.uk/infections/topics_az/tb/links/guidelines.htm
UK data and advice ℳ http://www.hpa.org.uk/infections/topics_az/tb/menu.htm
WHO Tuberculosis site ℳ http://www.who.int/tb/en

Viral hepatitis

Summary

There are a number of specific viruses that lead to hepatitis, the most common ones being A, B and C.

Hepatitis A

The hepatitis A virus generally causes mild and transient illness but it is occasionally severe.

- *Incidence* An estimated 1.4 million cases of hepatitis A occur annually, often in large outbreaks.[1] There were 378 cases of hepatitis A reported in England and Wales in 2008[2] and >2500 cases reported in the USA,[3] although it is estimated that there were actually 22 000 new infections in the USA during the year.
- *Prevalence* It is estimated that around 30% of people in the USA have ever been infected with hepatitis A.[3]
- *Case fatality* Increases with age from <1% in young adults to 12% in over 70s. (UK).
- *Transmission* It is spread by faecal–oral transmission, usually person to person and occasionally through food. Most common in regions and populations where there is a lack of sanitation and poor hygiene. In the UK often occurs in institutions.
- *Prevention* Improved sanitation and hygiene; vaccination of those travelling to endemic areas; vulnerable groups (institutionalized people with special needs who may have poor hygiene); contacts in outbreaks; men who have sex with men; people at occupational risk; those with chronic liver disease.

Hepatitis B

The hepatitis B virus (HBV) causes both acute and chronic disease. It is transmitted through blood, sexual contact and other bodily fluids.

- *Incidence* There were 892 cases of hepatitis B reported in England and Wales in 2002.[2] In 2008 there were >4000 cases reported in the USA although it is estimated that there were actually 38 000 new infections.[3]
- *Prevalence* Approximately 2 billion worldwide have current or previous infection, 350 million have chronic infection.[1] In the UK the prevalence of chronic infection is 0.3%[2] and it is estimated that around 5% of people in the USA have ever been infected.[3]
- *Mortality* Worldwide there were 105 000 deaths from hepatitis B in 2004.[4]
- *Morbidity* Worldwide hepatitis B was responsible for 2.1 million DALYs in 2004.[4]
- *Case fatality* 25% of those who become chronically infected during childhood later die from liver cancer or cirrhosis.[1]
- *Prevention* There is a safe and effective vaccine. WHO recommends that this is given to all infants. Those who have not been vaccinated as infants should be offered the vaccine if they have multiple sexual partners; are partners or household contacts of HBV infected persons; inject drugs; frequently require blood or blood products; have received solid organ transplantation; have an occupational risk of HBV infection, including health care workers; travel to countries with high rates of HBV.

Hepatitis C

The hepatitis C virus (HCV), discovered in 1989, causes acute and chronic liver disease. 4 out of 5 acute cases lead to chronic infection.[2] In chronic infection approximately 20% will develop cirrhosis and 1–5% will develop liver cancer.[1]

- *Incidence* 3–4 million per year worldwide. In 2008, 8898 new cases were reported in England and Wales[2] and there were an estimated 18 000 new infections in the USA.[3]
- *Prevalence* Globally, 170 million people have chronic HCV.[1] Wide geographic variation from 1% in northern Europe to >10% in Egypt. In the UK prevalence is 0.4%.[2]
- *Mortality* Worldwide there were 54 000 deaths from hepatitis C in 2004.[4]
- *Morbidity* Worldwide hepatitis C was responsible for almost 1 million DALYs in 2004.[4]
- *Transmission* Unscreened blood transfusions/blood products; re-use of needles and syringes that have not been adequately sterilized; injection drug use (main route of transmission in UK); sexual transmission, particularly in men who have sex with men; mother to child transmission (risk about 5%).
- *Prevention* Screen blood, blood products and organs for donation; sterilization of equipment for medical procedures (injection, surgery); needle exchange programmes and drug treatment to reduce transmission among injection drug users. Treatment is available but not affordable in most of the world.

Other hepatitis viruses

- *Hepatitis D* A virus that can cause severe liver disease but only occurs alongside hepatitis B.
- *Hepatitis E* Identified in the 1980s as a cause of mild disease with occasional severe infection particularly in pregnant women. It is transmitted by the faecal–oral route. It is rare in the UK but endemic in parts of Asia, Africa and Central America where sanitation is poor.

References

1 WHO ⌀ http://www.who.int
2 HPA ⌀ http://www.hpa.org.uk
3 Centers for Disease Control and Prevention ⌀ http://www.cdc.gov
4 WHO *The global burden of disease: 2004 update*. Geneva: WHO; 2004. ⌀ http://www.who.int/healthinfo/global_burden_disease/GBD_report_2004update_full.pdf

Index